A forgotten generation: Long-term survivors' experiences of HIV and AIDS

Judith Mary Sagar

A forgotten generation: Long-term survivors' experiences of HIV and AIDS

This book is dedicated to Richard Craig Day – thank you for being my friend and I will see you on the other side.

Copyright © 2013 Judith Mary Sagar

All rights reserved.

ISBN:149421833X
ISBN-13: 978-1494218331

CONTENTS
∞

PREFACE

ACKNOWLEDGEMENTS

INTRODUCTION

CHAPTER ONE: CRITICAL REFLECTIONS:
Concepts, ideas and shared meanings

CHAPTER TWO: TESTING POSITIVE:
Diagnosis day

CHAPTER THREE: THE EARLY YEARS:
Where do I go from here?

CHAPTER FOUR: HIV BEFORE HAART:
In sickness and in health

CHAPTER FIVE: POSITIVELY LIVING AS SEXUAL BEINGS:
Intimate relationships

CHAPTER SIX: EXPERIENCING HAART:
Managing combination therapy

CHAPTER SEVEN: TAKING CONTROL:
Experiencing the medical profession

CHAPTER EIGHT: ME, MYSELF and HIV:
Exploring networks of support

CHAPTER NINE: LIVING LONG-TERM WITH HIV:
Positive and negative elements

CHAPTER TEN: ON BEING THERE:
A researcher's tale

GLOSSARY

PREFACE

"Doctors are men [sic] who prescribe medicines of which they know little, to cure diseases of which they know less, in human beings of whom they know nothing."

Voltaire

∞

This is the first book I have ever written and it has been an arduous yet rewarding journey. The driving force behind the telling of this story-of-stories was initially inspired by the personal experiences of a very close friend of mine who had lived with AIDS for many years. His perceptions and experiences of living long-term with HIV were complex and thought-provoking. Equally, I had witnessed pejorative social attitudes and behaviours towards people living with HIV and AIDS whilst working in the field. All these matters provoked an overpowering desire for me to understand as much about HIV and AIDS as possible. On this journey, I met some extraordinary women and men both within and outside of a range of institutions; all of whom impacted greatly on my personal life. This story-of-stories presented in this particular format, has taken just under five years to accomplish with long breaks in between writing. Arguably it is far too long overdue but as my beloved Granddad Laycock used to say: *it is better late than never*!

The construction of the 'AIDS epidemic' began in 1981 when I was 16 years old and only vaguely conscious of my own sexual being. In 1983 a virus named LAV was identified in France and was linked to AIDS – *the killer disease*. In the United States during 1984 the retrovirus thought to cause AIDS was identified and named as HTLV-III. In 1986 it became clear to scientists that LAV and HTLV-III were actually the same retrovirus, and so *Human Immunodeficiency virus* (HIV) became its new name. Most of this escaped my attention; I was 21 years old, the world was my oyster and I was busy carving out a secretarial career for myself during this period. It was not until 1994 when I started a full-time Higher Education programme of study in Social Science that I acquired a profound interest and fascination in matters relating to HIV and AIDS. Prior to this, my personal awareness was basically influenced by my friendship networks and the media hype, although I truly *never* felt totally detached in terms of "*it could never happen to me*". I do not know why!

At an academic level in the first year of my first degree in 1994, I designed a small-scale research study on HIV-awareness amid Higher Education students; this cultivated a scholarly curiosity in HIV-related research studies, HIV science and medicine - in fact any HIV or AIDS printed matter. As well as my academic interests in HIV, I was also fascinated with the topics of gender, sexuality, 'race' and ethnicity. Soon after starting university, I became actively involved in a local, non-governmental organisation (NGO) working voluntarily with people living with HIV and AIDS. It was here that I met my dear friend Richard, who had lived with an HIV-positive diagnosis since 1990 from the tender age of 21 years. A deep and meaningful friendship soon blossomed between us and went from strength to strength until he died in May 2009 whilst I was writing this book. His love, courage, strength and the private experiences we shared together will continue to live on in my memory. During the latter end of the year 2000, I decided that Richard's personal experiences of living with AIDS should be incorporated into my PhD study which was designed to focus on the experiences of living long-term with an HIV-positive diagnosis.

Going back to 1994, I was faintly aware that there was still very little effective HIV medicine available for people living with HIV or AIDS. In fact, living with HIV or AIDS was medically considered as life-threatening and often perceived as a 'death sentence'. Apart from the monotherapy Zidovudine (commonly known as AZT) licensed in 1987, and two other drugs which were later licensed in 1994 (Lamivudine and Didanosine), medical treatment did not inspire hope and optimism for many HIV-positive people. Then towards the end of 1996, we saw the introduction of combination therapies known as Highly Active Antiretroviral Therapy (HAART); this medical development brought with it a promise of longer life expectancy for people living with HIV and AIDS. Thereon after, almost all HIV research concentrated its gaze towards the medical and clinical aspects of HIV matters.

With few exceptions, after the advent of HAART the abundance of HIV-related literature struggled to make sense of, and failed to tackle the challenges, uncertainties and inconsistencies of living long-term with HIV or AIDS. There was limited social research that focussed on the personal experiences of women and men directly affected by HIV; human beings who, in everyday life, skilfully managed and negotiated the difficulties, contradictions and the changing medical uncertainties that arose in the process of making sense of life following an HIV-positive diagnosis. I wanted to know more about how individuals personally experienced living long-term with HIV and AIDS.

My involvement with the first voluntary HIV charitable organisation had given me a valuable insight into the tangible concerns relating to HIV and AIDS matters at a grass-roots level. It presented me with an awareness of how crucial voluntary HIV organisations and self-help groups had become in terms of the vital role they played in care-giving and support for people affected by HIV and AIDS. From late 1996 onwards, these medical advancements and the perceived optimism of improved health and extended longevity saw HIV-related matters start to rapidly tumble down the health care and political agendas. Many HIV charities and organisations closed down or were forced to merge with others due to budgets in Health Authority funding being dramatically reduced. Similarly, funding for social research projects seeking to explore personal or social aspects of HIV and AIDS became almost non-existent. Instead clinical and medical matters relating to HIV started to become the prevailing focus for any HIV researcher who required sponsorship or financial funding.

From an academic perspective, it was apparent that whilst HIV and AIDS-related research was plentiful, very few studies after 1996 could be considered as *valuable* for promoting effective care and support practices for people living with and affected by HIV or AIDS at a community level. The abundance of HIV literature revealed very little in terms of how we should understand the complexities of everyday challenges or the accomplishments achieved by human beings living with an HIV-positive diagnosis. It was certainly difficult to comprehend and conceptualise what it actually meant to live long-term with HIV and AIDS. Similarly, it was not easy to appreciate how health and illness is negotiated in the context of HIV and AIDS. There was scant academic research from 1996 onwards centring on the social aspects of HIV and AIDS and even less which explored personal experiences of women and men who had lived long-term with an HIV-positive diagnosis. These widening gaps in our knowledge and understanding suggest our attention is being diverted elsewhere. Has HIV become yesterday's news?

Many HIV-related studies I evaluated after 1996 were largely involved with medical advancements and issues of compliance and adherence to complex combination therapies amongst 'patients' within a clinical setting. Dominant forms of knowledge on HIV seemed to centre on: HIV-specialist consultants; HIV health practitioners; the HIV-scientific community and leading pharmaceutical companies conducting medical research and clinical trials. It appeared that the HIV scientific and medical communities in conjunction with the pharmaceutical industry purloined the role as 'HIV experts'. Yet how did the medical community initially gather their knowledge and turn this into some kind of 'expertise'? The simple answer is primarily from the people living with an HIV-positive diagnosis on a daily basis. Undoubtedly when medical practitioners confront disease they do not simply face a pathogen on a Petri dish; instead they gather together patients' reports about bodily experiences and, in turn, interpret these bodily symptoms as an underlying cause.

The ever-increasing widening gap in our knowledge and understanding leaves us without the tools we need to appreciate the experiences and complex practices of people living with HIV and AIDS over the past three decades. I believed it was crucial to enhance our knowledge and understanding of living with HIV by concentrating on human beings who had experienced HIV and AIDS for many years. This story-of-stories therefore focuses on long-term survivors who have lived with an HIV-positive diagnosis prior to the advancement of HIV medicine and, in some cases, prior to medical health checks for HIV, which comprise: the CD4 count and viral load test. For me, the women and men living long-term with HIV had become the significant experts.

Whilst reading the personal experiences of the story-tellers involved, we must appreciate the many tears that were shed during the *telling* of these stories. Without exception, every woman and man shared tears of joy, sadness and frustration during and sometimes after our conversations. The compassion, the courage and the turmoil situated in the lives of our story-tellers who came forward to share their personal experiences of everyday life must never be forgotten or understated. It is my sincere hope that every reader will actively engage with the stories as they unfold, and critically reflect on the context of each situation throughout this journey. All stories, I do believe, have instrumental functions and it is the lessons they teach us rather than the feelings they may invoke that are important. This is a serious attempt to rigorously capture the authenticity and crucial insights of the narratives that were shared, by using the words and recounting the personal experiences of the women and men involved in the original HIV study.

We are about to grasp a glimmer of insight and understanding into what it means to live with an HIV-positive diagnosis from the perspective of our long-term survivors who shared their personal and private experiences for the purpose of helping others: this is their gift. In recounting these narratives, we seek to raise public awareness by exploring personal experiences to connect and illustrate everyday problems, challenges and contradictions that occur. We present not only common and similar experiences but also divergent and unfamiliar lived realities which were shared during our journey.

By adopting an approach of active engagement, it is hoped that we might broaden knowledge and understanding of HIV-related issues which is politically and socially useful for not only persons affected by HIV and AIDS but these insights might also help: health practitioners; consultants; doctors; clinicians; therapists; social researchers; social workers; care workers; carers; policymakers; educators; students and, to be sure, anyone who actively engages in this story-of-stories. It is a further aim that this might also encourage future social researchers to return their gaze towards the personal and social aspects of living long-term with HIV... they are, after all, long overdue!

It is hoped that this story-of-stories sheds light on how our long-term survivors have negotiated and managed everyday life living with this unpredictable chronic illness condition. If nothing else, these poignant personal stories historically reflect upon long-term experiences of women and men living with HIV and AIDS-related illness; they show us how real people made sense of their lives and continue to 'live out' their everyday life in real terms. It is a thorough and passionate portrayal of personal experiences revealed to me by the spirited women and men who took time out of their own lives to offer a valuable contribution to further public understanding of this stigmatised disease. There is nothing authoritative or magical about this book; it purely gives voice to and makes visible those women and men who took part in this explorative research, including myself. Any errors or mistakes are my own. I hope you find this journey enlightening!

A forgotten generation: Long-term survivors' experiences of HIV and AIDS

ACKNOWLEDGEMENTS

∞

There are so many amazing human beings I would like to acknowledge but for reasons of anonymity you cannot be named. Nevertheless, you ALL know *who you are*, in more ways than one, of that I am sure! My massive appreciation and gratitude goes to all the women and men who shared with me their long-term experiences of living with HIV and AIDS-related illness. My fondest memories of those who are no longer with us will always remain. To particular women and men who worked in the following HIV and other non-government organisations (NGOs); without their invaluable support and contribution at the onset this journey might never have been accomplished:

BEGIN (Wakefield); Blackliners; Bradford Community Health Trust; Body Positive North West; George House Trust (Manchester); Haemophilia Society (London); International Community of Women (ICW, London); National AIDS Trust; National Long Term Survivors Group (NLTSG); North Yorkshire AIDS Action; Positive Action (Hampshire); +VE magazine; Positive Nation; Positively Women; RAFT; The Terrence Higgins Trust [THT in Leeds, London, Brighton); UK Coalition of People Living With HIV and AIDS (PLWHA in London). It saddens me to say that many of the above organisations are no longer in operation which is a great loss to all those who continue to need support

This story-of-stories could not have been primarily achieved without the initial research findings of my original PhD study that was funded by the Economic and Social Research Council [ESRC] from 2000-2003 at the University of Leeds in the Department of Sociology and Social Policy. Accordingly, it is crucial to acknowledge the importance of the ESRC funding in the making of this story-of-stories. I would also like to thank my supervisors who kept me on the *straight and narrow* during this time: Dr Carolyn Baylies (who sadly passed away during my research); Professor Sylvia Walby and Professor Sasha Roseneil.

I must mention the significant people in my life who have always been there for me constantly. In no particular order I would like to acknowledge my Mum, my Dad and my 'evil wicked' step-mum Julie who sadly passed away before I completed this book. I salute my beloved partner Chris (the Master of the Avalon) for his endurance with my bad moods and his total belief in me when times were difficult. His wonderful skills for proof-reading each chapter cannot go unacknowledged. To my beautiful friend who I consider as my 'wise-owl' Debbie Jolly for her dedication and belief in my ability to finish this journey; I could not have accomplished this without her wonderful editing skills and our brilliantly bizarre conversations. To an amazingly compassionate human being Jane Stuckey for her love and understanding and for providing a roof over my head - I am sorry I did not get the chance to tell you the book was completed before you died; Peter Ejedewe who has always been a great soul mate and a good critic. I would like to say 'thank you' to Mike Peters for making me into this critical and reflective person that I am now; Stephen Sayers; Lindsay El-Kadi for her lovely, comfortable bed and chocolate treats; Robert Fieldhouse from Baseline; Marshia Summerfield for her proof-reading skills at the last minute and her lovely food. There are so many others not mentioned here but never far from my mind; thank you to you all. In addition, I would like to thank David and everyone at Writer Motive (www.writermotive.com) – their professional services and prices are second to none. Thank you all so very much! I acknowledge also that any mistakes and errors in this story-of-stories are my own.

INTRODUCTION
∞

"The beginning of knowledge is the discovery of something we do not understand."

Frank Herbert

The many ways of misunderstanding HIV and AIDS

Specific concerns relating to AIDS has never been considered as 'neutral' or fully inclusive due in part to the powerful and evocative images and representations which have persisted in the public domain since its 'discovery'; it is often considered as one of the most destructive global pandemics in history. For over thirty years there has been an assortment of social constructions of AIDS and HIV which have gathered momentum to engender a wide-range of meanings to numerous audiences. I believe HIV-related matters have generated more global meetings, scientific publications and political and governmental responses than any other disease in human history. In the past, the imagery and symbolism of HIV and AIDS carried with it a high media and public profile which became the subject of an unprecedented level of news stories, television and radio documentaries as well as attracting scientific, political, legal, ethical and moral profiles across cultures on a global scale. Few other diseases have involved individuals from such a multitude of backgrounds, bringing together medical and scientific researchers, health professionals, voluntary organisations, AIDS activists, politicians and policy makers in a constant array of meetings, conferences and publications worldwide.

One of the drawbacks of having such a high public profile is the unrelenting circulation of myths and misconceptions about HIV and AIDS which have equally gathered momentum. The lethal combination of fear, denial, prejudice, racism and homophobia across cultures has ensured dominant misunderstandings and misconceptions remain so deep-rooted and widespread that they continue to perpetuate in spite of emerging evidence to the contrary. In some cases, these misguided and false conceptions have prompted the very behaviours that have led human beings to become HIV-positive. Possibly one of the most striking features of HIV and AIDS are the ways in which societal and public reactions towards people living with HIV have led to fear, moral panic, and scapegoating of those affected by this disease. Yet is this a new phenomenon?

Historically, when there is a problem, hardship or a disaster across cultural societies, we have a tendency to cast blame on others as opposed to tackling the crisis itself. Blaming others is very much a human characteristic which can have catastrophic consequences for those being blamed. When faced with adversity which is inexplicable or beyond our control, the process of attributing blame tends to focus on people who are considered as 'outsiders' or marginalised individuals who are deemed as 'different' to the majority: particularly minority groups or 'foreigners'. When the Austrian-born German politician and leader of the Nazi Party Adolf Hitler blamed the Jewish community, disabled people, communists, gypsies, homosexuals and other 'undesirable' social groups for the economic hardship of 1920s Nazi Germany, this had catastrophic consequences resulting in the organisation of concentration camps and European war. Similarly epidemics of perilous contagious infections such as smallpox, the plague, syphilis, and even influenza have historically provoked social responses rooted in blaming others for spreading infections because of 'deviant' or 'undesirable behaviours'. Why does history continue to repeat itself and how can we learn from the past?

Like other contagious infections, HIV is not a disease of a particular type of person or group of people. It is an infectious disease that can potentially affect almost any human being regardless of life history, gender, ethnicity, social status and cultural and sub-cultural affiliation. We are forced to recognise and acknowledge this because HIV has affected and killed women, men, children, heterosexuals, homosexuals, bisexuals, asexuals, the sexually promiscuous and the sexually inexperienced, Black, Brown, Red, Yellow and White human beings, young, middle aged and old, rich and poor, injecting drug-users and non drug-users across the globe.

One thing that typically strikes me as profoundly unfathomable in contemporary society is when I meet people who are non-specialists in HIV; many seem to *know* something about AIDS or HIV yet more often than not what they seem to know is bound up in urban myths or dominant misconceptions of HIV or AIDS. Whilst working in the field of HIV, I have come across women and men who continue to believe there are innocent people who have contracted HIV through no fault of their own, in contrast to those who can be blamed for being HIV-positive. Not many years ago I received an e-mail from a close personal friend and I was dumbfounded. This HIV hoax had been sent to more than twenty other people including myself and falsely claimed that people were placing HIV-infected needles in cinemas and theatres in the UK to cause injury and 'revenge' transmission of HIV. Alongside the needle poking out of a seat rests a note stating 'you have just been infected by HIV'. The e-mail urges its recipients to pass this on to as many people as possible in order to save lives. These scaremongering stories shrouded in myth have emerged in the UK, United States, Australia, Canada and elsewhere. Why would any individual be inclined to believe in the existence of HIV-positive people going around town seeking revenge?

Another widely popular HIV myth which exists as a cautionary tale proposes that after a one-night stand of casual sex with an unknown woman, a man awakens and goes to the bathroom to find a message: 'Welcome to the AIDS club' written in lipstick on the mirror. Supposedly, there is an 'AIDS Mary' on the loose, as she has famously become known, who had contracted AIDS from her lover and swore she would pass it on to every man she could seduce. This is a new version of a very old myth or folk invention about 'revenge infection' and in reality there is no such person as 'AIDS Mary'. These myths and others like them are an imaginative expression of the fear and ignorance that prevailed in the beginning of the AIDS pandemic in the early 1980s. These HIV hoax e-mails usually end by stating: *This is not a joke! These people are everywhere. Please forward this on to everybody you care about.*

New variants circulating in the 1990s in the UK stayed with the same punch line 'welcome to the world of AIDS' but took a more sinister turn. No longer is the pleasure of casual sex with a stranger going to seal your doom; it is simply a matter of being in the wrong place at the wrong time. Nothing is safe anymore! Human beings are being randomly chosen for revenge infection by anonymous rogues by way of 'stealth injection'. The story unfolds usually in an e-mail that gangs are moving around the UK sticking HIV-infected needles into people and then giving them a card stating 'welcome to the world of AIDS'. The hoax tale goes on to suggest that "this is not a joke or an urban myth as the sender has seen these occurrences in Brighton and Crawley. The gangs do not operate only in nightclubs but are on the streets and in shopping centres; in fact they could be anywhere. This IS happening..."

Urban myths and legends tend to focus on contemporary public fears and social unease and many are rooted in underlying sexual themes which emphasise the innocence of the 'victims' in the narrative. It is hardly surprising that HIV and AIDS has become a central theme for urban myths. Within the context of HIV and AIDS we have the popular dichotomy separating sexual partners into the innocent victims and the guilty promiscuous predator; additionally, we can also include the already marginalised and degraded stereotypical characters of people living with HIV and AIDS, such as gay men, injecting drug users, commercial sex workers and Black Africans. These perpetuating myths and stories penetrate public consciousness and are widely circulated across cultures; of course they have been further amplified by popular news stories and high profile media coverage since earlier times concerning *'the truth about AIDS'*. During the 1980s popular and media constructions of AIDS and HIV were built upon already established prejudices, fears of contamination and widespread ignorance yet still these remain in contemporary society. How many stories do you know about the misconceptions of HIV and AIDS?

Why is this story-of-stories important?

The motivating force behind this story-of-stories aims to set the record straight and dispel these perpetuating misconceptions that permeate public consciousness. By offering an insight into the personal experiences of real people who have lived *long-term* with an HIV-positive diagnosis in the UK, it is hoped that readers will come to appreciate and recognise *the many ways of being HIV-positive*. When the AIDS pandemic began in the early 1980s, scientific knowledge and biomedical treatment had a limiting effect on the quality of life and life expectancy for people living with HIV and AIDS-related illness. During this era the very idea of AIDS signified fear, panic, stigma, prejudice, social rejection and isolation, acute chronic illness and the real threat of imminent death both within and outside of a UK context. As the global expansion of HIV scientific and biomedical knowledge continued to develop, we observed a dramatic change in terms of how the medical community came to define HIV as a disease; the term AIDS has been largely discarded and we resist the 'death sentence' scenario and instead approach HIV as a chronic illness condition. With effective HIV combination therapies becoming available to those who could afford them, the successful management of HIV was perceived to be within our reach. Does this mean that fear and prejudice, social rejection and uncertainty in conjunction with acute chronic illness had been eradicated?

Today, an HIV-positive diagnosis no longer carries with it the same meaning as it did in earlier times. Since 1996 and the advent of Highly Active Antiretroviral Therapy (HAART), the experiences of women and men living with HIV or AIDS diagnoses are perceived to have been transformed. We can now anticipate people living much longer with an HIV-positive diagnosis, as promises of an extended and improved quality of life become reality. Yet how this shift has affected women and men who have lived *long-term* with an HIV-positive diagnosis remains shrouded in mystery and silence. For example, it is unclear if there are new challenges and uncertainties that have been shaped by biomedical advances for people living long-term with HIV and AIDS. What are the on-going psychological and social implications that come into play following these medical advancements? In reality, how many individuals have actually been inclined to ask such questions since the advent of HAART in 1996? From extensive literature searches, I found there was limited research explaining how transformations in medical practices had impacted on the everyday lives of human beings living with an HIV-positive diagnosis. In particular, there was even less HIV research which focused its gaze towards a *long-term survivors' perspective* from 1996 onwards.

Changes in medical practices: what are the social consequences?

In light of new HIV scientific and medical developments, are we fully able to appreciate and comprehend the ways in which 'long-term survivors' living with HIV have managed and negotiated these fundamental changes? I developed a deep-rooted curiosity in wanting to know how we should understand the changing long-term experiences of living with HIV and AIDS over time. In particular, were there any new challenges and uncertainties to be managed since medicine promised longer life? What social factors might stay the same? How do unique human beings leading diverse lifestyles personally experience and live out their social lives in the context of HIV and AIDS? I was interested to determine how 'long-term survivors' managed their initial diagnoses and how life had been negotiated before-and-after the advent of more effective medicine became widely available. I wondered what it must be like to have to take complex medical regimes every day for the rest of your life. How intrusive would it be to have to take copious amounts of tablets every day? What about managing severe side effects of the medication? How would quality of life and health issues be affected by the medication? I wondered how people coped with a relatively new complex drug regimen on a daily basis. What might be the dominant issues that made some people resist medical treatment? There was scant research that could adequately answer these questions.

A long-term survivors' perspective

I considered it essential to approach the research journey from a long-term survivors' perspective as I believed the women and men who had lived long-term with HIV were the significant 'experts'. Deciding on how to define 'long term survivor' was problematic at the beginning; there were few meaningful social definitions that were appropriate and all-inclusive. Medical definitions such as: 'non-progressor'; 'long-term positives'; 'non-seroconverter', and 'slow progressor' somehow seemed unsuitable and somewhat clinical and restrictive. An alternative was the term 'long-term thriver'. However, the term *long term survivor* became the most appropriate term for the purpose of the original HIV study. In the first instance, I approached and sought valuable guidance from the National Long Term Survivors Group [NLTSG] situated in the UK. This remarkable self-help group was set up in the early 1990s to provide support and a safe place for people living with HIV for five years or more. To cut a long story short, after making simple calculations in terms of diagnosed years, I set a clear boundary of including only HIV-positive women and men who were diagnosed in 1994 or before. This calculation ensured that all our story-tellers had been diagnosed before the advent of Highly Active Antiretroviral Therapy [HAART] in 1996. The term 'survivor' is seen as an extremely constructive and optimistic term, and none of our story-tellers opposed the use of long-term survivor.

Introducing the characteristics of the story-tellers

The main aim of the original research journey was to be divided into two sections. First, I wanted to explore diverse personal experiences of living with an HIV-positive diagnosis before effective medical treatment was widely available. Second, it was crucial to explore how changing biomedical advancements following the advent of HAART in 1996 had impacted on the everyday lived experiences of long-term survivors. Consequently, each of our story-tellers shared the same characteristic in that they were diagnosed between 1981 and 1994 before the advent of HAART. At the time of diagnosis, many were either given a medical 'death sentence' or it was perceived that they would die very soon after discovering they were HIV-positive. I hold the belief that women and men living with HIV who had been diagnosed during the earliest times of the AIDS pandemic held a vast wealth of knowledge and expertise to share with us. Who else would know what it was like living with this 'terminal disease' and managing the challenges and medical uncertainties on a day-to-day basis during times of social ignorance and fear?

The original HIV research study involved in-depth conversations with twenty eight long-term survivors living with an HIV-positive diagnosis in the UK. This comprised: 19 gay men, 5 heterosexual women and 4 heterosexual men who were also living with Haemophilia. Eighteen story-tellers were medically defined as 'symptomatic', in other words showing clinical signs or symptoms associated with HIV and the remaining ten were showing no clinical signs or symptoms of HIV (medically defined as 'asymptomatic'). The differences in routes of transmission included: contaminated blood products, sexual transmission, sharing contaminated needles whilst injecting drugs and one unknown source. Our story-tellers were aged between 27 and 64 and lived across England.

Each long-term survivor was or had been to a greater or lesser extent a recipient of biomedical treatment and/or was under medical supervision for HIV health checks. Four story-tellers were diagnosed from 1981-1983; seven people were diagnosed during 1984-1986; a further four discovered their HIV-positive status during 1987-1989; nine story-tellers learned of their positive status from 1990-1992 and the remaining four were diagnosed during 1993-1994. At the time of diagnosis, fifteen long-term survivors were in intimate partnering relationships whilst the remaining thirteen were single. Five long-term sexual partnerships dissolved as a result of HIV and three intimate relationships were still enduring at the time of our interview. Three other intimate relationships just 'moved on' whilst four HIV-positive partners died of AIDS-related illness. At the time of our conversations in 2002, twelve story-tellers were in partnering relationships and fifteen of our story-tellers were single.

Five long-term survivors who were medically defined as asymptomatic had resisted taking any HIV medical treatments since the onset of diagnosis because of showing no clinical signs or symptoms associated with HIV. Two asymptomatic long-term survivors had previously taken the drug AZT (see glossary) in earlier times but were no longer on treatment at the time of our conversation. The remaining three story-tellers who were medically defined as asymptomatic were taking combination therapy as a preventative measure. Sixteen out of eighteen story-tellers who fell into the category of symptomatic were on combination therapies in 2002 at the time of our interview and two long-term survivors were awaiting 'salvage therapy' due to problems of resistance with past treatments.

Outlining the content of this book

The plan of this story-of-stories is straightforward and thematic. We begin in chapter one by critically reflecting on concepts, ideas and shared meanings relating to knowledge, health, illness and disease in order to ascertain what these terms mean and how they are understood in the public and private domain. We then touch upon aspects of our personal identities to explore what makes us who we are. To conclude, we expose how representations of AIDS and HIV in the mass media from the mid 1980s to early 1990s impacted on public beliefs and perceptions of people living with AIDS and HIV during these gloomy times. In chapter two we introduce all our story-tellers to readers and use their own voices and experiences to portray how each long-term survivor's personal situation led to the discovery of an HIV-positive diagnosis. Throughout the remaining chapters, with the exception of chapter ten, the collective voices, perceptions and personal experiences of our story-tellers have been used to create space for a long-term survivors' perspective on all the themes depicted in this story-of-stories.

In chapter three we explore how our long-term survivors primarily managed and took control over their everyday lives after discovering they were HIV-positive; in many cases our story-tellers had been given a medical 'death sentence' and perceived imminent death as a reality. In chapter four we unravel how health and illness was negotiated prior to Highly Active Antiretroviral Therapy (HAART) being introduced from 1996 onwards. We gain insight into the many fears, optimism, anxieties, hopes and uncertainties that were prevalent during this period of HIV before HAART. Throughout chapter five we examine how our story-tellers have been positively living as sexual beings in terms of intimate relationships with others in the context of HIV. This challenging chapter hopefully creates the space for readers to critically reflect upon divergent practices of sex as a defining feature of our own sexualities and sexual identities.

In chapters six and seven we reveal how our story-tellers have managed and/or resisted combination therapy and personally experienced the medical profession in the context of living with HIV and AIDS. We then move on to chapter eight to learn about networks of support and how living long-term with HIV has impacted on our story-tellers' sense of 'self'. Is HIV a big or small part of how our long-term survivors see themselves in terms of identity? Our story-tellers describe how family relationships and friendships have been maintained and negotiated and we discover whether these relationships have been affected by HIV. Finally, in chapter nine we gain insight into the positive and negative elements of living with HIV from a long-term survivors' perspective. There can be no conclusion to this story-of-stories as living long-term with an HIV or AIDS diagnosis is an everyday experience and is an on-going enterprise. Chapter ten allows space for me to reflect on my own experiences of *being there* throughout the original HIV research and permits the reader to understand in more depth the obstacles and highlights of this incredibly long and rewarding journey.

A conceptual framework for common understanding

It is crucial to establish a conceptual framework for shared meaning and common understanding, as we travel throughout the forthcoming chapters. For our specialist and non-specialist readers alike, basic information about HIV and AIDS is introduced to determine what we mean when we talk of HIV and AIDS. To conclude this introduction we shall explore some of the

A forgotten generation: Long-term survivors' experiences of HIV and AIDS

major and significant historical events in relation to AIDS and HIV over the past 30 years. Readers are directed to the glossary situated at the end of this book for terms associated with HIV and AIDS. This is an extensive glossary in which many of the terms may not be featured within the main body of this story-of-stories; it is however considered a necessary inclusion for readers who wish to learn more.

What is HIV and AIDS?

What does HIV and AIDS stand for? HIV stands for *Human Immunodeficiency Virus*. It is a retrovirus that almost all experts believe can lead to AIDS (*Acquired Immune Deficiency Syndrome*). There are two variants of HIV: these are HIV-1 and HIV-2 which are further divided into complex sub-types. HIV-1 group M is the most common type of HIV worldwide with over 90 per cent of cases deriving from this variant. HIV-1 group M is further subdivided into clades [see glossary] called subtypes which are allocated a letter from A to K. Also in the same variant HIV-1 are three other groups: N, O and P and a further HIV-1 RCV group. Not widely seen outside of West Africa is the variant HIV-2 which is relatively uncommon. Many testing kits for HIV-1 will also detect HIV-2.

Both variants of HIV damage the human body by destroying specific blood cells called CD4+ T-cells which are important cells that help the body fight against diseases. Occasionally, two viruses of different subtypes might merge in the cell of a person who is infected, mixing together the genetic material which presents a new hybrid virus. Many of these new strains do not survive for long and the classification of HIV strains into subtypes remains a complex issue and is subject to change as new discoveries unfold.

A small number of studies have shown how different subtypes can be associated with specific modes of transmission and can also affect disease progression. Nevertheless these findings remain inconclusive and are the subject of debate amongst scientists; no theory has been conclusively proven to date. Most HIV-1 antiretroviral drug treatments have been intended for specific subtypes; there is little evidence to suggest that these drugs are less effective for other subtypes. On the other hand, issues of resistance and problems associated with viral load testing for other subtypes are important factors for future pharmaceutical research to seriously consider if drugs are to be more effective long-term for various sub-types of the HIV retrovirus.

HIV routes of transmission: eradicating myths and rumours

Epidemiological research has recognised and clinically verified dominant routes of HIV transmission, as well as less common modes of transmission over time. Whilst widespread panic may still take place throughout many societies, it has been convincingly established that HIV transmission <u>cannot</u> occur by way of: air or water, insects, sneezing, spitting, social kissing, hugging, non-sexual touching or even sharing beds or household paraphernalia with people living with HIV. It should be noted that outside of the body HIV cannot reproduce as it does not survive well unlike the Hepatitis B Virus (HBV).

For the transmission of HIV to occur three conditions need to apply. First, the retrovirus has to be present in the body of a person already infected with HIV or in a contaminated bodily fluid or tissue. Second there has to be a sufficient quantity of the retrovirus present. Third, the retrovirus must enter the body of an uninfected person via an effective route for transmission. There must also be a plentiful supply of vulnerable cells, for example, susceptible receptor cells at the site of entry in conjunction with an inadequate defence system for HIV to be transmitted effectively.

The proven biological mechanisms widely acknowledged as the most common modes of HIV transmission include:

a) Unprotected sexual intercourse with someone who is infected; in other words, there is considerable risk involved when not using a condom or microbicide when having penetrative sex with a person who has HIV. Unprotected anal sex is more high risk than unprotected vaginal sex. The presence of other sexually transmitted infections can increase the risk of infection during sex. Unprotected oral sex can also be a risk for HIV transmission although this is recognised as a much lower risk than penetrative sex.

b) Sharing intravenous needles, syringes and other equipment used to prepare drugs for injection with multiple individuals is high risk behaviour for HIV transmission.

c) Mother-to-baby transmission: from a mother who is infected to her baby during the course of pregnancy, labour, delivery and by breast-feeding.

d) Receiving blood products, blood transfusions and organ and tissue transplants that are contaminated with the HIV retrovirus. Whilst the medical community consider this risk as remote due to the testing of blood, there is still risk attached in many countries.

HIV is not present in urine, faeces, vomit or sweat. However, it is present in many body fluids, such as saliva, blister fluid and tears. As there are only very low concentrations of HIV found in these body fluids, the presence of HIV does not constitute a risk for infection. In contrast to low concentrations of HIV found in the above bodily fluids, HIV is present in infectious quantities in blood and blood-derived products, semen, pre-seminal fluid (pre-cum – although this is low risk), rectal (anal) mucous, vaginal and cervical secretions or juices and breast milk (this is controversial and requires further scrutiny). HIV has also been detected in sufficient quantities in amniotic fluid, cerebrospinal fluid, tissue and organ donations, skin transplants and bone marrow transplants. These concentrations of HIV, however, are only a potential risk in invasive surgical proceedings.

Less common modes of HIV transmission are included below. Whilst I feel ethically obliged to include these potentially rare modes of transmission I have no desire to reawaken widespread panic, particularly in the case of biting and kissing. I therefore urge readers to consider these as extremely rare and pay particular attention to the lack of empirical evidence of these routes:

a) Being 'stuck' by a recently contaminated needle or sharp object.

b) Eating food that has been pre-chewed by an HIV-positive human being. Contamination may occur when <u>infected blood</u> from a caregiver mixes with food whilst chewing; this is extremely rare and has only been documented amongst small children who were teething or had unsophisticated immune systems in societies where pre-chewing is considered a widespread cultural habit.

c) Being bitten by a person with HIV which incorporates extensive tissue damage and the presence of blood may transmit the virus yet blood to blood contact must occur. There are only a small number of reported cases and it is considerably difficult to prove this mode of transmission.

d) Unsafe or unsanitary injections and other medical and dental practices might also transmit HIV yet these risks are remote due to standard practices amid practitioners on a global scale.

e) Contact between broken skin, open wounds or mucous membranes and HIV-infected blood can pose a risk of infection, but it is considered extremely rare.

f) Body piercing and tattooing presents a potential risk if equipment is not sterile however there are <u>no cases reported</u> as a mode of HIV transmission.

g) Deep, open-mouth or 'French' kissing can pose a theoretical threat if both parties' gums and mouths are bleeding. Again, this is an extremely remote route of HIV transmission and <u>it is not the kiss</u> or the saliva transmitting HIV, it is <u>the exchange of infected blood</u> that poses the threat.

h) Across Europe and North Africa there have been a small number of documented cases where infants who have been infected by unsafe injections have then transmitted HIV to their mothers through breast-feeding. This is thought to have been transmitted by the exchange of infected blood from cracked nipples.

The vast majority of people living with HIV have contracted the disease by means of unprotected penetrative sexual intercourse with a partner who already has HIV. Other HIV-positive individuals may have shared needles whilst intravenously injecting drugs using non-sterilised needles and syringes that have been contaminated by others already infected with HIV. In contrast, most babies born to mothers who are infected with HIV will not always become HIV-positive, particularly as current technology and medical practices and treatment advances. Finally, a smaller minority of HIV-positive individuals has been exposed to contaminated blood products prior to blood screening and heat treatments being carried out to safeguard against the spread of HIV. After 1985, all UK blood products were tested and heat-treated to destroy known viral contaminations of HIV infection. By 1989 the UK was allegedly largely self-sufficient in voluntarily donated heat-treated blood products. Any blood imported (by clinical choice) from international pharmaceutical operations is tested and/or treated before use in the UK. This is not the case for the Hepatitis C Virus (HCV) as will be revealed in the forthcoming chapters.

According to the <u>National Aids Trust</u> in 2011 there were 73,659 people in the UK living with an HIV-positive diagnosis and receiving medical care. Two thirds of people receiving HIV specialist care were male (49,083 men and 24,576 women). In the UK more people have contracted HIV through sex between men as opposed to heterosexual sex; however this is misleading. A large proportion of people infected via heterosexual transmission contracted HIV outside of the UK, whilst most men who have sex with men (MSM) acquired HIV infection within the UK. From the total HIV population in the UK, 36,355 people have contracted HIV through heterosexual contact which constitutes 49 per cent; HIV transmission via sex between men identified 31,825 reported cases (43 per cent). People injecting drugs represent approximately 2 per cent of the HIV population (1,636) and 1,488 have been exposed from mother-to-baby transmission. There were 533 individuals who had been exposed to contaminated blood products. In terms of ethnicity, 52 per cent of HIV-positive women and men living in the UK are White, whilst 35 per cent are Black African and 3 per cent are Black Caribbean. Mixed and other ethnic origins constitute 9 per cent of the total HIV population with 1 per cent unknown (this information is based on the Health Protection Agency's calculations for 2011).

In relation to intravenous drug use and HIV transmission, education and prevention programmes have been implemented to promote 'safer' drug use across cultures. Many governmental and other voluntary-based projects have emerged to promote wider harm reduction and primary health care services for injecting drug users, for example: needle exchanges, outreach facilities, community drug teams (CDT) and street agencies. It has become a priority for many countries to encourage as many injecting drug users into using these services and prevention programmes to prevent the spread of HIV infection and minimize drug related harm.

A brief history of AIDS and HIV: documenting 30 years

We conclude this introduction by outlining a brief history of HIV and AIDS over the past 30 years to remind ourselves of some of the main events of this relatively new disease. The syndrome known as AIDS [although not yet defined] was first identified in June 1981 when United States [US] scientists reported in the *Morbidity and Mortality Weekly Report* (MMWR) the first clinical evidence of a rare illness known as Pneumocystis Carinii Pneumonia (PCP) which killed five young gay men in Los Angeles. At the Centers for Disease Control and Prevention (CDC) in the United States, attention had been drawn towards an upsurge in demand for the drug pentamidine used in the treatment of PCP. In San Francisco and New York there was another unusually high occurrence of Kaposi's sarcoma (KS) amid gay men which typically only affected older men in Mediterranean climates. A scientific search began for the causative agent of these unusual immunological failures.

It took two years to isolate and identify a causative agent which much later came to be known as HIV. Since this time, clinical records and reviews of medical literature have exposed a somewhat disconcerting array of inexplicable AIDS-like cases dating way back to the 1940s in the United States and across Europe. Some researchers even argue that AIDS-like cases have occurred within populations well before the 1940s, albeit at much lower levels without stimulating suspicion or curiosity because of the rising incidence of infectious diseases.

During 1982 it became clear that this 'syndrome' or collection of symptoms had to be caused by an infectious agent, possibly a virus that might spread through blood. Scientists started to call this syndrome GRID (Gay-Related Immune Deficiency) and in the course of the year had identified three modes of transmission: sexual intercourse, blood transfusion and mother-to-baby. Clearly new cases were emerging which affected women, male heterosexual injecting drug users, Haitian refugees in Miami and also people living with Haemophilia; the syndrome was therefore renamed as AIDS [Acquired Immune Deficiency Syndrome]. In the UK one of the earliest male patients to die of AIDS was 37 year old Terry Higgins. Five months after Higgins' death, a group of friends founded a new charity to raise money for research: this was the Terrence Higgins Trust. By the end of 1982 AIDS had been reported in fourteen countries world wide.

In early 1983, the discovery of a retrovirus thought to be the cause of AIDS was isolated by Francoise Barré-Sinouss at the Pasteur Institute in France: this retrovirus was called lymphadenopathy-associated virus or LAV. During 1983 across Europe it became evident that there were two AIDS epidemics: one linked to Africa and the other linked to gay men who had been to the United States. In the States different patterns were emerging across different states amid Injecting drug users and gay men. The number of children diagnosed with AIDS had substantially increased towards the latter end of the year. The rise of AIDS amongst children prompted a report which falsely suggested that this increase might be due to the possibility of contracting AIDS through having contact with contaminated household paraphernalia, door knobs, cups, cutlery, and so on. This invoked fear and panic in a number of countries including the UK and became a major issue in the United States. At the end of 1983 two British people living with Haemophilia had been diagnosed with AIDS, and AIDS had been reported in thirty three countries.

In 1984 the US Government announced that the National Cancer Institute (NCI) led by Dr Robert Gallo had isolated the retrovirus which caused AIDS called HTLV III. This quickly prompted blood testing to detect antibodies to the retrovirus. During the same year, the death of a Canadian airline steward called Gaetan Dugas prompted widespread speculation that Dugas was responsible for 'bringing' HIV to North America. An early study by William Darrow of the CDC referred to Dugas as 'patient zero' which was later mentioned in Randy Shilts' (1987) book: 'And the Band Played On'. These rumours are considered to be unfounded as HIV had spread long before Dugas embarked upon his career. Neither the book nor the movie made reference to Dugas being responsible for bringing the retrovirus to North America.

By 1985 the Food and Drug Administration (FDA) in the US approved Robert Gallo's diagnostic kit based on the Western Blot technique. Later we saw the first commercial testing kit for HTLV III (HIV) antibody tests being licensed. In Atlanta the first international conference on AIDS was organised. The World Health Organisation (WHO) adopted a new clinical definition of AIDS in Africa to enable African countries to accurately identify and report the number of people who had contracted AIDS in these countries. In Uganda AIDS became known locally as 'slim disease' and across Central Africa large numbers of people were being identified as infected with AIDS. The declaration which shocked the world was when Rock Hudson, the first major celebrity, died of AIDS. In the UK, Dr Peter Jones, Director of Newcastle Haemophilia Reference Centre tested 99 of his patients living with Haemophilia A for HIV; 98 of which had received Factor VIII blood clotting agent and 76 patients tested positive for HTLV III (the precursor to HIV). At the end of 1985 AIDS had been reported in 51 countries.

In 1986 it emerged that the viruses LAV and HTLV III were actually the same retrovirus. It was ruled by an International Committee that both terms should be replaced by the name Human Immunodeficiency Virus (HIV). The World Health Organisation (WHO) introduced a global strategy for AIDS and in the UK the Government set up a Cabinet Committee on AIDS. In March 1986 the UK launched its first AIDS campaign in the form of a full page newspaper advertisement over one weekend. The charity Crusaid was formed to assist in funding for people living with HIV and HIV-related projects. By the end of 1986 there were 1,062 reports of HIV infection amongst people living with Haemophilia and others who had been recipients of a blood transfusion and tissue replacement in the UK. In Edinburgh a vast number of injecting drug users were testing positive for HIV. A second international AIDS conference was held in Paris and reported preliminary findings of the use of the drug Zidovudine (AZT) for the treatment of AIDS. Uganda and other African countries declared that its country had AIDS and asked for assistance from the World Health Authority. Zambia launched a national AIDS education campaign, promoting AIDS education in schools and rural areas using drama, dance and song.

In 1987 the Federal Drug Agency (FDA) approved AZT as the first antiretroviral drug for the treatment of AIDS within the United States. The Centers for Disease Control and Prevention (CDC) revised its definition of AIDS and placed a greater emphasis on the status of HIV. The International Council for AIDS Service Organisations (ICASO) was founded alongside the Global Network of People Living with HIV & AIDS. The World Health Organisation established a Special Programme on AIDS which later became known as the Global Programme on AIDS. In Uganda, Africa's first community-based response to AIDS was established (TASO) which became the role model for similar activities across the globe. In the US, Randy Shilts publishes *'And the Band Played on'* and activist Larry Kramer establishes the AIDS Coalition to Unleash Power (ACT UP), a non-violent activist movement which actively protested throughout the 1990s. In the UK the Government launched its 'Don't Die of Ignorance' advertising campaign and delivered leaflets to every household. Princess Diana met people living with AIDS whilst opening the first specialist hospital ward for AIDS patients. She did not wear gloves, which was widely reported in the national press and it was perceived to have helped change public attitudes towards people living with this disease. By November of 1987 AIDS had been reported in 127 countries across the world.

In 1988 health ministers from around the world met for the first time in London to discuss a common strategy for the AIDS epidemic. Delegates from 148 countries met to discuss *AIDS prevention* with the emphasis on education and the free exchange of information and experience; in addition they focussed on the need to protect human rights and dignity. The World Health Organisation's Global Programme on AIDS put forward World AIDS Day as an annual event to be held on the 1st December each year. In the UK the provision of funding for the expansion of needle exchange schemes was set in place to prevent HIV transmission amongst injecting drug users. In the US, the FDA put forward new regulations that would shorten the time taken for the development of new medicines for HIV and AIDS.

In 1989 the UK Government Cabinet Committee on AIDS was disbanded. The clinical trial for AZT in the US ended prematurely following the discovery that those taking AZT in the trial were effectively combating HIV as opposed to those taking only the placebo. AZT was to become available for everyone on the basis of this impulsive discovery. There were a number of new drugs available for the treatment of opportunistic infections and Didanosine (ddI) was authorised by the Federal Drugs Agency (FDA) for use by individuals intolerant to AZT.

In 1990 it was reported that a large number of Romanian orphans were HIV-positive as a result of contaminated blood products. The sixth international conference on AIDS was held in San Francisco amid global protests regarding the US immigration rules relating to not allowing HIV-positive people to enter the US. During 1991 the red ribbon was introduced as an international symbol of AIDS awareness and tolerance; actor Jeremy Irons became one of the first celebrities to wear a red ribbon at the Tony Awards ceremony. In the same year Freddie Mercury confirmed that he had AIDS and died a few hours after this announcement. Two weeks earlier, the professional basketball player, Earvin (Magic) Johnson declared he was HIV-positive and retired from the game. He then became a spokesperson for AIDS awareness and safer sex campaigns. A third drug belonging to the group known as nucleoside analogues called dideoxycytidine (Zalcitabine or ddC) was authorised by the FDA again for use by patients intolerant to AZT. During this year it became evident that AZT and other recently approved drugs were limited in efficacy over a prolonged period of time. Clinical evidence of resistance to these drugs started to emerge.

In 1992 we saw the drug known as ddC used in combination with AZT being approved by the FDA for adult patients who were showing clinical signs of immunological deterioration. This became the first successful use of a combination of drugs to treat AIDS-related illness. In 1993 the Concorde trial discovered that AZT was not an effective therapy for people living with HIV who were asymptomatic. In 1994 actor Tom Hanks won an Oscar for portraying a gay man living with AIDS in the film entitled: *Philadelphia*. In the same year, Elizabeth Glaser, wife of actor Paul Glaser who featured in the American cop series of Starsky and Hutch, died. She contracted HIV during childbirth and unknowingly passed this on to her daughter and son. During 1995 the results of the Delta trial demonstrated that combining AZT with ddI or ddC was a more effective treatment compared with AZT as monotherapy. Other studies confirmed this success and dual combination therapy became a standard medical approach to the treatment of HIV. In the same year, the FDA approved the first of a new group of medicines known as Protease Inhibitor antiretroviral drugs: this was Saquinavir. Also approved was the use of 3TC combined with AZT. Towards the end of 1995 the use of Saquinavir with nucleoside analogue antiretroviral drugs was further authorised.

A forgotten generation: Long-term survivors' experiences of HIV and AIDS

In 1996 it was a time of great optimism for people living with HIV as more effective medical treatment promised to successfully manage HIV and offer longer life expectancy. An increasing number of drugs had been approved by the FDA for use on their own and as a dual or triple combination with other drugs. Interestingly, the viral load test had been developed to provide information relating to the potential risk of disease progression around the same time. The advent of Highly Active Antiretroviral Therapy (HAART) was born towards the end of this year and was presented for the first time at the 11th International AIDS conference in Vancouver. The Joint United Nations (UN) Programme on AIDS or UNAIDS was set up in January 1996 which was designed to combine and replace other Programmes such as the work of WHO Global Programme on AIDS; the UN Children's Fund; the UN Population Fund; the UN Education Scientific and Cultural Organisation; the UN Development Programme and the World Bank. At the end of 1996, UNAIDS reported that new incidents of HIV infections had declined in many countries although the overall global rate of new infections had risen rapidly. Those countries that had shown a successful decline in new infections included: the US; New Zealand; Australia; northern European countries and parts of sub-Saharan Africa.

The history of HIV does not stop at the end of 1996 although this is questionable in terms of research on people living with HIV. We continue to explore other significant events within the 30 year history of HV and AIDS. It became apparent in 1997 that adverse side effects of taking protease inhibitor drugs had been widely reported. These effects were serious and could lead to diabetes and hyperglycaemia; the Federal Drug Agency (FDA) was forced to issue warnings. In 1998 doctors in San Francisco embarked on a new trial of post-exposure prevention. This is a treatment that aims to prevent the transmission of HIV after possible exposure before the virus takes hold in the body. During this year, more people were reporting severe side effects of the drugs, in particular Lipodystrophy [see glossary], which began to cast doubt on the long-term safety and efficacy of the combination therapies. The FDA continued to approve HIV drug treatments by endorsing the drug Sustiva [Efavirenz] as another NNRTI drug. In the UK, London Lighthouse closed its residential unit. The company AIDSvax began its first human trial using 5,000 volunteers across the United States for an AIDS vaccine in June 1998.

In 1999, US researchers from the University of Alabama, Birmingham reported the discovery of HIV-1 in a sub-species of chimpanzee, once common in Central Africa. They theorised that human hunters may have contracted this when exposed to the blood of the chimpanzee. A UK judge ordered that a five month old baby girl should be tested for HIV against her parents' wishes. According to the annual World Health Authority Report, AIDS had become the fourth biggest killer on a global scale.

For the first time, in 2000, the Clinton administration declared that AIDS was a threat to national security and to global stability. In 2001, following an announcement that generic drug manufacturers will offer to produce discounted generic forms of HIV medicine for developing countries, several major pharmaceutical companies agreed to offer further reduced drug prices to these countries. In 2002 the first rapid HIV test which reveals results in just 20 minutes using a finger prick test is approved by the Federal Drug Agency (FDA). In 2005 the FDA approves a generic AIDS drug produced outside of the USA which allowed the President's Emergency Plan for AIDS Relief [PEPFAR] to provide cheaper medications outside of the US. During the same year the AZT patent ran out which allowed further generic versions of the drug to be produced at a much lower cost.

In 2006, the head of Microsoft, Bill Gates stepped down from his role in the company to donate time to the Gates Foundation, which has become a large private source of funding in the fight against AIDS. The travel ban in the US was removed in 2009 which prevented HIV-positive individuals entering the country. A microbicide gel trial revealed that the gel reduces the risk of women becoming infected with HIV during sexual intercourse by nearly 40 per cent. This breakthrough took place in 2010. Some thirty years after the first case of AIDS was reported, in 2011 the National Institute of Health (NIH) publishes results of a study which stated that taking HIV antiretroviral drugs at the onset of infection leads to a dramatic reduction in HIV transmission. These results reinforced the importance of people knowing their HIV status and this was seen as another significant step forward.

Reaching the end of the introduction

Today, being told you are HIV-positive can bring with it a lot of uncertainty and anxiety. How you cope with a diagnosis such as this is largely dependent on your own personal circumstances and your personality and character. There are many ways in which HIV can affect lives and the medical diagnosis is only a small part of it. Coping with HIV has never been simply as issue of dealing with the physiological consequences of this retrovirus. The ways in which our story-tellers have faced uncertainty, ignorance and adversity and have preserved an optimistic and positive mental attitude in spite of everything is incredible. These narratives offer not only a backward glance on how each story-teller initially coped with and negotiated everyday life since discovering their positive status. In addition, these stories present a wealth of creative responses and coping mechanisms whilst managing the uncertainty of health and illness in the context of HIV and AIDS. We are offered a collective voice from a long-term survivors' perspective which is long overdue and it is to these we now turn.

CHAPTER ONE

Critical reflections: concepts, ideas and shared meanings

∞

"Intuition and concepts constitute... the elements of all our knowledge, so that neither concepts without an intuition in some way corresponding to them, nor intuition without concepts, can yield knowledge."

Immanuel Kant

Introduction

I want you to think for a moment about what you know and how you came to know it. What counts as knowledge? What do we mean when we say we *know* something? Where does our knowledge come from? We are incapable of understanding or making sense of our social world without language, information and ideas that organize, classify and categorise our experiences and what we observe around us into meaningful expressions. In general, knowledge can often be regarded as a set of ideas or 'facts' that seek to accurately or positively describe our world or parts of it in real terms. Yet how do we distinguish between knowing and believing? What do we know about our social world and is it truly knowable? It is essential to reflect on ideas about knowledge and other related concepts so that we can effectively interact with the HIV-related experiences we are about to reveal within this story-of-stories. At this stage I ask: What do you know about HIV and AIDS and where did you acquire your knowledge?

In brief, this chapter starts by exploring ideas on how we might think about the term 'knowledge' before critically examining how certain *concepts*, *ideas* and *shared values* might impact on our personal lives and dominant belief systems. We shall open up concepts pertaining to ideas and knowledge of 'health', 'illness' and 'disease' to see how we ourselves might view health and illness. How do we as human beings perceive our own health status and what happens to us when we become ill? We then shift our focus to ideas that might help shape our personal identities making us *who we are*, and briefly touch upon matters that might change how people see us and how we view ourselves in relation to others. We, as human beings, are constantly seeking answers to questions concerning the nature of our environment and the way it affects our personal lives and our social and personal identities. What makes us who we are? How do others perceive us? How do we see others around us? I ask you, the reader, to engage with and reflect on what you know and believe. What do we understand about how we come to acquire or develop knowledge about ourselves, others and our social world?

The final part of this chapter explores representations of AIDS and HIV in the mass media from the mid 1980s to early 1990s to reflect on how this impacted on public beliefs and perceptions of people living with AIDS and HIV. We predominantly focus our gaze on media reporting of HIV and AIDS during this era because it is the time when many of the story-tellers were initially diagnosed. It is intended, in some way, to remind the reader of the media coverage back then and set the backdrop for the narratives of personal experiences we are about to expose.

On Knowledge: critical reflections on a taken-for-granted term

Before we begin exploring ideas of health, disease and illness it is shrewd to critically reflect on what we mean we when use the term *knowledge*. What counts as knowledge and how is it to be conceptualised? What is the status of different forms of knowledge? Where do we find our sources of knowledge? Knowledge can refer to 'common-sense' or what we might perceive as expert knowledge; it can apply to existing information and specialised instruction that is known. We may also view knowledge as intelligence or enlightenment on a particular subject matter which might incorporate forms of knowledge on: individuals and groups; institutions; social relations; shared values and norms; cultural and sub-cultural practices; social and political structures in our societies and so on. Being well-informed can count as a form of personal knowledge. Whilst all of these do count as different kinds of knowledge, there does not appear to be an appropriate or precise definition of what we mean by knowledge that is all-encompassing as a shared or common understanding. Knowledge has different meanings for different people and carries with it a different status within particular social contexts.

I, like many others, argue that how we think about different types of knowledge depends on how we situate ourselves in our own social environment and how our social world is socially and culturally organised. Why do we accept one form of knowledge as legitimate and valid over another? For example: why does the majority of the world accept the prevailing HIV science as a legitimate form of knowledge over that of the AIDS dissidents who are also scientists? I am being provocative here.

Instead of searching for an all-encompassing definition of knowledge, it is far more important to examine how different forms of knowledge are socially or culturally organised. In other words, we must understand the relationship between how we construct, organise and convey knowledge using various media and the extent to which specific forms of knowledge carries with it a higher status than others. The importance of understanding this relationship is based on the belief that the way dominant forms of organised and expert knowledge is conveyed and socially practiced largely influences and shapes our own ideas, shared values and cultural and sub-cultural practices and becomes almost authoritative in essence.

What assumptions do we have about our social world? At one stage we assumed our world to be flat rather than round. How do we understand our social world in terms of the kinds of things that exist and do not exist? There is so much speculation about matters pertaining to life after death [afterlife], yet how much evidence is there to suggest that when we die we simply die rather than to the contrary? How does our world operate and how is it structured? Is our social world so fragmented with its multiple realities to be universally knowable? How you answer these questions depends of what you purport to know about your social world. This is called *ontology* – a way of understanding or *knowing* our world or parts of it based on explicit or implicit assumptions we have about the nature of our world. In order to know our social world we need to apply appropriate theories of knowledge that tells us *how we know what we know*. This is referred to as *epistemology* which focuses on how adequate our theories of knowledge are in relation to the social realities they are attempting to represent.

All of this may seem unnecessary and overly complex for the examination of what counts as knowledge. Yet we, as human beings, often employ ontological and epistemological deliberations when we make decisions on what forms of knowledge we accept as legitimate and those we reject. In everyday life we believe things that suit us; we often come to know things based on our beliefs and our interests. Members within unified social groups can and do develop genuinely held beliefs which subsequently support and legitimate their own interests. Beliefs and interests are connected in a mutually supporting way: beliefs tend to legitimate our interests and our interests support the sub-cultures within which these beliefs flourish and prosper. Certainly we do not talk openly about our own beliefs in this way. Instead we vehemently argue that our beliefs are justified and endorsed by 'facts' or based on knowledge or personal experiences that give testimony to this belief. If we are honest, we all believe things that suit us. Let us look at a couple of examples.

A forgotten generation: Long-term survivors' experiences of HIV and AIDS

Many rich and prosperous members of society commonly believe that income tax rates should be kept to a low minimum. Why is this? Not because it would make them even more affluent, although this would most certainly be true. Instead they argue and sincerely believe that it is the best policy for society. Low tax rates will motivate talented entrepreneurs to work even harder, thus expanding the economy and benefiting us all. Such a belief in low taxation, argues the affluent member, is clearly supported by economic debate and by the evidence of thriving economies in our global world. Holding such beliefs support particular interests and these interests support the affluent members of this sub-culture within which the beliefs flourish and prosper. Undoubtedly, there are those members of society who are not so rich or prosperous who also support this belief which is acknowledged here.

In the context of HIV and AIDS in the mid 1980s, the medical stance on AIDS was based on the accepted belief that heterosexual or homosexual, male or female everyone is at risk of contracting AIDS from sexual intercourse. In the absence of a vaccine, the best strategy was to educate the public about AIDS; it was a simple matter of common sense. Despite prevailing medical orthodoxy and public education campaigns, members who affiliated themselves with conservative moral politics believed that this was not so. AIDS was a homosexual phenomenon and was quite literally a godsend: a stroke of luck which provided an opportunity to go on the offensive against permissiveness. The only way of avoiding AIDS was heterosexuality, chastity and monogamy. Government public education campaigns on AIDS awareness was seen as promoting sex and promiscuity within a permissive society. Such divergent beliefs supported their own interests and their interests supported their political affiliation within which these divergent beliefs prospered. I believe we are getting the picture here! We can see more examples of this in the last section of this chapter.

In contrast, the libertarian viewpoint was rather different to that of conservative moralists. Libertarians focussed on the Government and perceived health education campaigns on AIDS as an attempt by the 'nanny state' to regulate matters pertaining to sexual morality. The AIDS campaigns on public education were seen as anti-sex propaganda; it was a way for the Government to legitimate state intervention and reclaim or take back our sexual freedoms given to us by the 1960s. Libertarians further believed that the Government had not only bowed down to the 'militant gay' lobbyists but had, at the same time, submitted to the influences of the conservative moralists: a kind of conspiracy or unholy alliance between the two affiliations. What a terrorising thought!

Whilst these arguments are perhaps complex, they do illustrate how beliefs and interests are inextricably connected. We must recognise that the privileging of certain forms of knowledge over another can be reliant upon how it affects social interests which simultaneously impact on dominant beliefs in terms of what we already believe we know about our social environment. Often we do not pay particular attention to these matters, but I ask that you reflect on these concerns as we proceed throughout this story-of-stories. What do you believe that suits you?

In today's society, we are completely inundated with information, technologies, ideas, beliefs and insights derived from scientific knowledge, these include: communication networks across the globe, mobile phones; laptops and computers; specialist and fad diet regimes; beauty products, treatments and cosmetic surgery; hair science; food technologies; health insights into calorific and optimum nutrition - *you are what you eat*; new reproductive technologies such as IVF and global vaccination programmes seeking to eradicate diseases forever: the list is endless. Without a doubt, we often think about ourselves and our lives through the lens of science. For example, we may explain our own personal habits, behaviours and appearances as genetic: our inheritance.

Alcoholism, intelligence, even homosexuality have all been described by some scientists as having a genetic component. It is in our genes! Increasingly, many societal problems are being explained by genetic influences which scientists continue to attempt to understand, predict, manipulate and control. A person's genetic make-up, for example, might be seen as a significant determining factor for certain diseases, such as heart disease and diabetes. This type of knowledge is potentially dangerous on many levels, is extremely contentious and has yet to be fully confirmed in research. There is much debate amid scientists, ethicists and the general public as to how genetic knowledge should be used. Is this form of knowledge good or bad science? Whatever we choose to believe, science and medical knowledge envelops our everyday life in so many ways.

It is widely accepted that expert and specialist forms of knowledge, such as scientific and medical knowledge carries with it a higher status and authority than other bodies of knowledge. These knowledge sources have a perceived legitimacy over others and are reliant upon our shared beliefs and values in conjunction with dominant cultural practices within our social world. Where we locate our sources of knowledge depends upon what it is we want or need to know and for what purpose. We draw upon multiple sources of knowledge when we wish to obtain information, become more well-informed or require more specialist forms of knowledge. We can access classificatory systems of knowledge pertaining to our social world currently in existence, for example: International Classification of Diseases (ICD). We might locate forms of knowledge from a variety of sources which include: TV, newspapers, books, journals and specialist magazines; the internet has now become an important source of knowledge; specific organisations and social network groups. We might approach socially certified professionals who we believe can offer or access expert knowledge that we, as unqualified individuals, do not have: such as a solicitor, a medical practitioner, a counsellor or a leading professor in their field. So, what do we do when we need to access sources of knowledge on health and illness?

Authoritative bodies of knowledge have to be socially sanctioned in order to retain a legitimate status. I pay particular attention here to scientific and medical knowledge as the most authoritative source of knowledge on matters of health, illness and disease. Yet one obvious source of knowledge in matters pertaining to our health is the experience of our own bodies. The personal knowledge we have of the subjective experiences of pleasure, pain or physical distress and bodily changes are of particular significance to us. At the same time we must be aware that our subjective experiences are influenced by other forms of knowledge such as words and language which in itself produces meaning.

When we go to a medical practitioner we expect that they have access to expert knowledge that we do not have. In the UK, for example, medical knowledge carries a very different status to that of common-sense or personal knowledge on matters of health, disease and illness; it has the socially sanctioned status of authority and legitimacy.

Let us stay with medical knowledge since this relates to our story. How do we *know* when we are ill? This is not as silly as it might sound. We might perhaps *feel* ill, as our bodies tell us that we are experiencing symptoms of illness but our bodies can not always interpret the underlying cause. We have a bad cough or a sore throat. It could be an infection. We have been experiencing severe headaches. Could it be a brain tumour? We might have pains in our chest. It might be angina or the onset of a heart attack. We might be feeling persistently tired, experiencing pain and discomfort but these bodily experiences do not necessarily mean that we *know* we are ill. So what measures do we have to take in order to *know* when we are ill?

Could our bodily experiences simply mean that we are hung over from the night before after copious amounts of alcohol and cigarettes? Could we be stressed or over-worked? Might we be worried about debt or how to make ends-meet and therefore interpret our bodily experiences as being 'under the weather'? We experience symptoms of illness or discomfort that make us question our health status but knowing we are ill can be far more complex. We go to a medical practitioner and speak of our symptoms. We undergo a medical examination to check out our bodies; the doctor takes our temperature and checks our blood pressure and then the heart and listens to the chest. Finally we are offered a course of antibiotics for the bad cough in case of infection.

We take the prescribed medication but our symptoms persist. We try to rationalise this and believe things will improve in time, maybe when the workload improves and we get paid. Our symptoms do not improve. We go back to the medical practitioner but this time after more rigorous medical tests we are diagnosed with bronchial pneumonia. We get a sick note for time off work, more prescribed medication and require complete bed rest. Our situation has completely changed. We have a medical diagnosis and authenticated proof that we are seriously ill. Personal knowledge of our own bodily experiences has considerably lower status than that of expert knowledge, although without experiencing symptoms of illness we would not have gone to see the medical practitioner. Having been given a medically authenticated diagnosis from a person who holds the status of medical expert means that we *know* we are ill and equally others *know* this too. This is the foundation of medical knowledge.

On the other hand, what happens when our bodily experiences do not reveal any symptoms of illness or discomfort? We could be totally unaware of living with a disease and be experiencing good health. We may only learn about our illness condition by accident or when it has reached a stage in its development when a visit to a medical practitioner reveals we have been ill for a long period of time. So how we know we are ill is a complex process. We require an expert medical diagnosis in order to obtain time away from work; we cannot authorize this ourselves. Medical practitioners are socially sanctioned to legally prescribe medicines and appropriate treatments to which we do not have access. Certainly, the knowledge of medical science is privileged and has the authority to validate what counts as medical knowledge. Yet existing medical knowledge does not mean that new knowledge cannot be constructed within this framework, as we shall see in this story-of-stories about HIV and AIDS-related illness. Let us now focus our gaze towards how we think about health.

Reflections of health: what is health?

As with the term *knowledge*, there are so many other terminologies we use on a daily basis without paying too much attention to what they embody in terms of shared meaning. At first, we might think we share a mutual understanding of the terms we use when we talk to each other but in reality is this always so? Until we begin to question what familiar terms actually do mean to us, it is not always straightforward. *How are you feeling nowadays? Oh, I am in rude health*! What does this actually mean? As soon as we attempt to characterize or describe everyday terms or familiar concepts, we are usually faced with an assortment of very different and divergent meanings amongst ourselves. What do we mean when we talk about *health*? We all have our own attitudes and beliefs when we refer to matters of our own health; these are significant to us in many ways and are often built on our subjective bodily experiences. Yet how do we know what others mean when they talk about their own health?

If I were a sports enthusiast, which I am not, I might consider my own health in terms of physical fitness: the ability to run so many miles or swim a great distance in a short period of time. If I were young, I might associate health with being able to dance all night or do karate or cycle everyday to work instead of using the car. If I were older I might simply consider health in terms of being able to get up in the mornings without too many aches and pains and walk to the local library or bingo hall. Some people may associate health with a varied and balanced diet with limited exercise, whilst others might believe a healthy start to the day is a full English breakfast. There is little consensus about what health is and probably even less when we come to examine how we might achieve health. How are we to understand the multiple dimensions of health?

Once you start to question ideas about the dimensions of health, it is clear that this depends on a variety of measures that we use to assess whether or not we and others around us are healthy. At first glance, we often associate health simply in terms of physical health: what we can and cannot physically achieve. Yet what about matters of mental health? Being healthy surely does not solely rely upon our functional ability to carry out a wide range of physical abilities; what about the demands of everyday life and our abilities to cope and manage psychologically? Imagine if you are athletic in build and run 5 miles every morning before your cup of black coffee without sugar for breakfast. You do not eat too much because you cannot be bothered; you are extremely depressed with life: you go to work every day but you hate it. You go for 5 or 6 pints of beer at the end of the day because you live alone. You outwardly laugh and joke with your work colleagues but you cry yourself to sleep every night. Are you healthy?

We need to have some kind of agreement as to what we mean when we use terms such as *health*, in order to communicate effectively with each other. Of course, beliefs about health do vary from place to place and have changed dramatically throughout periods of history. Some common attitudes and beliefs around health might often be expressed as:

1.   Something money cannot buy;

2.   A desirable state of psychological well-being and physical fitness;

3.   A personal state of strength, weakness or exhaustion;

4.   An absence of sickness, illness or *disease*;

5.   A blessing from God.

There are certainly many ways of characterising health yet for the purpose of clarity and common understanding we might want to separate how we approach the concept of health into two broader categories: *medical definitions* of health and *lay knowledge and beliefs*. [The term 'lay knowledge' is often used to characterise unqualified or untrained knowledge as opposed to specialist or expert knowledge; it is a term I dislike and use under duress]. Medical definitions emanate from medical practitioners and health-related organisations which are usually formulated on scientific and medical constructions of knowledge. Lay knowledge refers to ideas and perspectives we, as individuals, might have when we interpret our experiences of health in everyday life. This form of personal knowledge provides a way of understanding our own beliefs about health which are, without doubt, influenced by our existing social circumstances and prevailing medical forms of knowledge and are most certainly subject to change. Whilst medical knowledge of health carries with it a more privileged status, this is not to say that our own 'lay' beliefs about health are any less important as they influence how we understand and respond to health matters. Medical definitions and lay knowledge are therefore mutually dependent when it comes to matters of health.

One of the prevailing definitions put forward by the medical community is that health is *an absence of disease or bodily abnormality.* This is referred to as a negative definition of health and it raises important questions concerning how health is subjectively experienced as a relative quality. Regardless of how we feel, as long as we show no signs of bodily abnormality or disease then we are to be considered healthy. This definition assumes that our bodies must function to some form of 'normality'; there is a universal norm or standard in existence that our bodies should aspire to in order to be 'healthy'. This is problematic; how do you measure normality? Equally, there is no space for subjective experiences of illness which may or may not be linked to disease or bodily abnormality. So, in an attempt to rectify this flawed and unsatisfactory view, an alternative medical definition sees health as *the absence of illness or feelings of pain, anxiety and distress*. This similarly negative definition allows for experiences of illness but has its own problems in relation to its implication that health is purely a subjective experience which arguably it is not.

As health is such a multi-faceted phenomenon it is almost impossible to define in a socially useful way. But we still need to consider how we understand our own health status. For example, how are we to recognise or know when our bodies are absent of disease and bodily abnormalities? As we briefly explored earlier, not all diseases and illnesses are immediately accompanied by feelings and experiences of anxiety, distress or pain. This is certainly true in relation to HIV, as we will learn from the personal accounts of people who shared their long-term experiences of living with an HIV-positive diagnosis. It is worth pausing a moment to think about how we think about health, in particular our own health status. Are you currently experiencing good or poor health? How are you measuring your current health status?

Challenging the medical definition of health is a more socially-centred perspective proposed by the World Health Organisation (WHO: 1974): *health is a state of complete physical, mental and social well-being and not merely the absence of disease or infirmity*. Adopting a positive stance using a social rather than a medical approach, WHO associates health with the idea of an all-encompassing and balanced state of well-being. It is an extremely optimistic and ambitious proposition that undoubtedly departs from the negative view of health. All the same, it is open to widespread interpretation and raises almost as many new problems as it attempts to solve. How does one, for example, achieve and maintain a state of complete health? How can we reliably measure social well-being? What kind of individual and societal changes are necessary to achieve this (idealistic) healthy state?

If we were to write down our own subjective ideas and attempt to describe what constitutes *health*, what words would we use? What is not health?

What is not illness? What do we mean when we speak of being ill or sick? Virtually everyone has been ill at some point in their life. We come to accept that within any given society, almost all members encounter illness, injury, sickness and disease at some stage in our lifetime. Yet how are we to measure good health? How is the state of good health to be commonly understood and achieved? The dominant and underlying assumption for most people is that health represents the absence of injury, illness or disease or the absence of pain and bodily discomfort. What about matters of emotional and psychological differences between us in terms of our mental health? Many of us can identify for ourselves when we are miserable, sad or unduly worried and anxious; we can recognise and identify our own mental distress during times in our lives. What characteristics must we include in our considerations in order to accurately assess our state of health?

I make no attempt whatsoever to define health but instead critically reflect on what we mean when we talk about issues of health to demonstrate the complexity of such a familiar and taken-for-granted term. People's beliefs and attitudes on health matters are the consequences of trying to make sense of the various sources of knowledge and information to which we have access. There is a huge variety of sources of knowledge relating to health and illness at our fingertips. Many of our popular perceptions of health arise from our attempts to seek order where there is chaos and confusion in our social lives. Our own perceptions allow us to cope with the complexity of health issues as we attempt to make sense of our lives in relation to our selves and our everyday life choices.

Matters pertaining to our health and healthy life choices are given extensive coverage within the media: radio, television, newspapers, magazines and DVDs all devote space and time to current health matters. Accordingly, not all information and specialist knowledge pertaining to health and illness remain the property of medical and health professionals. The Internet now provides us with a massive explosion of diverse forms of expert and personal knowledge within seconds. Thirty years ago, access to such diverse sources of knowledge would have been unattainable. Ideas and forms of knowledge located by way of the Internet shape and influence our own beliefs and are literally available at the touch of a button. These technological advancements have stimulated debate into how instant access to various ideas and forms of knowledge has changed our social environment into an 'information society'. Our divergent beliefs about health do vary between us all and have dramatically changed over time. Scientific knowledge and its endeavours will, without doubt, however continue to influence and dominate our beliefs and values and impact on our social lives.

Yet, I believe that differing beliefs about health and well-being are further rooted in wider social and cultural contexts. How we live our lives and how we adopt our personal lifestyles cannot be separated from the social and economic structures in which we live out our lives. In other words, our understandings and interpretations of health are embedded in our social environments and are shaped by dominant social institutions, cultural affiliations, personal biographies and social identities. There is a tendency to view notions of health through our own cultural and sub-cultural lens which influences and shapes the way we come to understand, interpret and perceive health and health matters. The complexities and divergent understandings of what we mean when we use the term health cannot simply to be understood at an individual level.

How does our own health, well-being and experiences of illness impact on who we are and on our sense of 'self'? What do others think about us? As we develop as human beings from an early age, we come to recognise ourselves as individuals. We learn about aspects of our social identity such as gender (being male or female), social class (working class, middle class or upper middle class), the problematic distinction of 'race' (whether we are Black, Asian, Caucasian or of mixed heritage) and ethnicity (British, Jewish, Irish, English). We soon learn to recognise who we are and how we are similar to or different from other people within the social environment that we live in. Our personal identities then start to develop over time and as human beings we transform ourselves from babyhood to adulthood embracing physical and mental changes as a natural process.

The physical changes that do occur relate to our bodies. The commonsense notion of *the body* is that of a natural, biological entity. The experience of our own bodies is a source of personal knowledge we consider to be significant when we seek to know about matters of health and illness. Yet the body has become more than just a biological entity in today's society. Dominant intellectual traditions have, in the past, considered the body as something external to the mind; a natural reality. Our bodies have largely been constructed as a physical entity and as a functioning system that has been analysed and examined by anatomists and medical practitioners. Nowadays, however, there are many developments and ideas with reference to our bodies and, to be sure, medical, surgical and technological innovations concerned with changing our bodies and those associated with human reproduction are abundant. It is now possible to change a body from male to female and vice versa.

It is important to be aware of how the changing nature of human bodies and consumer culture tells us how ideas have shifted from our bodies being the producers of things, to our bodies as consumers of things. For example, keeping fit, keeping slim and maintaining youth clearly shows a commercial and cosmetic interest in our bodies. How we view health and how we view our bodies then is an important factor to consider. Our health, psychological wellbeing and our bodies are an important part of who we are. Once we are labelled as seriously 'ill' or when we become sick or injured this potentially impacts on our sense of self; it can permanently or temporarily change who we are and how we think about ourselves and can impact on how we are viewed by others around us. Being labelled as sick, injured or disabled can also have political connotations which can have positive and negative components attached to them.

Understanding disease: the medical model

If we view health simply in terms of the absence of disease or bodily abnormalities, then how do we understand disease? The term *disease* is widely used to represent a particular conception of illness amid the medical community. The term 'medical model' refers to the conception of disease established in the late nineteenth and early twentieth centuries and is based on an anatomical-pathological perspective of the individual body. Using this approach, disease can be understood as the presence of some pathology (see glossary) or irregularity that has typically invaded part(s) of the human body from the outside. Germs, bacteria and viruses, known as pathogenic agents, which are found in our bodies *may* cause disease. When disease is present, specific physical organs risk being attacked and bodily functions become impaired. The restoration of health can only be achieved by external physical intervention by way of medical practices such as surgery or drug therapies. In other words, disease is essentially a mechanical defect of our bodies which is largely independent of our minds and personalities.

The medical orthodox of disease is not as straightforward as it might first appear. The development of the medical model is not always met with acceptance by all members of the medical profession. There are some, especially members who work within public health, psychiatry and General Practitioners, who argue against the complete application of the medical model for medical practices. Epidemiologists (see glossary) in public health argue that there is an over-reliance on curative medicines by the public and too great an influence on the part of the medical community. Psychiatrists argue against the use of the medical model of disease for matters pertaining to mental illness. Disagreement and controversy remains widespread amid the medical community as to how far it is the appropriate and proper way to conceptualise insurmountable diseases such as cancer using this model.

The medical model is also distinguished from other models of health, illness and sickness. For example, holistic medicine and psychosomatic models of sickness are alternative approaches which regard illness as incorporating an expression of the mental state of the person who is sick. Holistic medicine acknowledges *malaise* of the whole organism: the body and the mind. Healing is, to some extent, dependent on the co-operation of the sick person in order to achieve good health. Yet the medical model of disease continues to be justified and vindicated by the perceived unremitting success of scientific advancements in medicine that conquer and manage infectious diseases with the use of pharmaceutical drugs and other treatments. We will explore how advancements in medical treatments have impacted on long-term survivors living with HIV in later chapters. How might you describe disease and its characteristics?

We continue to focus on the medical conception of disease and examine how medical practitioners come to establish disease in our bodies. Evidently, we must first of all seek medical attention before any disease can be medically established. The task of the person seeking medical attention is to recognise signs and symptoms and convey our subjective experiences to the medical practitioner who then searches for significant signs of alterations or abnormalities in the body. Our medical practitioner then undertakes extensive investigations consisting of objective tests measured by medical technologies and devices, or alternative specialised medical procedures to identify abnormalities; bodily irregularities are recognised by the medical profession as having a coherent and separate existence or origin. It is important to remember however that disease may or may not be accompanied by feelings of discomfort, distress or anxiety. We mentioned earlier that some people have diseases without even knowing or experiencing physical pain and discomfort. On the other hand, it may take a while for disturbances or abnormalities in our bodies to make their presence known and thus affect our health status. So, whether it is by accident or at a time when we experience symptoms indicating severe disruptions to our health, the identification of disease by way of extensive medical observations leads us to an expert diagnosis. We are then labelled as being ill.

The medical model assumes a clear separation of the mind and the body. Physical diseases are perceived to be located in our bodies and illness is reduced to disordered bodily functions, for example, biochemical or neuro-physiological disturbances. As a consequence, biomedicine attempts to understand, control and treat parts of the body in isolation from other parts of it. Illness is isolated to a certain part of the body and the rest of our body and indeed our minds are often overlooked, and at worst ignored. Medical knowledge, I believe, is not merely a description of disease and neither is it simply an attempt to effectively treat disease and illness. Cultural differences in medical practice and amid practitioners trained in medicine reveals variations in diagnoses and therapies.

Medical knowledge is also used to reproduce and reinforce existing social structures and common cultural values. This is certainly evident in the medical construction of HIV which can be transmitted via the most intimate of human contact. HIV strikes at the very heart of individual and social interactions and reveals the fragility of social order. Strictly speaking, AIDS is not the name of a disease and it cannot be transmitted from person to person. It describes a condition that requires the presence of other illnesses, namely opportunistic infections brought about by a compromised immune system that leaves the body vulnerable to cancers, fungal infections, viruses, Pneumocystis Carinii Pneumonia [hereinafter referred to as PCP] and so on. HIV is believed to be the virus that damages the immune system to such an extent that it may lead a person to later develop AIDS. The clinical diagnosis of AIDS has been subject to continual redefinition and clinicians tend to use the term HIV rather than AIDS today. What do we know about diseases? How many diseases are there across the globe? Alcoholism is a disease. Cancer is a disease. Diabetes is a disease. Epilepsy is a disease. Measles is a disease. Syphilis is a disease. HIV is a disease. Why do we view some diseases with more compassion than others?

Critical reflections on the meaning(s) of illness

Not surprisingly, health and illness is possibly discussed more often in everyday conversation that any other topic. Much of our private and public lives depend on us being physically, mentally and socially competent to function in everyday activities. Yet what do we mean when we talk about illness? Is illness merely the absence of health? How do we view others who are labelled as ill? We might think that illness is perhaps more straightforward to recognise and therefore less complex to characterize than health or disease. It is, after all something we largely feel or experience at a more personal level. One implication of illness is that it appears to be a departure from the 'norm' in terms of our bodily experiences: a departure from our normal or usual physical and mental feelings of well-being. Our subjective interpretation of problems we associate as health-related matters can be seen as an interaction between our bodies, our selves and our minds. As I keep repeating however, any identification of signs or symptoms of ill health may or may not accompany disease. For sure, we may be extremely uncertain about recognising significant signs and symptoms of severe illness conditions, as we may not have sufficient knowledge of diseases.

When we show signs or symptoms of illness what do we do? Some people immediately go and seek medical attention and reveal their symptoms. Some might research their symptoms on the Internet or consult The Family Health Encyclopaedia to glean some idea of what the illness condition might be and attempt to treat the problem themselves. Some ignore their symptoms and carry on with daily life until such a time when illness makes it impossible to continue with daily routine. Others might just take bed-rest for a short while and hope that whatever 'it' is goes away. Whatever we choose to do at the onset of symptoms, we are often forced to accept that something is wrong with us. Something is not functioning properly and we are not feeling how we usually feel. Clearly whatever we choose to do when we believe there is something wrong depends on the severity of our symptoms.

Let us reflect a moment on how we feel when we encounter minor ailments: perhaps the most common type of illness is a bad cold or a bout of the flu. When we have a blocked nose, sore throat, a headache, aches and pains in our joints and possibly a fever what do we do? Many of us do not seek help from a medical practitioner unless we are elderly or live with an underlying medical condition, such as HIV, that renders the cold or bout of flu as potentially hazardous. We may feel tempted to stay in bed and take complete rest rather than endure our daily activities, if this is practicably possible. We might choose to self-medicate and take aspirin or paracetamol, honey and lemon drinks, vitamin C or rely on other over-the-counter pharmaceutical remedies that we know will benefit a speedy recovery. Some of us also expect that those around us will show signs of sympathy and understanding whilst we are feeling ill. Being aware that our symptoms are most likely to be short-lived means we can look forward to feeling better very soon. This is not the case, however, if we live with a chronic illness condition. The impact on our experiences of illness and the effect on our identities and personal lives, and those around us who care are inevitably more profound.

Dependent upon the severity of our illness, being ill can mean that everyday activities and routines such as going to work, doing the cooking or cleaning or attending to other daily matters are, at varying degrees, disrupted. Illness can be a significant reminder to us that the usual, taken-for-granted functioning of our bodies and our minds is central to how we act and socially interact with those around us: our families, friends and work colleagues. When we are healthy or fully functioning we often overlook and undervalue these matters until something goes wrong and forces us to reflect on our selves and our social situation. If we cannot rely on our bodies or minds to function properly, then our involvement in everyday life within our social environment becomes more complex. An inability to take part in our usual everyday life and do everyday things means we may have to rely upon others to help out during periods of illness. Being ill and our experience of illness can essentially impact on our sense of *who we are* - our sense of 'self' and our self-esteem. Think about a time when you experienced an injury or a prolonged illness. How did you feel about yourself? In what ways did it stop you performing your usual routines or daily activities? Did you require help and assistance from others around you? What were the attitudes of others around you when you were ill?

To be sure, the very idea of being healthy and fully functioning is not only a personal desire but a social ideal which embodies a particular culture's notion of desired human qualities, social expectations, standards, norms and values. When we become ill it is socially accepted that during these times we might be unable to fulfil our normal social obligations and responsibilities in every day life. If we believe we have the flu, for example, we might feel unable to carry out our daily routines or familial obligations such as: going to work, attending school, college or university or picking up children from school because of severe aches and pains. But would it be the same if it is *only* a common cold? Prevailing social expectations that exist within our social environment can affect and influence our own attitudes and behaviour; the way we react to ideas about illness often reaffirms dominant core values and our own internalised expectations of ourselves.

Once illness has been identified and medically diagnosed as being an acute or chronic illness this can have a profound impact long term on our personal and social lives. In social terms the implications and consequences of being ill extend well beyond biological and physical disturbances: it affects our social role in society. The onset of a chronic illness can involve the severe disruption of a person's biography and often forces us to reassess how we will have to live out the rest of our lives. As human beings we have a unique ability of reflecting upon ourselves in terms of our social situation, our bodily experiences and perceptions about ourselves. Having this reflective ability means that we not only endure the disease within our bodies; we are also affected by our personal experiences of illness and how this impacts on others around us who might attach a significant meaning to it. A person living with HIV or AIDS-related illness does not only have to endure the physical discomforts associated with the disease; the personal experiences of being ill in conjunction with how others in society might react to their illness is equally significant and has serious implications and consequences for that person.

If we study illness a little closer we see how the presence of illness significantly shapes and changes how we socially interact within our cultural society. I am now going to separate the term 'sickness' and 'illness' to explore how being ill and being sick might be conceptualised in different ways. For clarity of meaning, when I use the term 'sickness' I am referring to the social functioning of a person who is labelled as being ill within their own cultural environment. When I use 'illness', I am referring to the personal experiences of being ill. It will make sense to the reader shortly when we explore the important concept of the 'sick role' which cannot be overlooked.

The notion of the 'sick role' is a concept originally popularised by Talcott Parsons (1951) which puts forward the idea that whilst the medical model of disease incorporates bodily abnormalities and dysfunction, *being sick* [i.e.: being labelled and accepted by others as ill] involves us taking on a role governed by social expectations within our cultural society; this incorporates certain responsibilities, a set of rights and privileges. This concept draws our attention towards the social regulation of illness as a form of social control, compliance and moral authority. When we are ill, we are often incapable of performing certain duties and roles. If our sickness is recognised as unintentional and is therefore not a deliberate attempt to excuse ourselves from our social obligations and is further legitimated by a medical practitioner then we are not held responsible. If you have contracted flu or have been medically diagnosed with an illness that is not considered as deliberate then you have the right to remove yourself from your social obligations. However if you go out and get blind drunk and are unable to attend work the next morning, this is seen as an act of deviance and therefore social privileges and rights are removed.

Sickness can be seen as a legitimate excuse for being exempt from your normal obligations, however rights and privileges depends on the sick person's intent on getting well. The sick must attempt to get well as quickly as possible and this implies that you seek appropriate medical help and co-operate with those helping to treat your illness. A sick person is also expected to 'act sick': so a trip to the shops or down to the pub whilst you are exempt from social obligations is not considered as acceptable behaviour.

Sickness then is not merely the condition of an individual but relates to the wider social order. It is connected to moral issues and prevailing social norms and social regulation. Sickness is often related to the ability to work and fulfil social obligations. The concept of the sick role is an ideal type and does not always reflect our social realities; I am sure we can think of situations where the sick role does not apply.

By identifying the concept of the sick role it does, however, help us to highlight how forms of social control do operate in society and distinguishes ways in which we deal with sickness. How we think in terms of what constitutes illness reflects dominant and prevailing norms, standards and shared cultural values. What happens when you are ill and cannot go to work over a prolonged period of time? What social expectations must you fulfil to retain your social status? Does your illness become part of your identity? We can certainly agree that people do react differently to someone who has a serious illness, such as cancer, than someone who lives with diabetes.

The nature of some chronic illness conditions, however, does not fit too neatly with the ideal of the sick role. Being chronically ill usually means that medical treatment is aimed at controlling and managing the illness over a prolonged period of time. Any intent to get well can be irrelevant for people living with certain chronic illnesses, such as Parkinson's disease, some types of cancer, heart disease and dementia. However people living with chronic illnesses such as: asthma, diabetes and epilepsy may vigorously avoid being socially identified as being ill because adopting the sick role could be considered a threat to their identity and self-worth: indeed some people cannot afford to withdraw from social obligations. Many people living with a chronic illness have no desire to be exempt from normal obligations yet they often experience considerable difficulty negotiating their roles and social status in society. As we will see in chapter two, the experiences of long-term survivors living with HIV clearly touches upon these matters. The idea of being exempt from social obligations on a temporary basis is not always applicable for chronically ill members of our society and so the benefits of adopting the sick role become meaningless and futile.

As we have established, there is a biological and a social foundation to sickness. Being ill affects us at a personal level, but being sick is a socially altered state. When we are viewed by others as being sick, our social status alters from being healthy to being ill and our function and roles within cultural society subsequently change. Dominant cultural ideas around *sickness* are attached to particular social meanings which can involve sickness as being seen as a threat to social order. Different people respond differently to particular illnesses or diseases; the implications of treating some diseases more favourably than others have profound consequences.

HIV as a disease is certainly no stranger to the idea that as a disease it is perceived to threaten social order. Some diseases carry with them a negative connotation which can stigmatise the disease: HIV again fits the criteria here in terms of potential discrimination and prejudice. The very definition of illness is socially constructed and social groups often assign responsibility for illness to the sick person. Illness conditions and diseases that might be transmitted sexually or involve substance abuse are often treated as being the responsibility of the sick person. As we have witnessed with HIV, there are those who are seen as responsible for their HIV-positive status: homosexuals, the promiscuous and injecting drug users. Then there are those who are considered the 'innocents': people living with Haemophilia, those who contracted HIV via blood transfusions and so on. We examine media representations of the 'innocent' and 'guilty' towards the end of this chapter. Can you think of any diseases that assign the responsibility for illness to the sick person?

When we become severely ill, we are often reminded of our own mortality. Human beings face two causes of death: untimely and tragic death and death due to the exhaustion of our natural life span. There is no way of avoiding death by attempting to cheat your way out of it; death is an inevitable part of life itself. We all ought to prepare ourselves and get ready to die at some stage in our lifetime. Yet many of us choose to ignore death; we often fear death; we refuse to talk amongst ourselves about issues of death and dying. How many of us realistically think about our own mortality? If we drink large amounts of alcohol every day do we consider the likelihood of cirrhosis of the liver and premature death? If we are overweight do we think about heart disease, heart attacks and ultimately death? Many women and men living with HIV and AIDS-related illness in this story-of-stories have had to face the challenges associated with the reality of imminent death following an HIV-positive diagnosis. How many of us think about death and the process of dying? What are our overriding fears and anxieties associated with death and dying?

Meanings and interpretations of illness are shaped by our individual personal experiences and a wider social and cultural context. When we are ill our lives can be seriously disrupted either temporarily or for a prolonged period of time. Ordinarily we do not reflect on our health status until something goes wrong; our health and our abilities to function in everyday life are often taken for granted. Following the onset of symptoms and a diagnosis of a chronic illness, we often experience a process of loss; we start to critically reflect on our sense of self: who are we? We can be affected by how others react around us. Illness impacts on our personal experiences and identities: some illnesses, like HIV, are perceived to threaten the social order and thus promote stigma, discriminatory practices and HIV prejudice. Living with chronic illness can also place a strain on our personal and social relationships with others. We may experience a crisis in terms of our sense of self, our identity and our self-image when illness threatens and disturbs our stable and established sense of who we are; it is to these matters we now turn.

What makes us 'who we are'? – reflecting on identity

How do we define ourselves? How do we know who we are? How do others identify us? How can we have a sense of our own unique identity when we share aspects of our own identities with others? Who we are and how we see ourselves is a complex process. Our identity is not just out *there* for the taking, it must always be negotiated and established: identity is about meaning, about *being* and *becoming* and is a continual process. Our experiences of *who we are* can be deeply affected by our social or cultural environment as well as our own capacity to create ourselves in our social world. Our sense of identity is confirmed in our significant relationships with others: we feel in harmony with ourselves when we have a role to play and we have a recognised place in our cultural society. If aspects of our identity are shaped by being HIV-positive how might this impact on our relationships, social roles and our identification with others?

The question of 'self-identity' that is being the same as, rather than being different from others, involves defining our selves rather than others and comes from many different sources, such as: gender identity – experiencing ourselves as masculine or feminine; sexuality identity – homosexual, bisexual or heterosexual; social class identity – working class, middle class or upper-middle class; ethnic identity; national identity; age; occupation; religious identity; cultural and sub-cultural affiliations. Identifying ourselves individually and collectively is certainly not straightforward to categorise. For example, a male, heterosexual, middle class, White, Catholic British man in his mid 30s might have different life experiences and a different sense of *who he is* to that of a male, homosexual, working class, Black, Anglican British man in his mid 30s. What I am suggesting here is how we come to know who we are largely depends on how we identify ourselves in relation to others and how we experience and situate ourselves within our own cultural environment. How might you describe yourself in terms of your own identity to another person?

Identity does appear to be incredibly important to us all both at an individual and collective level wherever we might be situated. We, as human beings, are not born with a single identity; our identities evolve and change over time. Our identities are rooted in our own identifications: in what we associate ourselves with. A person born in Britain might identify as *being* 'British'; this becomes part of their national identity. The same person might then identify as *being* gay, lesbian or heterosexual; this becomes part of their sexual identity. They might have an occupational status of *being* a solicitor, teacher, medical practitioner or traffic warden and therefore identify with a particular social class. They might be affiliated with a particular orthodox or fundamentalist religion or particular political party which significantly impacts on their self-identity and contributes to their own personal politics and ways of being in the world.

At a more personal level, the same person might identify as someone who needs to hate a particular religious or ethnic group because that is the perceived idea that other members of their own religious and ethnic group are 'supposed' to do. Although such personal beliefs have no basis in reality, they are often taken at face value by those who adopt such beliefs. This often creates problems for those who act on their mistaken and irrational belief systems. Identity is not simply based on what you know but is grounded in how you know what you know. This goes back to the ideas we discussed earlier about knowledge: we believe what suits us.

Without a doubt how we think about ourselves and how we experience our social lives deeply influences our sense of who we are. When we talk about our 'true selves' or look at our own reflection in the mirror what do we really see? If we were to describe who we are, what words would we use? How we think of ourselves in relation to others helps us create our own social world. We are aware of ourselves in two ways: as *being* ourselves and *thinking or reflecting* about ourselves. Our 'self image' is constructed in the ways in which we define who we are to ourselves and to others around us.

There is a common belief, for example, that we are what we are because of our genes [discussed earlier]. This established belief in biology being our destiny is often contrasted with notions of identity that stem from how we socially interact within our environment. How we develop our personal identities and notions of who we are is undoubtedly complex and can be determined by many factors including: genes, social roles, cultural and sub-cultural affiliations and the social institutions we interact with. Nevertheless, we must allow space for human agency and our capacity to create ourselves and live out our lives in our social world.

Human agency involves basic questions about social action (how we act in our social world), the moral choices we make and notions of our own free-will (independence). This is known as the debate between the 'individual' and 'society' and is multi-faceted. Depending on what you believe, often greater emphasis is given to one over the other; however the two are inextricably linked and cannot be separated. Ask yourself: do individuals create their own social worlds or is it society that shapes its members through socialisation, education and forms of social control? [Socialisation is a term that refers to the social processes by which children develop an awareness of social norms and values and attain a distinct sense of self] If individuals are shaped by society, how can society change so much, as it has done over the past 30 years? Similarly, how do individuals change society? These are very complex questions to consider and many of us go through life without engaging with such considerations. It is, however, something I have thought about for many years. The notion that there is a dividing wall between the individual and society, I believe, is a nonsense; but it is a popular nonsense that appears quite plausible. Perhaps the issues involved are so tricky to conceptualise that it requires some kind of simplification.

Until we critically reflect upon our own personal identities in more detail, and establish what factors help shape our notions of selfhood (who we are), we fail to notice how our personal experiences are an assembly of different bits and pieces; our social roles and identities are not singular or clear-cut in everyday life. A woman, for example, may find herself in varying roles and relationships in different social or cultural contexts in every day life. She might be a daughter, a mother, an aunt, a niece, a partner, a lover, a teacher, a traffic warden, a sister, a close friend, a writer, a manager, a supervisor, a counsellor or a neighbour and all of this may be daunting at times. Each of her roles incorporates sub-roles that bring with them certain restrictions and boundaries or they might even overlap with other roles and relationships. What I am suggesting here is as individuals our personal identities can become fractured; they are fluid and multi-dimensional and we often fail to acknowledge this when we think about who we are.

Once we begin to examine our selves and our personal identities in terms of patterns of roles and relationships that connect us to our social world and prevailing social expectations, this draws attention to the ways in which identities are created and formed out of social action. People create and change their social roles and regardless of how dominant social expectations might be, we are continually re-shaping our characters. There is always room for interpretation and negotiation. Yet frequently we do not acknowledge ourselves as an assembly of different bits and pieces in everyday social action. We do, however, feel the need to have a certain amount of control over our own lives so that we are able to manage difficult situations, or make appropriate decisions in the face of challenges that we might encounter in our everyday lives. A desire to control aspects of our lives is diminished when we are diagnosed with a chronic illness, such as HIV. How much control do you consider you have over important aspects of your life?

As mentioned earlier, we feel in harmony with our selves when we have a significant role to play, when our sense of identity is confirmed in our relationships with others, and when we have a recognised position or status within our own social world. For example, if we are unemployed because of chronic illness, this does not simply imply financial hardship. It shapes and undermines our social role, our sense of identity and brings into question our value and place in wider society. In cultures that favour heterosexuality, coupling and the family as a social norm, gay, lesbian and single people without children may struggle with their own sense of identity and self-worth. Similarly, if we are chronically ill and unable to function in everyday life, this too has an impact on how we see ourselves and also how others might see us. The more we seek out the characteristics of our 'true selves' the more we find our own culture with its expectations and patterns deeply embedded in our sense of selves.

Yet what about physical and mental changes which occur in our bodies and minds when we come to think of ourselves as being ill? How does this alter notions of who we are and impact on our personal identity and notions of self-worth? Only when we begin to question particular sets of beliefs about social norms, roles and cultural values that exist in our social world do we come to understand how these affect ideas about our sense of self. Adhering to social expectations and social norms can lead us to adopt certain attitudes which impacts on how we react and behave. Once our health is compromised by illness and the biophysical changes to our bodies, aspects of our everyday life can be severely disrupted. Our experience of illness can change how we see ourselves and force us to reassess who we are and where we are going from now on. Being ill might mean we have to significantly modify our daily routines and activities,' it can alter the relationships we have with others around us and it may severely disturb our sense of 'self. Illness is not merely a personal or individual condition, but can affect our social roles and relationships.

A forgotten generation: Long-term survivors' experiences of HIV and AIDS

Serious chronic illness conditions, like HIV and AIDS-related illness, can undermine the unity between our bodies, our minds and our sense of self and force, to a degree, identity changes. When we have to adapt to a chronic illness condition, this can mean totally altering our social and personal lives to accommodate bodily losses and physical limitations. For some it means struggling with rather than against illness whilst, for others, there is a battle to fight against bodily losses imposed upon them. Living with an HIV-positive diagnosis long term can involve a total disturbance of a person's taken-for-granted sense of identity at its very roots: it can become a complete transformation into 'another world' as being HIV-positive changes that person's life. But this is not always the case!

Representations of HIV and AIDS in the mass media: a disease of lifestyle?

From the mid 1980s to early 1990s, our perceptions of life expectancy for people living with AIDS and HIV was only a matter of years; unquestionably the sorrow and emptiness created by the untimely departure of friends, relatives and lovers during this era cannot be denied and should never be ignored or forgotten. Many news variations and other mass media representations of AIDS and HIV failed to acknowledge or cover this loss. A pause for thought for all our lost loved ones ... yet we must also spare some thought for all those women and men, namely our very own long-term survivors, who have lived with and successfully negotiated HIV and AIDS-related illness over many decades. AIDS is no longer presented as an apocalyptic threat – the end of the world is not nigh! And since AIDS has now become a relatively incoherent medical term, does its cultural significance still remain as potent? After all, HIV is now medically defined as just another chronic illness condition. Can it really be reduced to such simplicity? No, I believe the cultural significance is still potent and matters in relation to HIV are never simple.

For many people, HIV has always been perceived as the result of deviant and undesirable behaviour: a problem of morality more than a viral disease and a problem of medicine. This, I am sad to say, is still fairly prevalent in 2013 in some dark corners of our society regardless of the advancement of knowledge and public awareness on the subject. We have to appreciate that HIV and AIDS had to be recognised publicly before it could become a 'social problem' and, at the same time, it had to be recognised personally before it became an illness. Imagine for a moment if AIDS or HIV had a more positive social meaning attached to it... It is probably too difficult to imagine.

A forgotten generation: Long-term survivors' experiences of HIV and AIDS

All of our story-tellers were diagnosed between 1981 and 1994, so in order to at least try to appreciate the impact of an HIV-positive diagnosis during these murky times, it is crucial to remind ourselves how HIV and AIDS had been publicly recognised through the constructions of the mass media. We must, for sure, acknowledge and recognise that the mass media is an extremely effective mode of communication for raising awareness and educating the public on health-related matters as well as being a powerful tool of governments, conservative values and propaganda. The media coverage of AIDS has been credited with, and condemned for, a variety of constructions and perspectives on these matters. Nonetheless, glancing back, we must pay particular attention to the harmful ways the media misinformed the public in its reporting [and distorting] of medical and scientific matters in relation to HIV and AIDS. By paying selective attention to certain types of human and scientific evidence and, simply by getting things wrong in relation to HIV infection and the syndrome known as AIDS, this has had a profound impact on how we have come to think about AIDS and HIV: in terms of the negative social meanings associated with this stigmatised disease.

In the mid to late 80s, AIDS received an unprecedented amount of media and Government attention as it entered our public consciousness. During this era, living with AIDS was perceived to be inevitably fatal both within and outside of media reporting: AIDS the killer disease. In one sense, I suppose the media is to be forgiven for this, as medical and scientific perspectives also supported and confirmed this view: a medical diagnosis of AIDS did equate to imminent death. Yet despite continuous scientific debates and medical advancements in the construction of HIV and AIDS, its association with 'promiscuous' sub-cultures and deviant forms of [sexual] behaviour proved too tempting to disregard, as it helped create and elevate sensationalist and outrageously shameful headline stories.

From 1983, many papers associated AIDS with the term 'gay plague. For example: on 2nd May 1983 the *Daily Telegraph* posted headlines: *'gay plague may lead to blood ban on homosexuals'*. Other headlines such as *'gay plague sets off panic'* could be found in The Observer *(26 June 1983)*. The notion of the 'gay plague' appeared to dominate our national press in spite of incidents of infection amongst other identified 'high risk' social groups also being medically reported during these times, which included: injecting drug users, commercial sex workers and people living with Haemophilia. The term HIV did not come into play until 1986, before then the virus was scientifically known as either LAV or HTLV-III. In 1984 an article was published in Science magazine with the title: *HTLV-III in saliva of people with AIDS-related complex (ARC).* This led to an influx of panic stories in the press some months later about the contagious nature of AIDS. The *News of the World* ran an article: *'Kiss of death – Scientists now fear that the killer disease AIDS could be caught by just kissing.'* (20 January 1985). After this, the press ran stories about gay men being banned from work and barred from clubs and public houses.

'Hotel bans gay chef who took AIDS test' (*Sun*, 14 February 1985); *'Scared firemen ban the kiss of life'* (*Daily Mirror*, 19 February 1985);*'"Burn all your clothes" shock at AIDS hospital'* (*Sunday Mirror*, 10 February 1985). Not surprisingly, even the medical profession apparently became anxious: *'Doctor refuses to touch AIDS victim's body'* (*Daily Mail*, 16 January 1985). Interestingly, we do not pay much attention to how the press might influence the medical community, yet clearly this happens. Fortunately, not all members of the press jumped on the band wagon. In an attempt to put things right with public perceptions of the risks of contracting AIDS, the *Daily Telegraph* quoted the Chief Medical Officer for England, as saying:

> *'You cannot get it from sitting in the same room or sharing a meal with, a person with AIDS, since it is not transmitted through the air by coughing or sneezing… It is nonsense to say, as it has been suggested, that homosexuals should not eat in restaurants for fear of passing on the disease … Whilst it is true that the virus has been found in saliva, there is no evidence that the disease has been transmitted from plates and cups.'* (*Daily Telegraph*, 07 February, 1985).

The public perceptions of risk severely affected public attitudes and behaviour towards people living with AIDS and the stories kept flourishing. Around the same time, we see slight changes in attitudes in our national press, such as in the *Sunday Telegraph* (03 February 1985*)* when Mary Kennedy makes the comment: "*Of course people should not be persecuted or blamed for catching AIDS, because that is vindictive and uncharitable and anyway, it can be caught innocently."* Now let me see… … Well, any vindictive notion of contracting HIV 'innocently' can certainly be seen as uncharitable and speaks volumes.

Attitudes such as these create a very dangerous notion that there can be potential 'leakages' of infection from a culpable minority of people to a blame-free population: it is an attempt to distinguish between the 'guilty' and the 'innocent'. It implies that there are some people out there with AIDS who 'deserve' it. Any signs of compassion might appear to be reserved only for those perceived as 'the innocents'. One particular newspaper *The Daily Star* went even further some three years later and deliberately chose their time of attack. In 1988, the very next day after International AIDS Day (now known as World AIDS day) this newspaper proposed repressive measures against the perceived 'guilty victims':

> 'Surely, if the human race is under threat, it is entirely REASONABLE to segregate AIDS victims – otherwise the whole of mankind could be engulfed. Some experts have even suggested that offshore islands should be used for the colonies. Pro-homosexual groups like the Terrence Higgins Trust will scream that it is unfair. But they would. The truth is that promiscuous homosexuals are by far the biggest spawning ground for AIDS. They COULD curb the spread of the disease if they curbed their sexual appetites, but that does not seem to be happening, despite all the warnings and all the condom campaigns. Right now, ideas like AIDS colonies have got to be worth serious consideration.' (Daily Star, 2 December, 1988)

This type of attack on 'promiscuous homosexuals' was not unique but to propose segregation was exceptional. I am left wondering who the 'experts' were that suggested offshore islands should be used as colonies? How would you feel if you were HIV-positive after reading this? How many other chronic illnesses can you think of that carries with it such prejudice and widespread condemnation for the people living with a disease? It is evident that many journalists tended to adopt different styles of reporting dependent upon whether those who contracted the disease were gay or heterosexual. What was considered newsworthy in a positive light, during this era, tended to be the exception rather than the rule: in other words, we saw only those reports that offered contradictions to the dominant beliefs about AIDS. Personal biographies about those who might allow readers to empathise with their social plight filled our newspapers and magazines.

The human faces put to clinical cases of HIV tended to be innocent heterosexuals who had 'inadvertently' caught the disease via another route of transmission other than sexual. The 'innocent' and the 'guilty' are incidentally all deemed as 'victims' of this 'gay plague'. The innocents included: people living with Haemophilia; the recipients of blood transfusions; children, and the elderly who were all singled out for sympathetic attention by the media. We did not see, however, sympathetic reporting on the dilemmas that gay men faced or indeed reports on the thousands who had struggled with and subsequently died from AIDS during this period. The Daily Star printed this statement the following year:

> 'How many families have been sentenced to death by faceless blood donors who were drug addicts or permissive homosexuals? And how

long are we going to support spurious charities for those who brought this awful curse upon themselves? Sympathy is fine. But would not our support be better directed towards the innocents who received tainted blood through no fault of their own?' Daily Star, 29 August, 1989

On the whole, people who had died by contracting the disease by perceived 'illicit' or 'morally unacceptable' practices, that is those who died by being gay; by being bisexual; by being a commercial sex worker [prostitute], or by being an intravenous drug user were reported in a far more negative light than those who might have been infected 'accidentally' or iatrogenically (via blood transfusions or contaminated blood products). People who fell into the second category were reported as the 'innocent victims' of this 'abhorrent disease'.

In addition to newspaper reporting on AIDS, we also witnessed other advertising campaigns to promote education and public awareness on AIDS issues. During Christmas of 1986 an advertising poster campaign was launched nationally spelling out AIDS on Christmas wrapping paper with the question: *How many people will get it for Christmas?* Another poster conveyed the message *'Your next sexual partner could be that very special person'* framed inside a heart similar to a Valentine card, and beneath the heart it reads *'The one that gives you AIDS'.*

What is the message here? Who is the target audience? This was all very confusing as there was no information about AIDS or HIV. How many people 'did get it' - the message I mean? How much information were we able to glean about HIV and AIDS from such ambiguous campaigns? Did these posters merely spell out anti-sex messages that highlighted promiscuity as the cause of AIDS in order to terrorise people into abstinence or monogamy? Or did they tell us something else?

During December 1986, the British government was spurred into action as it launched the first television advertising campaign on AIDS. This, in part, was a reaction to the 'gay plague' coverage we had witnessed in the Press. This type of public education set out to increase knowledge and awareness that might lead to attitudinal change and shifts in public behaviour. But the Health Education Authority (HEA) had no real experience of promoting sexually explicit information and therefore terminology became problematic due to political sensitivities. The target audience were those perceived to be 'at risk' within the UK population – that is those who might contract HIV due to lifestyle choices. Yet who was to be included as *at risk* and who was not?

The television part of the campaign originally intended to highlight risk practices and how to avoid HIV transmission.

Interestingly, there were no campaigns, at this time, aimed at people who were already HIV-positive and similarly there were none aimed at changing general attitudes towards people living with HIV and AIDS or those perceived to be 'at risk'. This was the first governmental message on AIDS:

> *"There is now a danger that has become a threat to us all. It is a deadly disease and there is no known cure. The virus can be passed during sexual intercourse with an infected person. Anyone can get it, man or woman. So far it has been confined to small groups, but it is spreading. So protect yourself and read this leaflet when it arrives. If you ignore AIDS it could be the death of you. So, don't die of ignorance."*

Why was it *now* a danger and a threat to us all? What had changed? There was a distinct lack of information within this message: perhaps the idea that the public was in ignorance was directly related to the Government's own incompetence of relaying appropriate information to raise public awareness. How many of you remember the AIDS leaflets with the iceberg or the granite-like tome stones coming through your door? From this TV advertising campaign, we were invited to read a leaflet in private that was to be delivered to every household. Risk practices and how to avoid HIV transmission were covered but sexually explicit language was problematic and tended to water down the message intended.

At the same time in December 1986, whilst making a speech at a National Conference of police officers discussing measures of how to protect police forces from occupational exposure to HIV, a senior officer referred to 'obnoxious practices' and 'degenerate conduct' of sections of society. He described people living with HIV and AIDS as *'swirling around in a cesspit of their own making'*. Bernard Manning might have been proud of this speech, but how does this help the plight of those living with AIDS? We also saw poster campaigns which screamed out the following messages:

AIDS IS NOT PREJUDICED IT CAN KILL ANYONE!
THE LONGER YOU BELIEVE AIDS ONLY INFECTS OTHERS, THE FASTER IT'LL SPREAD
AIDS: HOW BIG DOES IT HAVE TO GET BEFORE YOU TAKE NOTICE?

In spite of the orthodox medical position, the varied attempts to educate the public with AIDS awareness campaigns, and the Health Education Authority campaigns, as late as 1989, *The Sun* newspaper recklessly printed this headline: 'STRAIGHT SEX CANNOT GIVE YOU AIDS – OFFICIAL.' Following on from this ridiculous, irresponsible statement, The Sun (17 November, 1989) then went on to declare:

> 'At last the truth can be told. The killer disease AIDS can only be caught by homosexuals, bisexuals, junkies or anyone who has received a tainted blood transfusion. FORGET the television adverts, FORGET the poster campaigns, FORGET the endless boring TV documentaries and FORGET the idea that ordinary heterosexual people can contract AIDS. They can't... the risk of catching AIDS if you are a heterosexual is 'statistically invisible'. In other words impossible. So now we know – anything else is just homosexual propaganda. And should be treated accordingly.'

This article was initially brought about by the Labour Peer, Lord Kilbracken in November 1989 who mistakenly claimed, whilst being a member of the All Party Parliamentary Group on AIDS, that there was only one case of heterosexually transmitted HIV in official statistics, and several newspapers ran this as a prominent feature. Under no circumstances can newspapers, like the *Sun*, be excused for this totally outrageous and irresponsible headline story.

Some five years ago, back in 1984, the *British Medical Journal* presented a published debate amongst scientists as to whether AIDS was a 'new' disease or an 'old' disease based on the problems that had largely gone unrecognised across central Africa. As this debate unfolded, it soon became clear that there were crucial differences between stories-about-AIDS within an African context and those found within Europe and North America. First, there was a completely different sex distribution between men and women who were medically diagnosed as having AIDS. Second, in most African cases people living with AIDS did not seem to emerge from specific 'risk groups', such as homosexual, bisexual men, injecting drug users, sex workers and so on. This evidence therefore widely challenged the dominant belief at the time that AIDS was a 'gay plague' which originated in Haiti amid gay men vacating there. This extensive debate was largely ignored by many journalists; it was probably 'too boring' for newspapers like the *Sun*.

Broadsheet newspapers did not always follow suit however and correspondents printed articles and viewpoints that clearly recognised and accepted the dominant orthodox views of the health professionals and government officials. In 1988 *The Times*, for example, welcomed government plans for anonymous testing and warned against complacency: *'AIDS will be here for a long time – longer than the reach of any public relations campaign. The more that is understood about its transmission the better. Too little is known about the epidemiology of AIDS'* (24 November, 1988). This was in opposition to what we had previously seen above. Specific sections within the *Independent* and *Guardian* highlighted their familiarity with social welfare, health, community, sexuality and gender. On the eve of World AIDS day in 1989, several weeks after The *Sun* declared 'STRAIGHT SEX CANNOT GIVE YOU AIDS – OFFICIAL' *The Times* wrote:

> *'AIDS is still seen as a sordid disease largely restricted to promiscuous homosexual men and intravenous drug abusers. The belief that 'normal' people are somehow immune to it is almost entrenched now as it was at the beginning of this epidemic. The evidence, human and scientific, tells a different story... Against this background, the insistence that AIDS is a 'gay plague' would be laughable were it not so tragically short-sighted. In the Western world, AIDS merely showed up among homosexual men first'* (30 November, 1989)

This article and others like it clearly reflect how newspapers can demonstrate responsibility in AIDS reporting. Many newspapers, however, enjoyed the power of the mass media without taking responsibility for their stories and its aftermath. Most, but thankfully not all, media coverage of AIDS and HIV we have identified here reveal messages suggesting that there is this HIV virus out there that selects its 'victims'. Imagine if there were diseases that deliberately selected 'victims': how might HIV and AIDS have been constructed if it were perceived as only selecting traffic wardens, single mothers, teenage adolescents, tax inspectors, newspaper journalists or police officers? For the sake of being ludicrous, why should any of us believe a disease belongs to any particular social group within contemporary cultural society?

There were many AIDS advertising and educational campaigns between 1986 and 1990 which involved a great number of public and governmental organisations and health officials. Yet there appeared to be very little substance to any of the messages at an informative level. Public Education Campaigns did, however, set out to inform the general population about HIV transmission and 'safer sex' practices but they took so long to produce, for a variety of complex reasons. As a consequence, many HIV-related and Non-Governmental Organisations (NGOs) had already achieved success in their own campaigns by highlighting specific concerns and raising public awareness about HIV and AIDS matters. Using sexually explicit language and identifying sexual practices that were more commonly understood amongst sexually-identified groups, these campaigns proved far more effective in raising public awareness.

Notwithstanding the above, other media forms that sought to draw attention to matters pertaining to HIV and AIDS did break certain barriers that no other public health campaigns had achieved in the past. Current affairs programmes, documentaries, audience participation shows, dramas and soap operas created space to show the complexities for alternative representations of HIV and AIDS. Some of these did impact on public beliefs about HIV and AIDS and caused many people to voluntarily seek out further information but there were limitations and often 'experts' were the key figures in many of these media productions.

One prominent dramatisation was brought to us in 1990 when we saw the HIV-positive diagnosis of a heterosexual central character, Mark Fowler, in the popularised BBC soap *Eastenders*. Following its airing, it has been quoted as resulting in the highest number of calls to the National AIDS Helpline after it was shown on TV (PHLS, 1993). The BBC's scriptwriters for *Eastenders* attempted to portray a more complex picture of a 22 year old fictitious person living with an HIV-positive diagnosis by giving a central character within the Soap a key HIV storyline. The scriptwriters sought advice and technical information from the Terrence Higgins Trust and the main characters in Eastenders were also able to use their resources and access counselling facilities. In return, the Terrence Higgins Trust received guarantees about the nature and the direction of the HIV storyline.

Here we saw Mark Fowler's fears about dying set out for the public during his counselling sessions. We also saw the dilemmas he encountered in negotiating sexual and intimate relationships with his new girlfriend and problems associated with him disclosing his HIV-positive status to significant others. There were also discussions about the possibility of him having children in the future. The HIV storyline explored the problems associated with HIV from the perspective of a person living with HIV, as well as those around him. We also witnessed how Dot Cotton changed her attitude towards Colin and Barry, when she learned that they were not flatmates but lovers. She starts to worry that she may be infected by drinking a cup of coffee from Barry's flask. She sought advice from Dr Legg who took on the role as teacher who advised other central Soap characters on a range of medical and psychological matters pertaining to HIV. Dr Legg informs Dot that she can only catch AIDS through sexual contact, a blood transfusion or sharing a syringe with someone who is already infected. This was a considerable advancement in the presentation of HIV and AIDS during this time. Well done, Eastenders!

It is not easy to imagine just how some of these media representations of AIDS and HIV impacted on people diagnosed with the disease during this time and afterwards. It is equally difficult to measure the extent to which public attitudes and behaviour started to positively change once knowledge and awareness of the medical realities of HIV became more firmly established. Twenty three of our story-tellers who speak about their experiences of living with HIV were diagnosed between 1981 and 1990. During this time: there was limited information on the virus; very few care and support mechanisms in operation, and no effective medical treatment available to them as there is today. In addition, many long-term survivors were told, at the time of diagnosis, that they were going to die within 5 years - some even earlier than 5 years. For those who were not given a medical 'death sentence' at the time of diagnosis, their own perceptions and beliefs were such that their life expectancy would be considerably cut short. For the vast majority of long-term survivors who tell us their story, pre-test counselling was non-existent and for some, HIV testing was carried out without their consent.

How do you think you would have managed an HIV-positive diagnosis in the 1980s? What would have been your reaction to the stories in the national press? To whom would you have disclosed your positive status? How do you think people around you would have reacted? Many matters concerning AIDS-related illness and HIV infection, sero-positivity and being infectious are, by their very nature, medically defined. From the mid 1980s onwards, the medical process of diagnosis for HIV infection has been relatively straightforward - by way of an ELISA blood test which identifies the presence of antibodies to the virus. However, *being* HIV-positive and living with an AIDS diagnosis is much more than just a medical matter. Living with and experiencing these conditions profoundly affect our sense of self, our relationships with others, our social roles and everyday social life. The personal, social and psychological realities of living everyday long-term with an HIV- positive diagnosis are, by far, more complex and much less understood. We turn now to the rest of the chapters to explore how our long-term survivors' have managed and negotiated everyday life living with HIV or AIDS from 1981 onwards.

CHAPTER TWO

Testing positive: Diagnosis day

∞

"AIDS is a problem of undesirable minorities – mainly sodomites and drug abusers, together with numbers of women who voluntarily associate with this sexual underworld."

Sir Alfred Sherman

Introduction

Consider for a moment how the above public statement might make you feel as a person living with an HIV-positive or AIDS diagnosis? This declaration by Sir Alfred Sherman, the co-founder of the Centre for Policy Studies, was cited in the *Independent* [Sunday 1st November 1994]. It is difficult to imagine the impact a statement such as this might have on a person living with HIV in terms of self-worth, self-confidence, potential stigma, secrecy and possible social rejection. Without doubt, HIV has been inextricably linked to stigma in that it has been connected to: a) stigmatised social groups, such as gay men, Black Africans, commercial sex workers and Intravenous [hereinafter IV] drug users; b) it can be sexually transmitted; and c) it was initially medically defined as a terminal disease. Managing an HIV-positive diagnosis is not only about coping with the physical consequences of chronic illness; HIV has become a public issue and involves negotiating social, personal and intimate relationships, dealing with negative attitudes and public beliefs and renegotiating a sense of self – *who I am*.

This chapter reveals how our story-tellers who took part in this HIV study discovered they were HIV-positive. Here we introduce all the women and men who made this story-of-stories happen, using their own voices and experiences to illustrate how each story-teller's personal situation led to 'diagnosis day'. We expose how some long-term survivors were tested for HIV involuntarily without their consent; this occurred either by mass-screening programmes for people living with Haemophilia or as a result of seeking medical attention for minor illnesses. Other personal accounts reveal to us how story-tellers decided to voluntarily test for HIV because of embarking on new relationships, or living with a partner who was already

HIV-positive. A few of our story-tellers were experiencing symptoms of illness associated with HIV or AIDS and decided to voluntarily test for HIV; others acknowledged certain risk behaviours associated with HIV and therefore believed it was necessary to voluntarily take the test.

Not all of our story-tellers were experiencing signs of illness at the time of their HIV-positive diagnosis. It is perhaps difficult to comprehend how you might feel when you consider you are healthy and then suddenly discover you have a 'fatal disease'. For those who were tested without their consent it must have been a tremendous shock that would have impacted enormously on their sense of self and their social world. Twenty two of our long-term survivors were tested and diagnosed with HIV between 1981 and 1990 and the remaining six long-term survivors who shared their personal experiences were diagnosed between 1992 and 1994. All story-tellers were diagnosed at a time when there was little effective HIV medicine available in the UK and 'imminent death' was very much a reality, especially for those diagnosed in earlier years.

Let us remind ourselves that the personal experiences we are about to read were told to me during the year 2002. As with all the chapters that unfold, I ask that you actively engage with and reflect upon how these personal stories might impact on your own thoughts, feelings and beliefs. As we have seen in chapter one, there are some who might publicly view AIDS and HIV as some sort of retribution for a questionable or immoral life style; ask yourself is this your own belief either now or in the past? Throughout this story-of-stories my aim is to stimulate and promote further enquiry and critical reflection from within us all. By doing this, it will facilitate an appreciation and develop a deeper understanding of ourselves and the matters we are about to reveal.

Experiencing the HIV-positive diagnosis: mass screening and haemophilia

In the early 1980s, people living with haemophilia were drawn into in a mass screening process across the UK which tested for the presence of HTLVIII (now known as HIV). Some people were tested voluntarily following discussions with their Haemophilia consultant whilst others were tested involuntarily and learned of their diagnosis from their medical practitioner or Haemophilia centre.

Many people often think of Haemophilia as a disease; it should be acknowledged that Haemophilia is not a disease but a disorder of blood clotting (see glossary). Children are born with it and if parents are aware of any family history, haemophilia can be diagnosed in the womb or at birth.

A forgotten generation: Long-term survivors' experiences of HIV and AIDS

There are many levels of severity ranging from very mild haemophilia to severe forms. For an in-depth and complete guide to haemophilia and related bleeding disorders see Jones, Peter (1998) *Living with Haemophilia*. Fourth edition, Oxford University Press.

It is worth noting here that for many people living with Haemophilia, dependent upon the severity of their illness condition, medical treatment and hospitalisation has been part of their everyday lives since childhood. During the 1980s in the UK, we should also acknowledge how newspaper coverage of HIV and Haemophilia potentially risked exposing people living with Haemophilia to significant others around them; by associating HIV with Haemophilia the public became aware of the possibility of people with Haemophilia having the HIV virus that causes AIDS. By reporting the relationship between HIV and Haemophilia in the Press, family members or friends of people living with Haemophilia were able to make assumptions or question whether or not someone with Haemophilia was HIV-positive. Such an invasion of privacy had the potentiality to cause widespread anxiety and distress to people living with haemophilia in relation to their family, friends and social relationships.

GLYNN

Glynn, a self-identified heterosexual man aged 37 was diagnosed with HTLV III back in 1983 when he was about 17 or 18 years old. He was included in a mass screening programme at his Haemophilia centre and voluntarily took the test. He recalled:

"... there were 65 of us and we all got told at the same time. We got told individually but there were 65 of us. They didn't really know anything about it so they just said *'you've got this thing'*, I don't even think they called it HIV at that time, and basically *'it was terminal'*... that was how they left it because it was so early on. We just said *'yeah ok'* because we were only 17 or 18 at the time. It was pretty strange to be told this... there were 80 odd Haemophiliacs tested at the centre and about 20 of them didn't have it: I mean we knew for a fact that the Christmas disease Haemophilia B group, they didn't have it because they have a different factor batch to us, factor IX and we have factor VIII."

Glynn remembers how at that age he didn't really think much about the diagnosis and put it to the back of his mind. He recalls having to tell his parents and how there was a lot going on because nobody knew of treatments and outcomes during this time. He further mentions how out of

65 people who were diagnosed as positive during the same time as himself, he is only one of three survivors left. When asked about his feelings in relation to this he told me:

"… I felt pretty crap really. It is difficult to put into words why some people have died, well actually, the majority of them are dead and I am one of three left. I cannot tell you why that is. I am upset about it and sad because they were all the people I grew up with from when I was 10 years old up until I left college – so all my school mates basically."

SPIKE

Spike, a self-identified heterosexual man aged 27 is the youngest member of this study and was only a child when he learned of his HIV-positive status – it was HTLV III at that time. As a consequence, he does not remember the exact date of his diagnosis but believes it was between 1981 and 1983. He states how his Mum had always been active in his Haemophilia care and remembers how HIV was never really spoken about within the family, as there was never any real need during his childhood. He tells us:

"I don't know when I was first told because I was so young when I would have contracted HIV... I can't remember sitting down with my consultant but I know it has always been there. I remember being told to mop up my own blood if I had a cut and stuff so … when you're a kid it's like water off a duck's back but even so I knew I was going to die like those kids in hospital who were probably dying. It was like… so what? You know it's going to happen ... before I started High School I knew I was positive and I knew that I would be dead within a few years. I always knew I would die young and even when I was 18 I knew that I wouldn't live for much longer."

Spike talks about getting on with life and 'sorting things out' in terms of making a Will and always having a clear idea of what he wanted to happen to things he possessed and how he wanted his own funeral arrangements and says "it was never a sad sort of thing to think about." Spike's story is somewhat different to others, as he was only 8 or 10 years old at the time of his diagnosis.

PAUL

Paul, a self-identified heterosexual man aged 38 was tested involuntarily and was informed by his Haematologist at a routine visit for his Haemophilia condition back in 1985, at the age of 21 years. He recalls:

"I was simply told I had been diagnosed with the antibody positive to the HTLVIII virus; that is what HIV was called at the time. I remember saying *'antibody positive, so that means I have got antibodies to it and am ok'*. Obviously it was explained to me that 'no it does not mean this' and that I have 'actually got the virus that causes AIDS'... I had no counselling... they tested without my authority or consent... I felt completely and utterly unsupported. I had no way of getting my head around it beforehand and I just went in there cold... I went to a doctor's appointment, came out being told I was positive and, with only a quarter of an hour in there, I was told I had 4 or 5 years to live. I had only taken an hour off work."

Paul is not alone with this type of experience. Whilst media coverage on HIV and Haemophilia was featured in the National Press, Paul spoke of his awareness in the news but he had not seriously thought it all through in relation to his own circumstances. For Paul, this positive diagnosis completely changed his entire outlook on life from current relationships to his life prospects to which we will turn to in later chapters.

MARTIN

Martin, a self-identified heterosexual man aged 38 recalls living at home during the time he discovered his HIV-positive status in 1985. Following coverage within the tabloid papers concerning the link between people living with Haemophilia and contaminated blood products, Martin voluntarily took the test; he was in his early 20s at the time. He tells us:

"I went for a blood test back in 1985 and on Friday 13th September I saw the doctor and he said "you are positive and don't tell anybody" and that was it. I went back to work and carried on working. I only knew what I had read in the papers that it was the gay plague and it was also affecting Haemophiliacs and my life expectancy was one year. I was only 21 or 22 at the time and you can't imagine dying at that age... my brother was a Haemophiliac too and he was HIV-positive. We didn't tell anybody... we didn't tell our parents or the rest of our family."

Martin had expected his test to be positive and had an idea what his result would reveal. He states that he didn't fall apart at the time and wasn't depressed. He recalls feeling that already some of his life choices were limited by his Haemophilia. Martin describes himself as *lucky* in terms of not experiencing many debilitating bleeds and not having bad reactions to his Haemophilia.

Voluntary testing: embarking on a new relationship

Three self-identified gay men revealed how, at the time of diagnosis, they had recently become involved in intimate relations with a new partner and therefore felt it was important to know their own and their partner's HIV status. Voluntarily testing, according to our story-tellers, was considered a matter of good practice when starting out in intimate relationships or 'falling in love'.

COLIN

Colin aged 42 decided to voluntarily take the test at his local sexual health clinic after meeting his partner, in July 1985; he was 25 years old. He talks of his limited knowledge about HIV at the time and makes mention of AIDS as 'the death sentence'. He told me:

"I had just fallen in love for the second time in my life. I can't remember whether he had just decided to take the test or he was actually awaiting the result… it came out positive. I thought I had better get one myself. My main concern was a practical one; if he is HIV-positive and I am not then we will have to use condoms and we will have to have safer sex… we were very into each other. Bizarrely my first reaction of getting a positive test was almost partially one of relief. I didn't know whether this was a death sentence or whether certain people wouldn't progress or wouldn't go on to get AIDS… I think I dealt with it with a certain amount of denial to start with… I essentially put my own diagnosis aside and simply didn't deal with it for four or five years."

Colin then told of how his partner soon developed AIDS and died in 1990. Colin stayed with him until his death and put all his energies into his care. Whilst talking about his partner's death, Colin broke down in tears:

"I only went out with him for a total of four and half years until his death. The first couple of years were fine and then by 1987 he was clearly ill and the last year he was dying with AIDS. I still cannot talk about it in depth without getting emotional because I think I learned so much about very rare issues about life and death."

DAVID

David aged 65 is the oldest member of the study and tells a remarkable story of how he discovered his HIV-positive status. He was 52 at the time of diagnosis in 1990 and recounted:

"I was a year into a new relationship and we both thought we were the luckiest people on earth… I changed my GP who was doing random blood testing and I was asked if I would like to know the results… I said yes of course, being quite confident that I wasn't infected, but the result came back positive. I had been having unsafe sex with my partner… I felt for the first time in my life that I was cheating somebody of something so important. I could have infected him or he could have infected me… we didn't know at that stage, it was dreadful… this anxiety of having been five years without a relationship because I have always been in a relationship, one after another, all my life and then to meet somebody and then a year into it, find this… He proved not to be positive… he was absolutely marvellous and he said 'I want to stay with you so that was hurdle number one over."

He then relates how his GP gave him the news:

"He was a very nice man but he told me, I was 52 and that I could expect to be dying by the time I was 54. Oh, and I thought I am not going to die as I have got too much to do… that inspired me as well because I became involved with the HIV community in London."

David goes on to describe how, during his involvement in the HIV Community, he witnessed many young men who were being diagnosed with HIV simply giving up and claiming benefits because they had given up work. He states these young men were sitting at home in their flats, watching TV and waiting to die. David says: "I wasn't going to do that because my personality isn't just to sit around… I am accused of being a fidget, you know."

WOODY

Woody aged 45 remembers how he was diagnosed back in 1992 at the age of 35, after voluntary testing at his local clinic. He had undergone pre-counselling prior to the HIV test and told me how he had previously lived in New York for three years. He says:

"I'd been putting off getting diagnosed because I had no symptoms; but then I just decided that it was about time I ought to know… I was actually seeing somebody at the time and he wanted to have sex without condoms… Thinking back I'd actually been seeing somebody who was HIV-positive and whose ex-lover had died from AIDS… I knew it at the time but my mind didn't actually connect the two… I didn't think "Oh my God! I've had unprotected sex with him" I can't explain that! I just sort of shut it out completely… there was a 50/50 chance that I might be. When I got the result I remember thinking for days, weeks, months "I'm HIV-positive! I'm HIV-positive! I'm HIV-positive! I wasn't surprised or shocked but I was upset and being HIV-positive is like 'I've got cancer, I've got cancer."

Woody later reflects on why he failed to make earlier connections relating to his previous sexual practices and his failure to acknowledge that his ex-lover had died from AIDS during his time in the States; he believes he had always put matters such as this to the back of his mind, despite his awareness of HIV and AIDS. As Woody tells us: it was simply "it won't happen to me" type of thing.

Living with a positive partner: a need to know

We reveal here personal experiences of story-tellers who decided to voluntarily take an HIV test as a result of already being in established sexual relationships with an HIV-positive partner. Four story-tellers reveal the circumstances in which they discovered their HIV-positive status and for some it was almost a relief; to be in a sero-discordant relationship would have created further problems and dilemmas and it is to these narratives we now turn.

CLAIR

Clair was diagnosed in 1987 and was married to a man living with Haemophilia and HIV. Whilst trying for children under the medical supervision of her late husband's Haemophilia doctor, Clair, a self-identified heterosexual woman aged 40, contracted the HIV virus at the age of 25. She tells us:

"In September 1987 it came back as positive... I didn't find out personally... I went into a strange sort of state and we decided to go to America on a holiday... we were flying actually across the Atlantic and I said to my husband, "Ooooh, you know we forgot to get the results." He then told me the result. It was actually positive; they told my husband rather than me... which I think was really bad even though he was part of the process."

Clair's personal experiences were astounding. She tells us that whilst trying for children under medical supervision, neither Clair nor her husband knew they were, in fact, fertile; this was never questioned by the medical practitioner at the time. Clair was taking an enormous risk to have a child and engaging in unprotected sex with her HIV-positive husband and yet neither of them had been examined to see if they were both fertile. The advice of the specialist, Clair told me, was confusing and he seemed ignorant of basic medical matters. Clair recalled how she was questioning just how transmissible HIV actually is, as a direct result of her own personal experiences:

"... my husband was diagnosed in 1985 but it was just like confusion. I mean like you are going to die, you've got AIDS and then the hysteria that was around... but the transmission I queried because I was negative for so many years. We had been having sex since 1979 and there was talk about how long blood products had been contaminated. We had been having unprotected sex; we never used a condom so I thought just how transmissible is this... it always seemed a bit odd."

Clair recalled how her initial awareness of HIV was based upon the lines of the leaflets that came through people's doors and the newspapers such as The Sun, back in 1985, and the gravestone article, alongside notions of the 'gay plague'. Clair describes all of this as 'horrendous' and a 'witch hunt'. She was aware of stories in the Press of little boys living with Haemophilia that were being denied education in school because of the infectious nature of the HIV infection. Clair's husband died a few years later following her own diagnosis.

JAY

Jay is a self-identified gay man of 35 years and learned of his HIV-positive status back in 1992 at the age of 25. For Jay, being HIV-positive has had very little impact on his life or lifestyle and is only a very small part of his extremely laid-back character. He recalls:

"I was living with a guy and we had been together for about 8 or 9 months and we'd been having unprotected sex… then it came out of the blue and he told me that he'd been positive for about two or three years. I never used to suffer from many colds or flu and I just started getting them and they were lasting longer. So, I went to my GP and it came back a week later positive. So they re-did it three months later and I was positive… I mean we'd had that much unprotected sex; the chances of my having it were steep… So I had actually prepared myself for it… it wasn't much of a shock."

Jay told me how he had prepared for the positive diagnosis in his own head when the nurse was to come back to give him the results. He laughs out loud as he remembers:

"I just reacted in the way I did because I expected it to be positive. I mean, I think they were more shocked than I was really… I took it calm and relaxed and I smiled and said 'thank you' and got up and left… to be quite honest, people say that I am strange when I say this but it really hasn't made much of a big difference… I don't think it has, it probably has in ways but I don't realise them."

His knowledge around HIV and AIDS issues at the time were limited and he admits that he knows even less now. Jay states that this is his own choice.

RICK

Rick, a self-identified gay man of 32 years, told a very touching and illuminating story of how he learned about his positive diagnosis. In 1987 he went for an anonymous test in London using a false name; he was 18 at the time. He did this because within his friendship circle he knew of many who had already tested positive. He re-tested in 1990 and, of course, knew the result would be the same as in 1987. He was in a long-term sexual relationship and his partner was HIV-positive but didn't tell him for a long time. He recalled:

"I just kept on going as normal and went to normal appointments. My partner got poorly and I gave up work to look after him. I did all his transfusions and everything so I had to look after him 24 hours a day... my partner actually gave me HIV and he did apologise to all my family before he died, but not to me. My partner told me 'I think you ought to go for a test' and the reason he gave was that he loved me that much he wanted to keep me and didn't want to lose me and that way, by giving me HIV, he thought he could keep me... I would never have left him anyway... but I was only 18 you know... I thought about it later and perhaps I should have protected myself against other things anyway... but none of us really used anything during those days... no-one ever thought of HIV and AIDS in those days."

Rick pushed aside his own diagnosis and instead cared for his partner until his death; he recalls how 'chuffed' he was when the medical profession told him that his partner only had 24 hours to live, and he lived a further eight months. Rick believes he kept his partner alive during this period with love and care only he could give. Rick managed to take his partner to the pub and other places he wanted to go before he died. This was a very touching story and a recurrent theme amongst many gay men during this time, who lovingly cared for their partners until their death.

RACHEL

Rachel, a self-identified heterosexual married woman of 37 years, spoke of her relief when she was diagnosed as being HIV-positive in March of 1993 at the age of 28. Her husband had fallen ill and after a battery of tests, the medics tested him for HIV infection. Rachel's story is very interesting, as her HIV awareness was extensive at this time, as she had lived and worked across many parts of Africa during her lifetime. She tells us:

"It is a totally different context than the UK context... you don't apply it to yourself in that situation... I never ever thought about it in relation to myself, so when I was actually faced with it... everything I ever knew went out of the window... I had my suspicions for a long time, so I wasn't surprised by it, but the thoughts that went through my mind was "Oh, well! That puts paid to any idea of having children'. This was pretty devastating because although I had never wanted children before I met my husband, once I had got together with him I very much wanted his children and to feel that I was never going to be able to have them... it was hard"

Rachel tells of how she had to give up work to look after her husband, as he was told he was going to die and had less than 18 months to live.

Rachel's husband was still alive and in good health at the time of this interview after responding well to treatment; they now have two daughters. Rachel and her husband felt that there was a distinct lack of information in their local community and therefore started providing a basic information pack and a newsletter for newly diagnosed people. As they had both 'picked up on being isolated', they wanted to make a positive, practical contribution to the local community based on their own knowledge and experiences and the information they subsequently gathered on issues pertaining to HIV and AIDS.

Testing involuntarily without consent

Imagine for a moment going for a routine blood test at your local health centre or your own GP for something you think is only a minor ailment. You return for your results only to be faced with an HIV-positive diagnosis out-of-the-blue. The shock and devastation at the news, despite perhaps knowing that you might, at some point within your life, have engaged in risk behaviour can be overwhelming. The personal accounts that follow tell us how story-tellers learned of their HIV-positive diagnoses after being tested without their consent.

MINNIE

Minnie is a self-identified gay man of 42 years, who was diagnosed early in 1981 at the age of 21. As a blood donor with a particularly rare blood group, Minnie was often called to donate 'an extra pint' and would usually receive a letter from the Regional Blood Transfusion Unit in his area. After receiving such a letter he tells us:

"... I thought it was for one of these appointments where they wanted more blood. I went to meet the doctor and they said: *'do* you know why we have asked you here?'... And I said 'presumably for blood' and they replied 'no'... the doctor proceeded to tell me "*you've got the virus HTLVIII which leads to AIDS*". I was presented with the 'do's and don'ts' by way of an old-fashioned gestetner copy of a leaflet stapled together...I went back to work, carried on with my life, learned about the disease as information developed and didn't go back for medical treatment until 1996."

Minnie speaks of how many of his contemporaries were diagnosed with the same virus and were dying having taken AZT treatment in earlier times. He recalls:

"… they were all being given AZT and I didn't believe it. I didn't believe that this drug was the answer and I wanted to know why all these people were taking AZT when they were not really ill… I lost many people with the illness. I myself was told categorically that, you know, three years at the most would be, well it led to AIDS. End of story! So I told my partner and I was in a monogamous relationship with him. My first worry was Oh my God! I might be dead in three years… I hope they have destroyed all my blood that I'd given to them… I know it [my blood] was not used in Factor VIII… Luckily, several months prior to my diagnosis, the police called at my house at 3 o'clock in the morning, taking me to hospital to 'live transfuse' a pregnant woman who was having a difficult labour who was of the same rare blood type as myself. Phew! She didn't need it in the end… but I could have laid next to this woman and passed it on as she was giving birth."

Minnie recalls going back to work and carrying on with his life and learning more about the disease as knowledge and information advanced. At the time of his diagnosis, he describes the information on HIV and AIDS as 'very very raw and basic'.

TYLER

Tyler, a self-identified gay man of 54 years, recalls how he discovered his positive status back in 1984 following a routine check up after a holiday. He had experienced a rash and went along for tests at his local sexual health clinic. When he went back for his results he tells us how his received the news. He was 38 years old at the time and living with his Mother:

"*We've got some bad news for you. You haven't got long to live.* And that was it really: there wasn't any counselling it was just left like that. It wasn't HIV at that time, it was HTLVIII and I mean I didn't know anything about it, no-one did. I just knew I was told that I hadn't long to live and there was no treatment… I couldn't concentrate on anything."

There was little information available at the time of Tyler's diagnosis and the diagnosis totally changed his life leaving him spending much of his time thinking 'this is the end'.

NEIL

Neil is a self-identified gay man of 42, who was diagnosed back in January 1985 at the age of 24 years old. In 1984 he had a re-occurrence of a childhood illness and had gone to his GP; as a matter of routine he had blood tests and he didn't think any more about it until he got a letter asking him to return for results of the blood screening. When he returned, the GP spoke of nothing relating to the reoccurring childhood illness Neil initially went to his GP about, but instead said, as Neil, recounted:

"... one of the things we've done is test for HIV, it was HTLVIII back then, and you're positive. He [GP] then said I had got, at best, about two years to live and there is nothing we can do except when you get ill treat some of the pain and he referred me to the hospital social worker... that was completely it. It was very homophobic and I was very scared. Now I would have kicked up a fuss but at the time, I think that was when there was the pre-AIDS hysteria in the 80s and I was very scared because I was still only 24... there was no information."

Neil had read small amounts about the illness in the Gay Press but still believed it was an 'American issue'. He recalls how he felt being given a medical 'death sentence':

"I was really fucked. I thought it would be a painful death: I didn't think it would be a clean death... I was very scared and I actually went back to work and told my employer... they were very good about it. My line manager was a lesbian and I got on very well with her... I felt quite confident about telling her. I didn't tell my family. When I 'came out' I was 18 and my parents found it hard to take. I still haven't told them. My main support was my partner."

CHRISTOPHER

Christopher a self-identified gay man aged 51 was diagnosed at 36 in 1988; he was in hospital for an arthritic condition when he learned of his HIV-positive diagnosis, which he described as 'a horrendous experience'. He recollects:

"I was in hospital... a nurse and a doctor walked into my room. I was in a private room because I was quite ill with this arthritic problem and I used to have a lot of pain and didn't sleep very well; so, they used to put me in a single room for my own benefit and for the benefit of other patients because

I could be quite noisy. And they came in fully gowned, masked and gloved and told me about my positive results. Then a practice nurse or a social worker or someone came in and talked about things like "don't worry you could get run over by a bus". Hmmm, I thought, cheers love! It was horrendous; it was really horrendous."

Christopher was in a long-term relationship at the time of diagnosis and remembers being totally devastated at the time. He knew very little about HIV and AIDS at the time and for twelve months remained convinced that every ailment he suffered, be it a cough, cold or new mark on his body was going to be the end for him.

PERRY

Perry, a self-identified gay man of 40 years learned of his HIV-positive status during 1990 whilst being treated for a sexually transmitted disease he had recently contracted; he was 28 at this time. He was asked if he would like to be tested for HIV and agreed, having already undertaken the test previously with a negative result outcome. He tells us:

"I did the test and it came back positive. I knew quite a lot about it 'cos there was a big advertising campaign on the telly around that time. I was still unprepared for it obviously. I didn't think it would happen to me just like everybody else. I was pretty shocked and stunned and I felt quite isolated. I remember thinking "Oh my God, I am going to die of AIDS". I had recently given up my job and I was sent to the hospital to meet a couple of other people who were HIV-positive and had had it for quite a few years. They were able to chat to me a bit so that was OK."

Perry remembers feelings of how he had not really had much out of life and wanted someone to blame for his HIV-positive diagnosis. He then describes various incidents that led to him being diagnosed with mental health problems. For Perry, it is difficult to separate his HIV and mental health issues.

Voluntary testing: showing signs of illness

Our story-tellers here reveal personal accounts of experiences of illness prior to making a decision to voluntarily test for HIV. These narratives are in date order starting with the earliest diagnosis.

JO

Jo, a self-identified gay man of 53, tested voluntarily in 1982 after experiencing severe pains under his arms and across his body at the age of 33. He went along to see his GP and describes how his GP examined his lymph nodes and did what was called a 'Sailor's Handshake'. This is where with one hand the GP takes hold of the person's hand and with the other hand feels the lymph nodes just by the elbow. Apparently, this was a common practice amongst sailors when they met 'molls' on the docks to see whether or not they had Syphilis. Interesting! She suggested that Jo went along to, as he put it, the 'clap clinic'. This he did and later discovered he had tested positive for HTLVIII, the precursor for HIV. Jo tells us:

"It was kind of a shock… I began to think, well is this something I have been carrying for a long time? I lived in New York in 1974 and at that time it was very steamy… I knew people in the States and therefore think I was pretty well informed and of course it was the 'death sentence' so I knew that this was it… I was living in a flat and had sort of become very isolated and I was very depressed and essentially come Christmas I tried to top myself… wasn't successful because when push came to shove, I couldn't do it because I just couldn't bear the thought of someone having to clear up after me [*here he laughs*]."

He goes on to describe how little information there was around at the time of his diagnosis; however his consultant was at the forefront of HIV research in his area and therefore Jo was given an 'amazing amount of support' in relation to his HIV and was asked go take part in an AZT clinical trial. Jo declined this offer:

"I wasn't prepared to go with this… I didn't like it. If anything, it was this kind of stubbornness that saved me because I watched AZT kill, I mean, there's no two other ways it killed people. I watched them taking the drug and just dying… and then of course we found out that the AZT was a failed chemotherapy drug that had been withdrawn. I was angry; I got real sort of rage so I wouldn't even think of antiretrovirals."

MARC

Marc, a self-identified gay man of 38 years decided after a period of ill health to voluntarily test for HIV in April 1990 aged 26. He describes finding some lumps under his arms and his glands being swollen, he knew that this was a symptom of infection and it took him six months to build up courage to go and get the test. However, he was pretty sure that the test would come back positive because he had had a lot of unprotected sex. Marc tells us:

"Well, the doctor thought I might be positive and was a bit uncomfortable giving me the diagnosis, so I challenged him. I was a bit confrontational and I got to see the counsellor... I was a bit upset and a bit sort of shocked after my diagnosis. I got out of there and went back to work to take my mind off of it. That evening I just went home and smoked loads and loads of cannabis and passed out. Later my cousin telephoned to tell me my Grandmother had just died so that was my diagnosis day."

Marc speaks of his awareness of the Concorde Trial (a joint French/British clinical trial of AZT in asymptomatic HIV-positive individuals) during this period and the only treatment options being AZT. He remembers being 'pissed off with my job' and so he gave in his notice six weeks following his diagnosis.

PABLO

Pablo, a self-identified gay male of 32 years speaks of generally being unwell and experiencing a sore throat and swollen glands under his arms back in 1990. He didn't really believe it was anything major and went to his GP for a general check up. He was tested for Glandular fever and other blood was taken. He went back to his GP one week later and was told that it wasn't glandular fever. The GP took further blood and asked him if he had been tested for HIV. Pablo stated that he tested on at least five occasions and these had come back negative and so consented to another HIV test. He got his results four weeks later and cut a vacation short to go and see his doctor, as the GP had requested to see him in person. Pablo was 20 years old at the time of his diagnosis. He tells us:

"The doctor called me through and I sat down. There was no emotion, it was awful; it was just a case of him saying: "Oh, I'm very sorry but we have got your results and I'm sorry to tell you you're HIV-positive" That was that. There was no sort of advice or offer of any additional information... it was so difficult for me. I didn't even tell anyone I had gone for this test... I didn't even tell the girl I was living with at the time... I was just numb... I didn't scream, shout or kick out. I didn't ball my eyes out... I just walked for about two hours around the village thinking: who do I tell first? To be perfectly honest I kept it to myself for a long time, perhaps four or five months before I told anybody."

He told me that during this time he couldn't sleep with his [then] female sexual partner because he was too frightened to do so. And he recalls:

"What really pissed me off was the fact that she already knew she was positive and never told me all the time we were together. I had been seeing her for about a year and a half and not having protective sex... I knew I wasn't totally gay when I was with her but I had never been with a man all the time I was with her. So I knew it couldn't have been anyone else... When I actually told her I was positive, she said "well I have something to tell you, I am HIV-positive too." Basically, she ruined my life. She was basically the 'death sentence' on me: when you were diagnosed with this you know you have only got a couple of years to live."

He goes on to say that about four or five days after this revelation, he could not look at his girlfriend again and so the relationship ended and soon afterwards Pablo's partner later died of an AIDS-related illness.

LISETTE

Lisette is a 51 year old, self-identified heterosexual mother and grandmother with a previous history of IV drug use and a former career in the porn industry. At the age of 39, whilst travelling in the USA to visit her daughter she became unwell, back in 1990. She was asked if she wanted testing for HIV as there was a 'drive on testing' and she thought she might as well, as she was quite convinced she hadn't got it. She had previously been to her local doctor and he had told her that *'HIV had nothing to do with her'* because despite her having taken drugs intravenously in the past, she had given them up. Lisette recalls:

"It took about six weeks to get the results, which was a bit of a strain and they delivered the results in person. So I think the minute I saw this woman come up the drive I knew there was something up... she came to tell me that I was positive. I didn't believe it. I was completely stunned and I had never considered the implications of being positive. I was about to leave the country and my 15 year old daughter lived here and I had to try to do something with her because she knew I had been tested. She totally believed that she would never see me again... that I was going to die and I had no idea what to do next. She knew that I had to go back home but within four months she came back to the UK. I had to go home... and that's what I did."

Lisette goes on to describe how she had seen the tombstone advertisements on the TV and the information she had gathered together came from 'that stuff'. She states:

"I was in shock and when I came back here [the UK] I went to the GP who told me I had to go to the GUM clinic. I was absolutely horrified because in the past the only people I knew that went to the GUM clinic were not very nice people. I felt that this was actually worse than being diagnosed (she laughs). In reality the people there were really nice... it's more of a shock if you're a heterosexual woman who really hasn't been to a GUM clinic or as it is known the 'clap clinic'. I think also that I thought I was probably going to die in the next six months... it was horrible really."

She remembers the confusion of thinking about dying soon and yet not feeling particularly unwell. She went on to contact Body Positive in London and believed that this was one of the best things she had done, as it put her in touch with other positive individuals. She no longer felt alone 'out there' because there were other people that she could relate to.

LARRY

Larry, a self-identified gay man aged 56 is the only person unable to identify the route of his HIV transmission. He asserted that he had never engaged in penetrative anal sex with other men and had voluntarily tested for HIV due to being gay and "having had, in the past, plenty of promiscuous sexual encounters". In 1992, he suddenly became very ill and thought he had got glandular fever. At 46, he recalls:

"I thought I am gonna go and have an HIV test, which I did. I was very blasé about it because I knew them all up there as I had worked as a volunteer... low and behold when the results came back I can't remember whether I was sitting down or standing up. Oh, my whole world just fell apart. The woman came in and said, "Larry, the test came back and it's positive." I thought to myself 'is this the best way to tell someone?' You can't beat about the bush I suppose... I felt it was the 'death sentence' when I was first told. I think I may have clutched at any straw that was offered at the time... I'm no youngster: I was 46 at the time so death had come into my life. I wasn't like one of these youngsters who feel that they're immortal but I don't think anyone expects that kind of news. It was a terrible shock. In fact, for the six years following my diagnosis I cut myself off completely. I didn't go out other than for shopping. I didn't go out on the gay scene I just kept myself to myself. I felt disgusted and dirty and thought I was gonna die."

Larry had been exposed to quite a lot of literature concerning HIV and AIDS, as he had been involved with a local HIV organisation in his area. He speaks of being aware of the monotherapy, known as AZT, as the only treatment at the time and believes: "AZT in my opinion killed everyone because they got the dosages wrong." For Larry, his whole world fell apart following his HIV-positive diagnosis.

TONY

Tony, a self-identified gay male aged 40 years became ill in 1991 and went into a period of denial for over 3 years about testing for HIV. He had friends who were HIV-positive and one of the last people he had slept with was HIV-positive; he describes his self-esteem as pretty low, was very 'skinny' at the time and attempted to block out anything to do with HIV or AIDS. In 1994, at the age of 32 years Tony learned he was HIV-positive and recalls:

"I wasn't very well and I'd gone to London with my boyfriend. I had never seen my legs so skinny and I had got some HIV friends. It was very scary seeing people who were ill and looked gaunt in terms of body size. My friend kept suggesting I go and get the test; so, I got my head around it and said OK. I went for the test but never went back for the result. I eventually was persuaded to go for the test result. I knew by their body language. I did cry but I was prepared for it and I didn't panic. I wasn't told that I only had so many years to live or anything like that. I was told that I would be financially better off if I had HIV but what is financial security worth when you are ill and lethargic all the time? Your whole self-esteem goes, you know, going to the bus stop and meeting people and thinking that they are pointing the finger at you. Paranoia is a big thing in HIV."

At the time of diagnosis, Tony recalls not knowing a lot about HIV apart from stuff on the television adverts and leaflets. He took all the information with a 'pinch of salt'

The last personal experience included in this section is rather unique in that the story-teller took the HIV test but was not actually showing signs of illness herself. She tested voluntarily because her five month old son was in hospital and was extremely ill.

SANDRA

Sandra, aged 37 is a self-identified heterosexual woman who discovered her HIV-positive status in 1994. She recalls how her five month old son had been extremely ill for several weeks and the medical team at the hospital were desperately trying to find out what was wrong with him. At the age of 29 at the time of diagnosis, Sandra recounted:

"Unbeknown to my husband and I, they [the medical team] had suspected HIV but hadn't told us. It was only when I went through my son's notes that I saw a query 'HIV'. I questioned them and they came out with it and so we decided to do a blood test on me so that they could find out what was wrong with my son... I didn't have any counselling... I consented to a blood test and on the same day it came back as positive... we knew that basically at that time there wasn't a hell of a lot they could do with my son."

She explains to me that she was numb after the diagnosis and speaks of her concern for her son who, at that time, was connected to 'all sorts of equipment' and was experiencing breathing difficulties. She tells us:

"I didn't at that time think that this sort of thing happened to people like me... so you know I was a bit shocked but then I thought well 'go ahead' I didn't really have anything to fear... the paramount thing was to find out what was wrong with my son and to do everything I could to help him. When the test came back positive I was in shock because I had seen the adverts on TV and I knew roughly what this meant... my son died. After the test came back positive we kept on top of everything... they asked if we wanted to use experimental drugs for my son. I refused to see him suffer and I remember saying that if they were going to override my wishes then I was going to leave them to it and they could get on with it and I was going home. They didn't. They took our wishes into consideration and then it was up to my husband and me to decide what we were going to do because we had a very good relationship. We both got a piece of paper, tore it in half, wrote down what we thought we should do and what we thought was best for our son... for the first time in weeks, we believed that we actually had control over our son's care... it wasn't the experts poking and prodding and finally we could have our son back."

Sandra explained that there wasn't much resistance from the medical profession in terms of what they wanted to do in relation to their son's care.

She told me how grateful she was of the team and the care they gave until the end. She does say about her own diagnosis however:

"As far as I was concerned, HIV was a disease that meant death and it happened to people who were promiscuous. People who were involved with strange sort of sexual practices, you know, that kind of thing. I had this stereotypical sort of attitude towards people affected and I didn't class myself as one of those people... For me it was prostitutes and gay people. I didn't know anyone in my family or friendship circle who was affected by AIDS so it was something quite alien... oh and drug users, and drugs never featured in my life so I don't know... I thought I had led a very decent lifestyle and things like that don't happen to people like me."

Voluntary testing: acknowledging risk behaviour

The last section of this chapter reveals personal accounts of long-term survivors who decided to voluntarily go for an HIV test as a result of acknowledging and making a personal risk assessment of their own personal lifestyle and/or previous behaviours. As mentioned earlier, all the women and men who took part in the original HIV study are included in this chapter to introduce to the reader how each of our story-tellers discovered their HIV-positive status following an HIV test.

ELISABETH

Elisabeth, aged 48, is a self-identified heterosexual, an ex-addict, mother and grandmother. She learned of her positive diagnosis during Christmas of 1985. At the time of diagnosis, she was an IV drug user and her awareness of AIDS was that it was something amid gay men in San Francisco. Elisabeth had no idea HIV could be passed on by sharing needles. Around 1984, she recalls a man from her home town being diagnosed with HTLV III. As it happened, she said, the guy was gay and an IV drug user. She knew this guy and had 'used' with him in the past. At the age of 31 at the time of her diagnosis, Elisabeth recounted:

"As it happened I had a small lump on my breast. I went to the local hospital and I said to the doctor, 'while I am here I might as well have this AIDS test'. The doctor was puzzled and asked why, so I told him 'I am an IV drug user and I've just found out that people like me can get it'. The poor little man jumped about six feet in the air and literally ran behind his desk because he'd been talking to me and I'd been lying on the couch. He put on a gown, two masks and two pairs of rubber gloves and took my blood."

This sounds preposterous but it is a recurrent theme throughout many personal experiences of our long-term survivors in this story. Elisabeth remembers being left wondering what on earth was going on and why this doctor was behaving in such a manner. This was back in July or August 1985 and he told Elisabeth that her local GP would pass on the results. She forgot all about the test until she received a letter from her GP in October informing her that she was to be removed from his list. She recalls:

"I wasn't an addict that went to the doctors. I never took prescribed drugs. If you couldn't get it in a syringe then I wasn't interested and, you know, I obviously had a GP for the kids and we never really bothered them. The kids are all quite healthy... I thought it was odd to strike me off his list and then bells began to ring... the alarm bells in the back of my head and I thought 'no it can't be'... So I went and got myself a 'junky doctor' that was what they called doctors who were sympathetic to addicts... we had been arrested for dealing and were looking at seven years in prison and my oldest son was suffering with stress... I asked the doctor to find out my results... on Christmas Eve whilst treating my son, the doctor told me 'I've found out your results... they're positive and you've got about two years to live'. I was in a state of shock and I went home."

Elisabeth remembers that there was very little information available to her at the time of her diagnosis. Nearby was a hospital that had set up a clinic with a doctor from London heading the clinical team; she accessed this clinic and recalls:

"There was a nurse there who told me that her husband was refusing to let her work there because of the people with AIDS. He believed that she could catch it from cups and stuff and he told her she was not allowed to work there anymore. She went against his wishes... even the doctors were expecting us to drop down dead... This clinic was at the top of a hill and, you know, if you were walking up that hill there was only one place you would be going. And so, I would stand at the bottom of that hill and wait until there was no-one in sight. It was horrible if someone saw you walking back down. That's when you got to know who was positive in my local area."

A forgotten generation: Long-term survivors' experiences of HIV and AIDS

TOM

Tom, a self-identified gay man of 55, voluntarily took the test and discovered he was HIV-positive in February 1986. He was 39 years old at the time, was still working and in an established intimate relationship. He decided to take the test after receiving a call from somebody he had been in a relationship with the year before who had just been diagnosed with Kaposi Sarcoma (see Glossary). The next day Tom went for the test and received his results approximately one week later. He recalls:

"I suppose most people don't really think it could be them... I was shocked to be told this was the case and as the prognosis was two years to live, I wanted to go and find out as much as I possibly could about this virus that was going to rob me of the next forty odd years... there was stuff out in the media about it being contagious and infectious to other people. I kind of turned into a hypochondriac at the time [he laughs] especially when I was discovering moles. I would actually chart all the moles on my body. I realise now how stupid and how unproductive it was."

It took Tom two years of stress and anxiety following his diagnosis before he felt any sense of relief that he had basically lived longer than his own prognosis. However, within six months of being diagnosed, Tom helped start up an HIV organisation in his local area to help others with the same diagnosis.

PETER

Peter, a self-identified gay man of 48 years, tells us of how he voluntarily tested very early in 1985 when he first heard about the virus. He agreed to take part in an AIDS-related trial at his local clinic for sexually transmitted diseases. Having given blood for the trial, he decided he did not want to know the result and told the medical team of his decision. He stated that providing he practised safer sex (and at that time information around safer sexual practices were limited) all would be well. This was agreed and he learned of his positive status some 18 months later, during Christmas 1987. He was 33 years old at the time of diagnosis and recalls:

"... the professionals at the clinic were very good... during the period of time, I became very concerned, anxious, worried because more and more publicity was being given about this illness that was killing people who were developing it...I was in a situation left wondering "am I or aren't I? Shall I find out the results?" It was a living hell until I realised that I had developed something called PGL (persistent generalised lymphadenopathy), which is swollen lymph nodes which people spoke a lot about during this time... it was something that people with HTLVIII were experiencing. I was pretty sure by now that I was positive so I rang up the hospital and the doctor did eventually tell me on the phone because I think he felt that I could handle it... I wasn't going to jump out of the window. He did have reservations at first; he wanted me to go three weeks actually wanting to know the result every single day. I went on for three weeks and there were some days I didn't want to know, but I didn't tell him and finally he confirmed the positive result over the phone... although I would have rather been negative, I breathed a sigh of relief because at least I knew where I stood and it was easier to live with the knowledge of being HIV rather than the fear that perhaps I might be or perhaps if I wasn't, that one day I would be."

Peter remembers his reluctance to take AZT at the time, which was the only treatment and so refused when doctors suggested he take the drug. He told me that he believed people were dying as a result of the AZT and that he believed that this drug was not a cure and did not kill off the virus.

JOHN

John, a self-identified gay man aged 48 years voluntarily tested back in 1987 and tested negative. Two years later, at the age of 35, he decided that he would go for another test and if that proved to be negative he would take precautions to protect himself and stay negative. In 1989, his second test was positive and even though he wasn't particularly surprised, at the time of diagnosis he recalls:

"It was quite upsetting. The woman who gave me the result was a lot older than myself and was extremely remote and middle class. I always remember her saying to me 'many people when they are given this news decide to become celibate.' I remember thinking to myself that this was very convenient and I am not going to do this. My awareness I think at the time was that those people who were infected developed AIDS and died quite quickly and quite nastily. I remember being told that on average people became ill and died within five years. So I went away with that sort of thought... I was thirty four or thirty five at the time and I remember wondering if I was going to ever see forty. So, you stop thinking about growing old and becoming sixty and retiring. You don't really think about life in the longer term at all."

John didn't recall being aware of any major developments in knowledge and awareness of HIV and AIDS at the time of his diagnosis but was referred to an Agency in his local area which dealt with people living with HIV and AIDS.

RICHARD

Richard, a self-identified gay man of 32 years tested positive when he was 21 years old back in 1990 whilst working away from his local area down in London. He took the test voluntarily because he knew he had put himself 'at risk' sexually in the past and had a close friend who was ill in hospital with AIDS. He recalls being very aware of people dying and no-one really wanting to talk about this. He believes he took many risks because of the reluctance to talk about what was going on. This prompted him to take the test. He recalls:

"Before I was diagnosed I was a happy 21 year old man. I had just had my birthday; I was a man in my own right and I was doing well with a good job and then all of a sudden my life just fell to bits. I found out I was positive and very shortly afterwards my best friend died... I felt guilty and I felt dirty and I felt that I had something to be ashamed of. Above all, I felt I might be putting other people at risk because there were still lots of people going around with many questions with regards to how HIV was actually transmitted. I lost my job and so I moved out of London... I moved back to my parents because no-one could really give me any length of time that they thought I might live... five years was considered pretty optimistic at this point."

Richard did not mention any previous knowledge of HIV or AIDS campaigns during this period but spoke of his awareness of risk in relation to engaging in receptive anal sex. He was also aware that AZT was available as a monotherapy but he didn't believe it was effective and thought the doses were rather large. He was, however, put on AZT immediately following his diagnosis.

The way in which many of our story-tellers learned of their HIV-positive status is rather shocking and dispassionate; scientific and medical knowledge was limited during this era and fear and uncertainty was widespread. It is somewhat difficult to comprehend how we might react to being told we have less than five years to live following a medical diagnosis of HIV. Many of our story-tellers actively decided to take the HIV test on the basis of starting a new relationship, or living with someone who was already

HIV-positive or acknowledging that they might have previously taken risks associated with AIDS and HIV. The knowledge of living with an HIV-positive diagnosis and how the virus progressed must have been quite frightening, especially for those who had already lost their friends to AIDS. Imagine being in a group of 65 people and being only one of three surviving members of that group. How many other chronic illnesses have led to experiences such as these?

Before we move on to the next chapter, let us reflect a moment on what we have just learned. How do the story-tellers' personal accounts of discovering an HIV-positive diagnosis impact on us? Who do you identify with and relate to within this chapter? How do these experiences connect to our own feelings? In what ways can you, the reader, empathise with the story-tellers' experiences? Who do you feel little empathy for and why? Can you identify any prejudices you might have towards specific personal experiences? Reflect a while, before moving on.

A forgotten generation: Long-term survivors' experiences of HIV and AIDS

CHAPTER THREE

The early years: Where do I go from here?

∞

"The uncertainty which seeps into every aspect of my life, from the mundane to the profound, is not insurmountable. It just reminds me, all the time, how strange the business of living is."
                               J MacLachlan, the Observer, January 13, 1991

Introduction

Uncertainty is and will always be a feature in our everyday lives, as it reveals a space between our knowing something and not knowing something. When matters are uncertain it becomes difficult to make decisions and negotiate everyday life whilst facing the unknown; this, in turn, can create doubt and confusion as well as raising our levels of anxiety and despair. Unquestionably, in the context of HIV, medical uncertainty brought with it fear, doubt, anxiety, stigma and the likelihood of imminent death for those faced with a positive diagnosis. Yet, at the same time, we acknowledge that facing uncertainty can also bring with it hope, optimism and opportunity for the future. The medical uncertainty of AIDS and HIV in earlier times is well documented and established. Yet whilst medical practitioners were clearly faced with managing clinical uncertainties associated with HIV and AIDS, it emerges many did not choose to share their uncertainty with patients. Instead, most medical practitioners chose to make known to their patients the probability and timing of an early death, in the face of such limitations of scientific and medical knowledge about HIV from the mid 1980s onwards. Why did this happen?

The onset of severe illness presents a profound threat to our personal and social existence; yet when we are faced with our own mortality, how do we cope with and negotiate everyday life in terms of our personal and social responsibilities and successfully deal with our emotions? HIV and AIDS have had a high media and public profile. The meanings associated to these conditions are not simply attached to scientific and medical knowledge; they are also attached to what our HIV status tells others about our private lives, who we are and how we behave. The public representation of HIV and AIDS has had a powerful influence on how people living with an HIV-positive diagnosis are viewed by others, including medical practitioners. The lack of medical certainty and scientific knowledge on AIDS and HIV in early times meant that once an HIV-positive diagnosis was established by the medical profession, the patient had to then go away and 'deal with it'.

This chapter explores how our long-term survivors primarily took control and managed their everyday lives after discovering they were living with an HIV or AIDS medical diagnosis. We draw attention to the dominant issues and diverse uncertainties and anxieties that emerged from the onset of diagnosis. What happens now? The first set of narratives uncovers the personal accounts of story-tellers who had been given a medical prognosis of life expectancy on 'diagnosis day'. Our story-tellers in this section were diagnosed between 1981 and 1994. What is interesting, however, is that Minnie was diagnosed in 1981 which was the earliest date in this study; some thirteen years later, with the advancement of HIV science and medical knowledge, Sandra was also given a medical 'death sentence' as late as 1994. Clearly, some medical practitioners continued to choose to tell newly diagnosed patients about the probability and timing of an early death.

The second set of narratives reveals how our long-term survivors perceived their own life expectancy as a result of the huge loss of lives of people living with AIDS and the AIDS public profile and media attention. Story-tellers included in this section were diagnosed between 1982 and 1992 and none of them were given a medical prognosis of life expectancy from medical practitioners at the time. Why did some medics chose to predict 'imminent death' whilst others did not? The final set of narratives reveals the personal experiences of our story-tellers who, at the time of diagnosis, were in an established intimate relationship and living with a positive partner. Our story-tellers were diagnosed between 1985 and 1993 and again, none were given a medical prognosis of life expectancy.

From these personal experiences you will see how some medical practitioners made huge errors by telling our story-tellers they were going to die within a given period of time, with little medical certainty to back up their prognosis. With 'imminent death' in mind, we are forced to wonder how this potentially impacts on our sense of mortality, identity and selfhood and how this disturbs our social world and biography. How long do I have to live? What shall I do? How will I live and who will care for me? Who should I tell? What does my future hold for me? How will I die? Instead of a person living with an illness you are transformed into a person who is dying from AIDS. Individual reactions and initial psychological and social challenges to be negotiated varied and were dependent upon on a number of factors and

A forgotten generation: Long-term survivors' experiences of HIV and AIDS

also where each person 'was at' in their life at the time of diagnosis. Starting with the earliest diagnosis we uncover the personal stories of experiences and coping strategies in everyday life after essentially being given a medical 'death sentence' following diagnosis.

Facing mortality: a medical 'death sentence'

MINNIE

Minnie, diagnosed in 1981 at the age of 21, was in a relationship when he discovered he was HIV-positive. He was told categorically that he had three years at the most to live. Minnie disclosed his positive status to his partner, who later took the test and was found to be HIV-negative. Minnie told me he learned as much about HIV and AIDS as knowledge developed over time. He tells us:

"I travelled an awful lot because I was told not to… I thought I want to travel. These were big plans of mine to do some travelling and if I am going to be dead in three years, I might as well do it now. So, I took off travelling and I did that for a long time. I was always able to work my way around one way or another and I knew my body well enough to know when it would be right to go and do something about my HIV if it became a problem."

He stated that he had few health problems associated with his HIV-positive diagnosis from 1981 up until 1996. He did, however, experience problems associated with insurance in relation to obtaining a mortgage because he would have had to declare his positive status and life insurance would be denied. Similarly, he could not obtain a pension for the same reason and, at the time of interview, he had no pension cover. Minnie carried on with his life in his usual way for many years; he spoke of losing many of his contemporaries to AIDS in spite of them taking AZT monotherapy (see glossary) at the time. Minnie was therefore doubtful that AZT was an effective treatment and therefore did not take the drug until 1996 when he became ill.

TYLER

In 1984 when Tyler was diagnosed at the age of 38, his GP told him he only had months to live. He was not in a relationship at the time; he lived with his mother and had built up a successful business. He described how facing his own mortality created 'a lot of pain and hardship' for him. He recalls:

"I couldn't concentrate on anything I was so depressed; I couldn't concentrate on work. I could not control my workforce and I thought 'what is the point of building up a business if I am going to be dead soon!' And then I started going around the world and seeing things I wanted to see. I lost the business and lost my houses. You know, you lose work, you lose money and then you can't pay bills."

Not surprisingly, for Tyler, being told he only had months to live changed his life entirely. He told me that if he had not been given a life expectancy of months and had received appropriate support he would not have spent so much time thinking 'this is the end' and he would have concentrated on his business and made it grow, so that he had financial security for later in life. During this time he lost interest in the positive side of life and his only concern was 'surviving the day'. Tyler also revealed that he made many attempts to take his own life and was left thinking in later years:

"Why am I still here when all my friends died years ago? This is some punishment… Why haven't I gone? Why didn't I go with everyone else? All my friends have gone. The friends I have now are through HIV-positive groups… this loss affected me very badly because the friends I had were people I chose to be with and people who chose to be with me. Those people who I surround myself with now aren't friends at that level. They are people I have met because of what is wrong with us all. That is what we have in common, not our lifestyles but our illness. So I have lost *lifestyle-friendships* and now I've replaced them with *illness-friendships* which is totally different… it makes you wonder when is it my turn? And when it doesn't come you go through a phase of wanting to end your life yourself. You know, there is this guilt thing and you don't ever come to terms with it. I am still here and they have all gone and many of them led much better lifestyles than I did. It makes you wonder where the logic in all of this is."

Tyler also told me that from discovering his positive-status and being told that he only had months to live, the loss of his business and income had left him financially poor.

A forgotten generation: Long-term survivors' experiences of HIV and AIDS

NEIL

It was 1985 when Neil learned of his HIV-positive diagnosis, at the age of 24. He was working full time, and in an intimate relationship and, at the time of interview in 2002, was still with his long-term partner who is HIV-negative. He tells us:

"I think that immediately after diagnosis I thought about it for certainly a few weeks maybe a month or so. As it went by, bit by bit, I started not thinking about it in a way... I did have a bout of Shingles fairly soon after diagnosis, but apart from that I had no illnesses at all. I concentrated on home, work and living well. I did see it as a battle and that I could beat it."

Neil told me how he became very work-focussed and went into a 'nest-building phase' with his partner building their own home, spending money and energy on their new flat. His main support was his long-term partner and he spoke of his secrecy in relation to his parents not knowing about his illness condition. His relationship had become somewhat strained with his parents when he 'came out' and told them he was gay at the age of 18. At the time of interview, Neil told me he had started getting on very well with his Mum and Dad and that they still didn't know of his HIV-positive status. He couldn't face telling them he was HIV-positive. The secrecy was a big issue for Neil. This is shared by many HIV-positive people in this study.

MARTIN

In 1985, at the age of 21, Martin learned of his HIV-positive status and recalls it was Friday 13th. He was single at the time of diagnosis and lived with his parents. He had presumed he might be HIV-positive as he had read in the papers how people living with Haemophilia were at risk from contaminated blood products. His doctor advised him to tell no-one of his positive diagnosis and his life expectancy was approximately one year. He tells us:

"I wasn't totally depressed and I didn't fall apart. It was just so hard to imagine that at 21 I was going to die. From a personal side, I never expected to meet a girl, marry a girl and I never expected to have children. In terms of picking up a pension, I was too young to think about pensions in any case. I felt my career prospects had certainly been hit, as I thought a lot of choices of what I could do were taken away... I felt that I couldn't apply for another job because when I applied to the Civil Service I had a medical, as anybody applying to the Civil Services does, and they took me on... if someone were to find out I was HIV-positive they would not employ me."

Martin told me of how his brother, also living with Haemophilia, had been diagnosed as HIV-positive and neither he nor his brother told their parents at the time. His brother later died and Martin moved South two years after diagnosis. He speaks of the secrecy of not telling people of his positive status and how difficult relationships were for him because of his perceived responsibility of being HIV-positive. When asked about how he coped with his one year life expectancy prognosis, he told me he adopted the 'ostrich method' of sticking his head in the sand but he did experience *black moments*.

PAUL

Similarly, in 1985 as part of the mass screening process for people living with Haemophilia, Paul, at the age of 21, discovered his HIV-positive status during a routine check up; he did not voluntarily take an HIV test. Paul was working at the time and was in an intimate relationship. Unlike Martin, Paul was given four to five years life expectancy which changed his whole outlook on life. He told his parents and recalls how his Mum could not handle the situation without crying. His father kept on saying 'Son, you will be alright.' He tells us more:

"My relationship with my girlfriend finished. We had been seeing each other for a few years and the sex stopped. Sex is an important part of your life and that was put on hold for quite a while. My job, my attitude to my job at the time also changed. I had good career prospects and I felt that I couldn't work anymore. I didn't think it was worth it anymore. My whole attitude to life changed. I think I just started to value my time because I didn't think I had much time left. Work was a waste of my life. I couldn't see the point in a lot of things in life. I think one of the significant things was the fact that I had always wanted to be a Dad. HIV stopped that... I didn't think I had long to live and I was dying. I couldn't see the point."

Paul spoke about the impact HIV had on his life early on; the way in which HIV was reported on the television in conjunction with many people dying of AIDS affected him in relation to disclosing his HIV-positive status to those around him. He tells us:

"I used to spend a lot of time in tears and crying myself to sleep at nights. I don't do this anymore. I am hard to it now, or have just developed coping mechanisms to deal with it...In the early days, I never told my friends about my status for a number of reasons. It was a very scary time in 1985/86 as there were many HIV stories, lots of tabloids covering stories about HIV, there were lots of people telling HIV jokes, people thought you could get it from toilet seats. I thought it was better not to tell anybody. I didn't want my friends to suddenly stop coming round for coffee... I didn't want people's fear or ignorance to spoil our friendship. I didn't think that anyone could actually help me and I didn't want people to feel sorry for me either. So, I basically got on with it on my own for a long, long time. The only people who knew were my mum and dad, my girlfriend, my brother and sister...it took me the best part of probably 12 years of living with this before I told any friends... I didn't want them to not have anything to do with me anymore because I was infectious. It was like two angles at opposing sides. It is one of those things. There are so many contradictions around my HIV that it makes your life like a Jekyll and Hyde, because of the two sides to everything. There is one story that you tell people and then there is another one that is the truth... I started lying to my friends. I started lying about my HIV. I started lying about my clinicians. I started lying about when I wasn't feeling well. I didn't like that."

Paul spoke of feeling isolated in the early years and felt unable to access appropriate HIV support from HIV-specific organisations. He told me that as a heterosexual man, many groups only catered for gay men and related to gay sexual practices. At his Haemophilia clinic, it was difficult to access effective HIV support, as people's status was kept secret and nobody wanted to talk about the HIV virus. It was four years after his diagnosis that Paul first met up with other people living with Haemophilia and HIV because of the secrecy and isolation. He told me:

"It was about 1989 when I first met the group. I was the youngest out of the lot but only by a few years. We used to meet once a month for a couple of years until about 1991 or 1992. But over that time, every single person who went to the group except me died... everyone died of different things. It was like that when there was only AZT and their symptoms got worse... initially I got so much support from others, feeling that I wasn't on my own. It was an absolutely brilliant experience... there were other guys out there that did the same things as I did and felt like their life had been robbed and all the rest. But everyone in my group died... everybody I knew died. I was the only one left alive. This did reinforce the fact that I had not got long to live... it just reinforced the fact that YES HIV kills people and there's no doubt about it... it just felt a bit unreal in my life at that point. I didn't have any contact with anybody with HIV for a number of years after that."

Paul spoke of his devastation and loss. The members of this group had become his friends and he had got to know their partners. Whilst it was empowering for Paul at the start, it became very traumatic towards the end. Paul made a conscious decision not to have any contact with any person living with HIV and just got on with his life until he became very ill and had to access appropriate support.

ELISABETH

It was the Christmas of 1985 when Elisabeth, at the age of 31, learned of her HIV-positive status. She was informed she had a life expectancy of two years. She was in a relationship at the time of diagnosis, had three children and was a practising IV drug user. She recalls:

"I was in a state of shock when I went home. I said to my boyfriend 'look what you have given me', as I had assumed that he had given it to me because I had only really shared (needles) with him and a couple of other people. He had lived in Thailand and had been in prison there. He was a real sort of bad boy. He used to carry a gun… he got tested and he was negative. We didn't really talk about it… obviously I told my boyfriend but we told no-one else. I didn't tell my children. I thought life was hard enough and they were only 7, 9 and 11 at the time. They wouldn't understand it. I mean I didn't understand it… I am glad I didn't tell them because there was actually nowhere for kids to go and get support."

Elisabeth told me of how she spent the next couple of months crying quite a lot and how she used a lot of heroin; more than she had ever used in her whole life. She remembers how she would make dinner and whilst cutting up vegetables if she cut herself, would look at the blood. She says:

"They tell you you've got this terminal illness but you've got no lumps, you have no outward signs, you have not lost a leg or a limb and I didn't look any different. I would look at myself in the mirror and try to see a difference but I couldn't. There is a virus inside me and it is killing me. I would have those kinds of thoughts."

Elisabeth went on to tell me of her determination to live for at least nine years in spite of the medical prognosis she was given. As she was separated from her husband, the children's father, she didn't want to die and leave her children in the care of their father who was also an addict. She described him as 'pretty useless'. She said to herself: 'I am not going to die until my youngest is 16.' Elisabeth never thought about it again and made this decision with conviction. She moved away from the area where she had been living, as she was 'on the run' from the Police; she finally got arrested and went to prison and hid her HIV-positive status. She told me with honesty and openness that 'I was an addict long before I was HIV-positive. That had been the overriding thing in my life that I have had to fight.'

TOM

Tom was diagnosed at the age of 39 in February of 1986. He tested voluntarily after discovering a past lover had been diagnosed with Kaposi Sarcoma [see glossary]. He was given a medical prognosis of 2 years life expectancy and was in an intimate relationship. Tom was working shifts at the time of diagnosis. He recalls:

"I kind of turned into a hypochondriac at the time... but then after it had gone on for two years there was a tremendous sense of relief as I had gone more than what was communicated to me. This lifted a huge amount of anxiety off me and I became reasonably brighter about the whole thing."

Tom kept journals of his thoughts and life after his diagnosis and was able to recall many issues after re-reading these in later years. He remembers having to spend three months living in isolation with his diagnosis before he finally met other HIV-positive people at Body Positive in Brighton [and later in London]. This gave him an opportunity of listening to other people's experiences and sharing his own which he said made him feel better about himself. Prior to this, he thought he was 'the only one in the world'. Three months later, Tom started a Body Positive in his own local area and he recalled 'in the process of helping other people, I more than helped myself'.

Tom told me of his paranoia and being uptight about bleeding at work. He had disclosed his HIV-positive status to other people on his work team and they were supportive and even told him to 'lighten up about it'. He became non-sexual for a year and had 'a huge hang-up about infecting other people.' This was terrifying for Tom. On the whole, however, Tom recalls being reasonably empowered and comfortable with his sexuality. He was determined to be as proud of being HIV-positive as he was of being gay.

Tom recalls becoming less materialistic and more concerned with his own well-being after living for over two years following diagnosis. He tells us:

"When somebody says that you are not going to have many tomorrows, the sensible thing to do is to try and look at today and see what you have got today and see how valuable that is... I dread to think if I hadn't have been forced into various situations which had led to the change in my persona, I would be somebody now that I didn't like... Every birthday became precious because it was like one more year; another big marker for survival really."

Tom later embarked on a working career in the HIV field in a professional capacity and accomplished many groundbreaking achievements, despite some of his friends thinking that this type of work was too close to his own personal situation. He remembers many friends suggesting this type of work was 'suicidal' and that Tom would soon be on course to 'burning himself out'.

JOHN

In 1989, at the age of 35, John was told of his HIV-positive status and recalls being told at the clinic that on average people became ill and died within five years. He was not in a relationship and was working full time. He recalls:

"I ran up £9,000 of debt and I thought 'that's fine because I won't be around to have to repay it. I don't care!' And then five years later I was still working and had to repay it. I remember wondering whether I was going to see 40, so I stopped thinking about growing old, becoming 60 and retiring and I suppose you don't really think about life in the longer term at all... I don't have a problem with death, just me being ill is a problem. I was afraid of being ill and not being independent. I haven't had any contact with my family since I was 17 years old, so I didn't know what would happen, or what will happen if and when I become unable to look after myself for whatever reason. One of the hardest things is that HIV is not predictable and is different for everybody... with AIDS, some people at this stage die of pneumonia, some go blind, some get dementia. So, you cannot prepare yourself in a way... the uncertainty is the worse thing!"

John went on to say that uncertainty was the worst factor of living with the HIV virus and this is shared by almost every person in the study. In the early years, every time he caught a cold or had the flu he would think: 'Oh, is this the start of something more serious?' and this would cause unnecessary worry and anxiety. He also told me:

"I know it is not really an issue, you know, I still go to the clinic every 3 or 4 months and my T-cell count is about 600 so I know that I am unlikely to get HIV-related infections at the moment... it could be, but I still get colds and flu like everybody else... I remember getting floaters in one of my eyes and I was thinking ooooooooooooohhhhhhhhhhh, this is, can't remember now what it is called... there is an eye condition related to HIV [*he means CMV*] I was thinking, Oh, God! So I went to the doctor and the eye hospital and it was perfectly fine and the last couple of years I have started wearing glasses, which is old age and nothing else [laughing]."

In later years, such tensions and anxieties have diminished due to him regularly attending HIV health checks at an HIV clinic which measure his T-cell count and viral load (see glossary). John therefore believes he is more likely to be aware of any illness condition that might be related to his HIV-positive status because of these routine medical tests.

DAVID

David was diagnosed in 1990 at the age of 52 and was in a relationship which, at the time of our interview, was still flourishing; his partner is HIV-negative. David continued to work until he took early retirement (not as a result of his HIV-positive status). At the time of diagnosis, David was told that he could expect to be dying at the age of 54, which was in two years time. David's story, like others, is inspiring because despite being told he had two years to live, David had his own ideas on his life expectancy. He tells us:

"My target was 60 and I am way past that target now. I thought I am not going to die, as I have far too much to do. I started looking at alternative and complementary therapies and alternative lifestyles... We (David and his partner) told three couples and no-one else: that was my two former lovers and their partners and another couple who I have been friendly with for over 40 years. We looked around for HIV support and found a group that led us into an Eastern way of thinking about things: learning to love and respect you... every day is precious and no day is wasted on being unhappy because you can just lift yourself out of the lows if you have all the right conditions and I have. I have a loving partner, financial security, a nice home and because of being gay all my life, I have made a family-of-friends. I take nothing for granted and I am aware of myself and other people and their needs and I try to learn from other people's mistakes."

David told me that he believed HIV was the best thing that happened to him because he didn't take everyday for granted and didn't believe he was going to live forever. He also learned that if people wanted to die and had a death wish then this was their right and choice. David had no desire to impose life onto somebody else. He learned this from overcoming his own anger and 'guilt complex' whilst he watched young people dying of AIDS during his voluntary work in the HIV field. David believed his own guilt emanated from his own thoughts of 'why am I living when these young people in their 20s and 30s are dying?' This was a problem he faced and subsequently conquered over time. This was also voiced by many other long-term survivors in this story-of-stories.

RICHARD

Richard was diagnosed in 1990 at the age of 21; he was not in an intimate relationship at this time. He was working full time in London and voluntarily took the test after a close friend of his had become ill with AIDS and was in hospital. Richard's account is unusual in that the consultant, at the time of diagnosis, told Richard that he had probably only recently contracted HIV. The consultant suggested that Richard might have 5, 10 or even 15 years to live but ultimately the medics did not know. Richard tells us:

"I felt I had to leave my place of work and where I lived and up sticks and move back up North. I am not so sure how wise that was with hindsight... I did this mainly so I would get support from my family. I might have been a lot wiser staying in London. I did get a flat of my own, however, so that was a good thing. One thing was that my confidence was completely in tatters. I was so frightened of being found out that I was HIV-positive. I got another job in the same field but I had hospital appointments... that might have had something to do with my short stay at work... I was living in a small town and HIV was relatively new. The consultant I went to see was an HIV specialist and I am sure everybody knew what he did. When I was asked, 'who did you see?' and I said his name, I felt vulnerable as if everyone knew what the consultant specialised in. I lost two jobs. I spent a long time thinking that people had the right to know... I am talking about people in general: employers, partners you are having sex with or anybody for that matter... HIV just happens to be a taboo for some people. Now, I think forcing people to test or forcing people to disclose their positive status is wrong... I am not ungrateful that I am still here but I never thought I would be here today. I am very vulnerable... I am aware of my status and my health."

Whilst Richard told me of his vulnerability, he also acknowledged his own bravery as he embarked on a career in the HIV field in the early years. He told me of the impact he hopes to have had on people's lives, with specific reference to his involvement in training and workshops around HIV issues. He tells us:

"... I allow myself to be vulnerable by sitting at the front of workshops and allowing people to ask me questions about my HIV and living with HIV. Taking part in HIV awareness training allows people to understand more and I hope I have impacted on people's lives; I am pretty sure I have. I hope I have offered people an opportunity to look for themselves at what HIV is and what it is not, and from that make choices for themselves."

SANDRA

At the age of 29, Sandra was diagnosed HIV-positive following her five month old son's severe illness condition in 1994. Her son died in hospital two weeks later with an AIDS-related condition and Sandra was given a five year life expectancy. At the time of her diagnosis, Sandra recalls how her concerns were predominantly with her son's funeral arrangements and her own concerns did not emerge for seven months. Following her son's death, Sandra worked 70 or 80 hours per week for agencies in order to cope with her loss. One morning she could not get up out of bed, as her body would not let her. She tells us:

"My husband was there for me. We stayed together through the death of our son and we got married because we had just been living together. So, we got married after my diagnosis and we spent four happy years together... He couldn't really understand what it was like. I started to have a lot of psychological problems, just dealing with the possibility of death and my perspective on life changed totally. We were very carefree people before this... for me all that ended when my son died, but my husband wanted to carry on with the life we had before. I couldn't understand how he could... I changed a hell of a lot. I became a different person. I became afraid of any sexual contact in case I infected my husband. I felt guilty enough that I had passed it on to my child and I just could not cope with the idea of the possibility that I could infect my husband because I loved him. I still do love him. I decided the best thing for me [and him] was for me to leave, so that he could have a life. At the time of my diagnosis there was a death sentence, as we didn't have the combination therapies that we have now. He was told that I would be lucky if I lived for five years... I knew there was no cure and people were dying. My son had died and I had watched him die."

Sandra told me of how she grieved for over three years for her son before facing her own situation and speaks of her anger. She recounts:
"I became very angry that this had happened to me. I hadn't done anything to deserve it and I wished I had. I had been so careful, well obviously not careful enough to wear a condom but I had never done anything dodgy as I saw it and it wasn't fair. I was very angry with everybody. I was angry with the professionals; I wouldn't let anybody see me. I became a recluse."

She also told me of how she felt she had lost her status in society. Sandra could no longer carry on with life as 'normal'. She could not tell anyone of her HIV-positive status, as she was so ashamed. Her concerns were around what people might think of her as a person. For two years, Sandra told no-one, other than her husband. Her fear of rejection was overwhelming and when she did tell a couple, who were Christian friends of her and her husband, her fears were substantiated. After telling the couple of her HIV-positive status, the couple then spoke to her husband alone. She tells us:

"I was so close to my husband, he told me everything. He came back and told me that he had had this conversation with our Christian friends and they had said to him, "this is God's way of telling you that you shouldn't be with this woman because God has saved you from catching the virus and you shouldn't be with her"._

Sandra then spoke of her anger and feelings of rejection. She cut the couple out of her life whilst her husband maintained a relationship with them. This was her first experience of telling someone whom she trusted of her HIV-positive status. She became cautious of telling anybody, which is understandable. Sandra's family live thousands of miles away and therefore are not aware of her HIV-positive status. After telling a second person of her status some time later, she faced rejection yet again. The person whom she confided in eventually asked her not to call again, as she felt an overriding sense of being burdened with the knowledge of Sandra's HIV-positive status. Sandra told me of her refusal to tell anyone else because these two experiences were too painful for her. She tells us more:

"Unless someone is prepared to cure me or help me, then I am not telling anyone... It is a burden to carry this dreadful secret. It is very difficult to live with and I feel like a prisoner. I have not moved on to a stage where HIV is an acceptable part of my life. For me, it is like an alien that has invaded my body and my mind."

A forgotten generation: Long-term survivors' experiences of HIV and AIDS

Facing up to mortality: perceptions of imminent death

The next set of narratives explores personal perceptions of how our long-term survivors understood their own mortality after discovering they were HIV-positive. None of our story-tellers featured in this section were given a medical prognosis of life expectancy by a medical practitioner on 'diagnosis day'; it is rather puzzling why some story-tellers were given a medical 'death sentence' whilst others were not. Nevertheless, our story-tellers reveal how they believed imminent death to be a reality because of media coverage and the extensive loss of lives to AIDS. Again, we start with those diagnosed earliest and explore the early years of everyday life after diagnosis:

JO

In 1982, at the age of 33, Jo was diagnosed HIV-positive after experiencing problems with his lymph nodes. He was not in a relationship at this time and had previously worked in the acting profession. Jo was not given a medical prognosis for life expectancy but was aware that being HIV-positive was essentially a 'death sentence'. He recalls:

"I went to a special clinic… they took a look at my lymph nodes which were enlarged and arranged for me to have a biopsy. It came out as HTLVIII which is the precursor of HIV. What was interesting was that when I was in the hospital in a side room, there were basically two beds. There was myself and this other person. This other person, it turned out, I had met when I was an actor on tour. We'd had a sort of fling for a week. He was there in the most terrible state and I can only assume that within weeks he was dead."

Jo told me of his failed attempt at his own life after feeling isolated and very depressed. After this, he decided to get on and piece his life back together. It was at a demonstration against Nuclear Power that he met his current partner. From the early days, Jo stated that he always tried to be upfront and honest about his status with friends. He did not tell his parents, as he did not want to distress them because of the 'misinformation' that was about at the time. Now his parents have both died, he speaks of extraordinary relief that lies and secrecy no longer have to be perpetuated.

A forgotten generation: Long-term survivors' experiences of HIV and AIDS

GLYNN

At the age of 17 or 18, Glynn was diagnosed with HTLVIII in 1983 as part of the mass screening process for people living with Haemophilia. Whilst he was not given a medical prognosis for life expectancy, he was told that it was terminal. He is one of three remaining survivors out of 65 people who were diagnosed at the same time. Because of his age and his youthful outlook, Glynn remembers just getting on with life but recalls how he felt about the thought of dying at a 'pretty young age'. He tells us:

"I was pretty pissed off I suppose because I didn't want to die young. I wanted to have a good life and then I suppose it went the other way. You've got to cram everything into what you've got now and things like that. I think that was how a lot of us thought. Then we got some compensation for it [*contracting HIV from contaminated blood products*] and we just thought that we may as well just enjoy it. Do what we want because in 10 years time we probably won't be here… I mean we went out, we had good times, we had drinks and I mean most of us blew the money we were given. At the time I got my money, I was leaving college and we were all going our separate ways. That was a bit more difficult to cope with, as well. You know, if you had a bit of money then you felt a bit sort of happier."

Glynn told me how he discovered that he and other people living with Haemophilia had further contracted Hepatitis C via contaminated blood products. He recounts:

"Well, I just laughed. I laughed and laughed because I just couldn't believe it. When they told me I just laughed and thought 'what the hell'. It didn't make me feel any worse or any better because I thought 'well I have already got HIV. You just think sod it!"

CHRISTOPHER

Christopher was diagnosed in 1988 at the age of 36 whilst being treated in hospital for an arthritic condition. He was in a long-term intimate relationship and was in full time employment. He was not given any time-scale for life expectancy yet for the first 12 months he thought he was dying. He tells us:

"I was convinced I was going to die and that I was going to die very soon… whether I got a cold or whether I got a cough, or if I had a mark on my body, I really thought it was going to be the 'Philadelphia' film for me... My partner wanted me not to tell people and if I became ill it had to be cancer or my heart or whatever, he was very ashamed... It made me feel ashamed as well for the first four or five years after diagnosis."

Christopher went on to tell me that after five years or more, the majority of time he does not think about his HIV-positive status. He believes he is not in denial but has a very positive mental attitude for physical and emotional illnesses. He told me 'I also feel that I am dying to live and not living to die'.

LISETTE

Lisette was diagnosed in 1990 whilst travelling and visiting her daughter in the USA at the age of 39. She was not in a relationship at the time and whilst she was not given a time-scale for life expectancy, she firmly believed she was going to die in six months. Before she returned to the UK she told me how a friend had obtained for her 'tons and tons of leaflets' pertaining to HIV information and on her return to the UK she waded through the literature. She tells us:

"I kind of felt worse. Thinking of the possibilities of what might happen to me, or in those days it was going to happen to you; there wasn't any maybe about it, you know... I just thought that it was all like a weird game that I am involved in, but the thing is they [*the medics*] didn't know anything. The woman that was my consultant, you know, by the time I had finished reading all the literature I knew more than she did. She was, however, very willing and really wanted to learn more about it. And then I remember going back to my GP and asking her to sign one of those DS1500 forms – you know if you are getting Income Support and you have an illness where you aren't going to live for more than five or six months, then you no longer have to put in sick notes. You just automatically get the money and it makes life easier. I remember going in and asking her about this and she was rather reluctant to sign it at first. I remember saying to her, "Well, can you guarantee that I'm going to be alive in five or six months?" and my GP said 'No!' To me, that was the time, if you like, when somebody was saying something about time and my life expectancy."

Lisette told me how she felt that she had a lot of 'unfinished stuff' in her life and how she had desperate urges to *finish things off*. She was also trying to enjoy each day for what it was. If she was only going to live for six months, then for Lisette, it seemed crazy for her to spend this time worrying about what was going to happen. Lisette was also not experiencing good health at this time, which made matters more difficult for her to enjoy each day. She later got in touch with Body Positive in London which 'was probably one of the best things I ever did'. She recounts:

"I met other people and I found out I was not alone. I also met another woman which was a big thing for me. It became obvious to me from reading the literature, and I couldn't get enough of it, that all of the published material was what they knew about men and not about women... so I was armed with all this information and when it came to making a decision, I couldn't make it because the information was only based on men. If you are asking me to take a drug, for instance, because you have such-and-such results, you can't show me that these results include women. So I would just dismiss the information entirely."

She told me she was grateful that she did not have small children and would console herself with the fact that her children were 15 and 18 when she was diagnosed and therefore were grown up in a sense. A big issue for Lisette, as was mentioned by others in the study, was the uncertainty around being HIV-positive and lack of knowledge available in the early years.

MARC

Marc was diagnosed in 1990 at the age of 26 after a period of ill health. He was working at the time and was not in relationship. He was not given a time-scale for life expectancy but believed his mortality was being challenged. He was aware of current information pertaining to HIV and AIDS at this time and prior to his test results, believed he might be HIV-positive because he had engaged in a lot of unprotected gay sex. He tells us:

"I was upset, I suppose, I just felt a bit phased and I was in shock. I didn't quite know what to do... it made planning for the future quite hard. I had some money at the time and because I was unsure about the future I just decided to spoil myself and now I am really annoyed as I could really use the cash... For the first year I dealt with the situation by just taking a lot of recreational drugs and then after a year I realised that was not a solution so I stopped... my efforts were more on just not using any drugs, that was in the second year of my diagnosis... and then in the third year of my diagnosis I just decided I needed to sort out my housing situation and I eventually got this place... around the same time I met someone and I wasn't working, only part-time but I then returned to full time work and that was kind of in year four. You know, lots of things happened."

Marc believed the major factor that affects people's attitudes the most is health. If you are well it is easier to maintain a positive attitude than if you are unwell. He recounts:

"I think HIV is like a big magnifying glass; you just sort of magnify things with feelings that you already have. I don't think it changes anything... I mean before I was diagnosed if I woke up with blotches on my face I would look in the mirror and think 'Oh my God! What is going on?' And today if I wake up in the morning and have blotches all over my face I would think 'Oh my God! I have got AIDS!' I don't think HIV has changed anything; it just makes you a bit more sensitive to probabilities... You know, we all know that we are going to die one day. It is just if you are HIV-positive you know that a bit more."

Marc told me that after a few years he realised that he was living as though he was expecting to die and this was an amazing revelation for him. He became rather upset at this revelation initially; however it soon became a turning point in his life. He realised that he actually had a choice in how he related to his own situation.

PABLO

In 1990, Pablo was diagnosed HIV-positive at the age of 20, following a period of ill health. He was in a relationship with a woman at the time. He told me that he had been bisexual but later self-identified as gay. He was not given a time-scale for life expectancy yet believed he only had a matter of years to live. He tells us:

"I will be honest, for the first couple of years after being diagnosed I didn't give a shit really... I just went out there, I drank myself silly. I slept with God knows how many people. Obviously protected, not unprotected. That only ever happened once and I told the person the next day that it shouldn't have happened. I told him to go for a test straight away, even though I didn't feel there would probably be any chance of him getting infected. It is better to be safe than sorry... it was like self-destruct really. It suddenly dawned on me that I had probably only got a couple of years to live and I might as well live my life to the full. So, I went out every night getting pissed. I went down the route of trying all bloody drugs out... I moved about various places. I didn't settle in one place very long. It was like being on a roller coaster. I was trying to get away from it but it was always there, if you understand what I mean."

Pablo told me that one day he looked at himself and decided to get his life in order and get to grips with things. The turning point, he revealed, was accessing a group in Brighton called Open Door, which was an HIV drop-in centre. He believed this helped him get back his positive attitude to life.

LARRY

Larry was diagnosed in 1992, at the age of 46, after he had experienced a period of ill health. He was not in a relationship at the time and was not working. He did not receive a time-scale for life expectancy but did believe it was a 'death sentence' when he was told; his whole world fell apart. He tells us:

"The first impact it had on me was crikey! I'm going to be dead this time next week. The death sentence... Obviously I don't think anyone really expects that kind of news and even if you are older you don't really want to die. You want to hang on to life. For the next six years I had this negative outlook on everything... my health suffered emotionally because of the shock, the horror, the anger and all the other things. I was grieving for myself. I just kept myself to myself. I felt as if horns were coming out of my head and everyone could see that I was HIV-positive. I just withdrew. First of all, my father died and then in quick succession about one month later I lost my job and then one month after that I was diagnosed with HIV... I never felt sorry for myself, I just felt bad about myself and I had thoughts that were not very healthy. Then one day I got to the end of my tether and realised this was not doing me any good. I wasn't dead. I wasn't dying and so I was wrong, wasn't I? I wasn't dying with it, I was living with it and it wasn't a death sentence but a life sentence. I have got it for life and that was what changed everything. It all made sense to me."

Larry told me that one of the main differences in his life, once he changed his attitude, was socialising again, as he hadn't socialised with his friends for six years. Going out and having fun on the gay scene gave Larry his life back. After this time, he was able to regard everything as natural again and life hadn't been natural for him when he was living in fear and isolation. He viewed life as a gift and another chance.

WOODY

In 1992, at the age of 35, Woody was diagnosed HIV-positive after voluntarily going for the test. He was embarking on a new intimate relationship and wanted to know his HIV status. He was working at the time and was not given a medical prognosis for life expectancy. When he was diagnosed, Woody had a CD4 count (see glossary) of 250 and was therefore put on AZT treatment immediately. He was told that because of his low CD4 count, he had probably been living with HIV for a considerable amount of time; his condition was deemed serious and advanced. He believed that his life expectancy was limited. He tells us:

"I wasn't given any length of time for survival… it was pointed out that everybody was completely different. Basically there was no way of telling, as it affects everybody differently and I remember thinking that I would not survive for five years at that point. This was my own perception. I used to think about it all the time. If I was at work with people who had colds, I would think 'Oh, don't cough near me because I am very susceptible'… I remember being given the name of a social worker and talking about benefits and not being able to work. We also talked about the implications of applying for a mortgage or life insurance and health insurance. We also went through the procedure for informing the GP and dentists and people like that and why these people should be informed. At one point I actually applied for something like Disability Living Allowance, but I don't think it was called that then, but its equivalent. This was on the basis of my CD4 count being low. What they did was take me through all the practical implications."

Woody was fortunate to get appropriate support around his HIV-positive status at the time. He spoke of having to think about adjusting his lifestyle and become a person with HIV rather than a person without HIV. His biggest fear was deteriorating slowly over a long period of time, wasting away and losing weight; basically he feared withering away until he died. Woody remembers his fears were not around actually death and dying but rather spending a prolonged period of time in hospital. He tells us:

"I wasn't fearful of dying but I was fearful of being ill. I thought of myself as a person with HIV. Suddenly I became a different person. I looked at things from the point of view of a person with HIV in terms of what I could do and what I couldn't do. Well, a different person is not quite right. I was the same person but I was a person with a transmittable disease so I had to look at everything differently."

Woody told me that he keeps his HIV-positive status a secret from most people around him. Apart from telling one or two close friends and his partner at the time of diagnosis who was HIV-negative, nobody else knows of his HIV-positive status; he does not want to be thought of as somebody who is HIV-positive in a way that might affect his ability to do everyday things, such as work and so on. The close friends he disclosed his status to are also HIV-positive; Woody told me that he knew of their HIV-positive status before he told them. Many of his family are deceased; however, Woody has two sisters who do not know.

On being positive and living with HIV-positive partners

The final set of narratives are personal experiences of long-term survivors who were living in established sero-concordant (see glossary) relationships at the time of diagnosis. Our story-tellers reveal how they experienced everyday life in terms of putting to one side their own problems to concentrate on caring for their HIV-positive partners during the first few years after 'diagnosis day'. Feelings of relief are expressed by some story-tellers in terms of discovering they were HIV-positive because the idea of one partner being positive whilst the other is negative would have been difficult to negotiate. Again, we begin with those story-tellers diagnosed the earliest.

COLIN

Colin learned of his HIV-positive status in 1985 at the age of 25, after testing voluntarily at his local sexual health clinic. He had just embarked on an intimate sexual relationship with his male partner and had fallen in love. Colin had worked voluntarily on the Gay Switchboard until 1984 and spoke of the limited knowledge and awareness of HIV and AIDS issues, or GRID (Gay-related Infection Disease) as it was known then. Colin's partner was also HIV-positive and two years into their relationship went on to develop AIDS. Colin told me how he put his own positive diagnosis on hold. He recounts:

"Bizarrely, my first reaction of getting a positive test was almost partially one of relief... I don't think I thought about my own status ... mainly because my partner became sick within a couple of years... so I ended up having to look after him. I think all my energies were involved in looking after and coping with him. I say *coping with* because he was a fiery young man with a drink problem and a very disturbed background, but a lovely guy, very intelligent, fiercely honest and a remarkable person… our relationship lasted four and half years until his death. The first couple of years were fine but by 1987/1988 he was clearly becoming ill and in the last year was dying with AIDS. I still can't talk about it in depth without getting emotional because I think I learned so much about very rare issues about life and death… You know, I looked after the guy, like many… I don't know if I looked after him as well as I could have, but I think I did my best. He dealt with his illness with extraordinary bravery; he turned into a very remarkable person. If you are looking after a person who is dying you have your nose rubbed into some very raw facts about illness and death, which most of us go around not thinking about a lot of the time. I am talking about actually witnessing the physical decay, witnessing cancers coming out on his skin and the poor guy being unable to hold down any food… and losing weight. Thank God he never got dementia. He was absolutely lucid all the way up to the last hour of his life. In the end, he was just this sort of walking shadow and I mean he was only 29 and he looked like a little shuffling old man. I was there when he died. I was sitting next to him on his bed. He insisted on coming home to die from the hospital ward."

Colin told me of how his partner was absolutely determined to live through Christmas. His partner had been in hospital for six weeks with various illness conditions; the hospital released him home and they went to Colin's parents over the festive period. Colin recalls:

"… He insisted he wanted a holiday, so we went off to Paris, him in his wheelchair. I knew it was a mad thing to do but he insisted on doing it. He was a very determined person when he wanted to be. He had a very bad temper and would shout and scream if he didn't get his own way. So we had two days in Paris before he came down with another bout of pneumonia and I had already had a bad experience in the previous May of being with him in the States and him coming down with pneumonia and us having to get him to hospital there. I took him back home; the hospital took one look at him and said, 'this is it! He is not going to get out of this one. I said to him, 'You are dying. What do you want to do?' He wanted to go home… there was an ambulance strike at the time and a couple of ambulance drivers came off the picket line and volunteered to drive him home and take care of his practical nursing needs. So we went back to our flat and he took only about 12 hours to die… his family came round… a whole bunch of friends turned up. It was quite remarkable and he was lying in bed almost holding court. I mean, he was desperately ill and half in and out of consciousness but he was still lucid at times. At one point the strangeness got to me so much that a friend of mine took me up to the pub.

I remember it is the only time I have ever just poured alcohol down my throat and stayed absolutely stone cold sober... I came back and he was sitting up in the sitting room having a Gin and Tonic. He said, 'Oh! Thank God you're back'. Then he went to bed. About 2 o'clock in the morning he woke me up because he was struggling out of bed to get to the loo. His Mum tried to help him and he wouldn't have any of it, he wanted to do it himself. Eventually he did and he came back to bed... he just fell down on the mattress like a dead thing and that was the last moment of consciousness. After that, he slipped into a coma and died about 11 that morning. It was an incredible experience."

Colin told me that he would not have missed this experience for the world, as it was a remarkable death. His partner died 'in style', surrounded by people who loved him and it was very real. After this, Colin stayed healthy for many years until 1995; he had sporadically taken treatments which had been available in 1989. He took part in the Concorde trial and had taken AZT. He gave it up after six weeks after experiencing horrendous side effects. Colin was determined to survive after his partner's death and says 'not for one moment did I operate like a person who thought he was going to die.'

CLAIR

In 1987, at the age of 25, Clair was diagnosed HIV-positive. Her husband was diagnosed as HIV-positive in 1985 and was living with Haemophilia. She did not receive a medical prognosis for life expectancy and was trying for a child, under medical supervision, prior to her testing positive. Clair did not believe in the certainty of death at the time because there was so little history or knowledge that had been grounded in substantial evidence. She believed it was inappropriate for the medical profession to be saying to people 'you are going to die within five years'. She tells us:

"I would like to see all of this go down as a huge medical fuck up, basically... well blunder [laughing]... It is appalling really... if it wasn't so serious it would make you laugh. It is laughable; the whole thing has been hype. First of all, the politics of it being a gay thing and all the other issues of anal sex, vaginal erosion... it's all been around sex, it hasn't worked, has it? HIV is a label... Certainly, my husband's experiences of what happened to him makes you realise that they [the medical profession] don't really know what they are doing. Just sitting in a hospital ward and watching what goes on at the bedside of somebody who is seriously ill. My husband got cancer, non-Hodgkin's lymphoma (see glossary) and that was the first sign that there was something wrong. They gave him AZT and he was on it for two years. He had to take it every six hours and I watched him. He said that he didn't like it but he took it because, well you were frightened not to because you had been told… he had to have chemotherapy to reduce the white blood cells to nought. You are so vulnerable to infection and if you get a temperature you must go back to hospital. He went to hospital, after having a temperature, on Sunday morning about 5 or 6 o'clock in the morning; and the doctor said he needed antibiotics. Hours went by and still he had not had the treatment. I spoke to a nurse and told her that my husband had not received his antibiotics and was told 'Oh no, no! We give them out at 12 o'clock'. He was suffering with a temperature and I realise that they have to have a routine. She was really snotty. The next day the doctor came by with 20 students and he was saying 'Yes, this is the chap with blah-de-blah, came in, low white blood count, what we did was get antibiotics into him; this is the first thing you must do, treat with antibiotics immediately.' I piped up and said that was not actually what happened and told them what had happened. The doctor could not believe it and was screaming at the door at the nurses. My husband could have died and that is just a minor example of things that went on… They don't like it when you try to tell them, you are seen as patronising. I was watching all these things going on."

Clair told me that her husband's experiences had affected her, whilst her own HIV-positive diagnosis had not affected her too much. She was relatively healthy. Clair did mention the uncertainty around the illness did create some challenges for her.

RICK

Rick was only 18 when he was diagnosed HIV-positive in 1987. He used a false name and later re-tested in 1990 when he was 21 years old. He was in an intimate relationship at the time, and his partner was also HIV-positive and had known this for quite a long time. Rick believes his partner 'gave him HIV to keep him'. He was not given a medical time-scale for life expectancy and was working at the time of diagnosis. He gave up his working career to look after his partner who had become very ill. Rick was extremely proud of the care he gave to his partner until his death. He recalls:

"We had one Marie Curie nurse in 8 months for 24 hours because I was absolutely exhausted… we had to carry him [his partner] around and there was diarrhoea everywhere. He wouldn't allow District Nurses in the house.

A forgotten generation: Long-term survivors' experiences of HIV and AIDS

The nurse we actually had was useless. I mean he walked straight in, you could see all the diarrhoea and he walked straight through with his Doc Marten boots on. A doctor who came a day and half before he died, he was an old doctor just said 'let him die'. I mean he was 'fitting' [having a seizure] and they had got spatulas and things to put down his throat and he just said, 'let him die'. He was jumping like a metre off the bed 'fitting' and it was me that put my hand in his mouth to stop him biting his tongue. So all my hand was cut open... yes, he was dying, but I promised him he could die at home. Because of the fits, he needed diamorphine which was the only thing they could not let me have at home. All other drug treatments, all the blood transfusions, his morphine transfusions were ok but diamorphine was pure heroin and they couldn't let me take this home. The doctor wouldn't do anything but said 'let him die'. He nearly swallowed his tongue, so it was my fingers that went down his throat. The doctor wouldn't take his temperature; he refused to give any anal paracetamol which he needed, as his temperature was absolutely sky high. I refused to see that doctor again."

As mentioned in chapter one, Rick was 'chuffed' when the medics said his partner had only got 24 hours to live and Rick managed to keep him alive for a further 8 months. He took his partner to places he wanted to go in his wheelchair and took him to Bingo. He told me:

"Oh yes, I was chuffed because we got him out to the pub and one of his friends who ran the pub got him a stool and we got him a cushion and we bought him his gin and tonic or his pint of lager and, you know, we did whatever he fancied doing."

I asked Rick if he had any issues about death and dying following his diagnosis and he told me:

"I have never been scared of dying. I sat and watched my partner die. All I hope is that if something did happen to me it would be something a little bit simpler than what happened to my partner. He had 13 complications. I would like a nice heart attack or pneumonia is one of the nicest ones. I always think something simple would be nice. You can't guarantee something simple I suppose. A few of my friends have died and the family sent letters out to people on the buddy list on the Internet saying 'so-and-so passed away peacefully in their sleep'. So I am not worried about dying but I just hope it is something quick and easy."

The last quote has been extremely difficult for me to recount, as Rick died a few years after our conversations. I visited him on several occasions in hospital whilst he was dying and I had a missed call on my mobile from him

15 minutes before he died. During our time together when I visited him, he was very open and honest and told me he was frightened of dying when the time came. His biggest fear was around the idea that he didn't want to cause his family unnecessary suffering by dying and leaving them to grieve. Rick very much needed permission to die when the time was right; he was experiencing extreme discomfort and had remained alive for the sake of his family. He needed to know that it was all right for him to die and leave his family behind. He got permission to die. At the end, Rick was very brave and died without my being there. He wanted me to be by his side and I missed him by several minutes. I am, unsurprisingly, so very proud of him.

RACHEL

In 1993, at the age of 28, Rachel was diagnosed HIV-positive. Her husband was HIV-positive and had contracted the virus in Africa from a contaminated needle. Rachel was relieved that they were both HIV-positive. She was working full time at the time of her diagnosis and did not receive a medical prognosis for life expectancy. Her husband however had become quite ill and was given less than 18 months to live. She gave up her working career to care for her husband, who was still alive and in good health at the time of her interview in 2002. She tells us:

"… I gave up work to look after him because he was very ill at the time. He was having difficulty going up and down the stairs and walking 20 yards and that sort of thing. Packing up work obviously had an enormous effect on me because I loved my job. He responded well to treatment and so we could start planning and starting looking ahead and start thinking well perhaps we don't need to be so negative about things. My health was fine and had been pretty much as far as HIV is concerned all the way along. Later on we had some fantastic guidance when we started looking at the possibility of having children… once we realised we could start actually looking forward we started looking at things positively."

Rachel and her husband went on to have two daughters and both children are HIV-negative. Whilst the children are quite young at present, Rachel told me that she would never lie to them about HIV. She tells us:

"I will tell them the truth at a level that they can understand at each stage. It is something that is not without risk; obviously I worry about if they say something out of hand or whether they are going to end up getting bullied. But ultimately we decided that the risk of losing their trust because we lied to them is much worse than the risk of somebody saying something out of hand and us having to handle that. So, they come to the clinic with us and we don't pretend it is something else. We just treat it as though it is normal and that it is not something that we should be frightened of."

The personal experiences that have unfolded in this chapter are, undeniably, pretty remarkable and extremely thought-provoking. We have witnessed how some story-tellers were given a life expectancy of between a few months, to 1 or 2 years, to 4 or 5 years or from 5, 10 or 15 years. How could the medical profession have gotten these crucial matters so wrong? Differences in life expectancy have been far-reaching yet the impact on the lives of those who received a medical 'death sentence' is incomprehensible. Our story-tellers have revealed to us how they negotiated life after 'diagnosis day' with some travelling the world, spending huge amounts of money, focusing on home life with loved ones, taking recreational drugs, or simply ignoring their HIV-positive status until such time they became ill. Many experienced the tragic loss of their friends to AIDS and HIV and few spoke of feelings of isolation and depression, which led to them attempting to take their own lives. We have learned about financial hardship and problems associated with insurance and mortgage policies and how 'living life to the full' has since left them financially poor. Yet without exception, all of our story-tellers have successfully renegotiated their lives in meaningful ways.

Some story-tellers reflected on why they were still alive whilst others were not. Lies and secrecy around being HIV-positive is clearly a problem for some story-tellers, whilst others are open and 'up front' about it. What is clear from some of the personal accounts is how valuable HIV support networks have been in helping people to understand and negotiate every day life after diagnosis. Thinking of HIV as a life sentence as opposed to a death sentence is a remarkable approach to everyday life. The levels of care our story-tellers have given to their HIV-positive partners is astounding; the experiences of losing your loved one who is living with the same illness condition as yourself must be a complex matter to internalise and deal with at an emotional level. Clearly, experiencing good health does effect how you look upon being HIV-positive as opposed to experiencing prolonged periods of ill health. The coping mechanisms and decision-making strategies our story-tellers have negotiated throughout these earlier times are, without doubt, something we can all learn from.

Once more I ask you, the reader, to consider how these personal experiences have impacted upon your own thoughts, beliefs and feelings before moving on. Has anything changed for you and in what way? Who can you relate to in these stories and truly empathise with? Are there any personal accounts that make you feel uncomfortable? If so, think about why this might be. There are so few certainties in our complex social lives today; however one given certainty that we can all be sure of is we will all die one day. We often do not consider our own mortality in everyday life and why should we? Yet many of our story-tellers were in their early twenties or thirties when they were forced to face their own mortality.

How do you think you might react if you were given a life expectancy of no more than five years or six months? If you cared for someone with the same medical condition as yourself how would this affect you? How might you negotiate an appropriate quality of life for yourself? There may be some personal accounts that are outside of your own experiences which you cannot fully appreciate, yet please consider these. I appreciate your time spent actively engaging with these narratives.

A forgotten generation: Long-term survivors' experiences of HIV and AIDS

CHAPTER FOUR

HIV before HAART: in sickness and in health

∞

"Uncertainty and mystery are energies of life. Don't let them scare you unduly, for they keep boredom at bay and spark creativity."
R. I. Fitzhenry

"Any idiot can face a crisis – it is day to day living that wears you out."
Anton Chekhov

Introduction

We all experience uncertainty, fear, hope, anxieties and aspirations within our daily lives; these are all part of the energy of life itself. To be in good health both physically and mentally is as an ideal state many of us aspire to, as explored in chapter one. Most of us are interested in how our body works and possibly more interested in why it sometimes does not work. How we come to view 'health' is essential for us to maintain a healthy state. Yet if we consider health in terms of the absence of illness or disease how is health to be understood in the context of HIV? Prior to the advent of Highly Active Antiretroviral Therapy (hereinafter referred to as HAART) in 1996, there were few effective medical treatments available for people living with HIV and AIDS. This alone presented an assortment of fears, anxieties and degrees of uncertainty for maintaining good health and potentially managing prolonged periods of ill health. How we are to understand degrees of HIV-related uncertainties in terms of health and illness is complex and requires more in-depth consideration.

First we must acknowledge the *medical uncertainty* of ambiguous symptom patterns, disease progression, and life expectancy as knowledge and awareness of HIV and AIDS developed in earlier times. Add to this the *personal uncertainties* that potentially occur in individual lives, and these might include: complex and conflicting roles and relationships with others around us; renegotiating a sense of our self, *who we are*; our fears and anxieties concerning prolonged illness and imminent death; and, our future prospects around the uncertainty of work and the financial consequences of living with an HIV-positive diagnosis. Thirdly, we must add to our considerations the *social uncertainty* that we might face from others around us; these uncertainties may arise from unpredictable social reactions pertaining to public beliefs about HIV and AIDS which are continually reinforced in our social structures (e.g. the media constructions of AIDS and HIV). At a glance, we are presented with a complex set of relations to consider and comprehend in relation to the uncertainties of living with HIV and AIDS.

Undeniably, the numerous levels and degrees of unease and uncertainties of living long-term with an HIV-positive diagnosis are ambiguous and extensive. This chapter explores how the uncertainty of health, illness and potential illness was experienced prior to 1996 when Highly Active Antiretroviral Therapy (HAART) was introduced as effective treatments for the management of HIV. We begin by exploring the personal experiences of our story-tellers who were ill at the time of diagnosis to gain insight into the many fears, anxieties, hopes and uncertainties that were prevalent during this period. We then move on to reveal and appreciate an assortment of fears and uncertainties based on the perceptions and personal experiences of the drug Zidovudine (ZDV, commonly known as AZT), a monotherapy for HIV and AIDS. We also gain knowledge and insight into how our long-term survivors attempted to manage and negotiate health and periods of illness during a challenging era when little effective treatment was available. As before, we start with story-tellers who were diagnosed during the earliest years.

Illness experiences at the time of diagnosis: fears, hopes and uncertainty

Our story-tellers in this section were diagnosed between 1982 and 1994, were experiencing ill health or presenting symptoms associated with HIV at the time of diagnosis. We explore their personal experiences of health and illness and reveal their fears, hopes and uncertainty for the future. We unravel how our long-term survivors perceived the drug AZT which was the only medical treatment for HIV during these times, and learn why many refused to take the treatment or participate in the Concorde trial.

JO

Jo was 33 years old at the time of diagnosis in 1982 and had been experiencing severe pain under his arms and across his body. He went to his GP and tested positive for HTLVIII (the precursor of HIV); he was then referred to a consultant who was working at the forefront of research in this field at the time. The consultant later asked Jo if he would like to take part in the Concorde Trial which was attempting to evaluate the efficacy of the drug known as Zidovudine (ZDV, AZT). Jo tells us:

"I was actually being given an amazing amount of support for what there was... there was very little that they did know at this time... my consultant wanted me to take part in a cohort where they were giving people AZT. Some people would get AZT and some people would only get the placebo and that drove me mad. I said 'I can't... I'm not prepared to go with this'. It seemed crazy that if there was something that could work for people then they should be given it. That's how I saw it... I thought that they should make sure within their trials that they had worked things out and that people were balanced. If I was going to get the placebo and someone else was going to get the AZT then that person should at least be the same weight as myself and have the same metabolism as me. I didn't know anything about genetics but metabolism was essential so that they could measure how it was working... As far as I was concerned what I needed them to do was put a line down the centre of my body, give one half the AZT and the other half the placebo and then they could measure the effect... I wasn't prepared to go with the trial. I didn't like it! I mean because of my stubbornness I believe that this saved me, because I watched AZT kill people. You know, there is no two ways about it, AZT killed people. I watched people taking the drugs and then dying... I mean of course when we found out that it was a failed chemotherapy drug that had been withdrawn, I was angry. I got real rage... so I wouldn't even think about taking antiretrovirals but I was always asymptomatic, I didn't present with symptoms or problems associated with my illness."

Jo told me that after he refused to take part in the Concorde trial he felt as though he was being 'side-lined' by his HIV consultant, as he saw less and less of him over time. He therefore decided to change and moved on to different HIV doctors who were new to the field. Jo was continually having medical consultations with new medical practitioners, some of whom were good and others who were impossible to relate to. Jo spoke of his desire to have continuity with just one HIV consultant due to the medical uncertainties of living with HIV and the distinct lack of knowledge at this time. Jo tells us:

"One of the biggest changes for me has actually been the huge loss of empowerment. During the early days there was me as the patient and those as the doctors and we were in the same boat. There was a lack of knowledge, we had discussions around HIV and you were treated on the same level as the doctor. They were learning from you and these discussions made a huge difference. When the combination treatments came along and were deemed to be more effective, they put pressure on you to take the medication and the patient was no longer in the loop."

Jo enjoyed a long period of good health; he did not take any treatments until many years later when he was experiencing severe fatigue. This was after the advent of HAART in 1996 which we explore in more detail with Jo in chapter six. He did recount, however, how in the early years he was expecting to die some time soon due to lack of effective treatments available. He spoke of how he watched close friends die and how this promoted 'terrible stress and strain to be dealing with this sort of thing' which had given Jo a kind of 'survivor guilt'.

Feelings of *survivor guilt* were not uncommon amongst other long-term survivors living with HIV who had experienced the loss of friends to AIDS. In the past, *survivor guilt* has been portrayed amid survivors of the Holocaust, veterans of war, recipients of organ transplants and family members who have failed to contract hereditary illness conditions. There has been little discussion of this state amid long-term survivors of chronic illnesses. The concept of 'survivor guilt' emerges from situations where women and men have been involved in life-threatening events and have lived to tell the tale. Tragedies that have caused multiple deaths can present survivor guilt amongst those who survived.

In the case of chronic illnesses, like AIDS, survivor guilt has, for some, emerged after the deaths of large numbers of people who had an AIDS diagnosis; there is an implicit association with human beings who have endured similar ordeals. Survivor guilt explores the other side of the coin of why me? In other words why not me? Tyler's experiences support this in chapter three when he asked why he had survived when others had not. People who struggle with this state often believe the 'wrong person survived', not dissimilar to Tyler who believed 'it just doesn't seem right'. There is a 'deserving' element to this guilt which can produce feelings of unworthiness in some cases, especially when 'surviving the odds' makes little sense to the person concerned: *I do not deserve to be still here when others are not.* A number of our story-tellers who had experienced the loss of their friends to AIDS were asking themselves: 'Why am I still here? Why are all my friends dead, and I am still alive?' Having lived long-term and experienced the loss of a large number of contemporaries to AIDS, often presented feelings of guilt and remorse and the idea of why not me?

MARC

Marc was 26 years old at the time of his diagnosis in 1990 and had been experiencing swollen glands under his arms. He was aware that this was a symptom of HIV and subsequently went for an HIV test. When asked about his knowledge and awareness of treatments prior to 1996, Marc recalled:

"There was no treatment around at this time. There was just AZT but that was only on a trial and the trial was called the Concorde Trial… I know a few people who have gone on that trial and they reported quite bad side effects because the doses were quite high and that put me off, so I didn't take it… I had a very good consultant and she said I was well and there was no reason for her to think that I wouldn't stay well because I was showing no signs of ill health and my CD4 count wasn't very low and I didn't show any symptoms. She said that the pharmacological advances were such that she was expecting drugs to be available in the near future, which would make living with HIV the same as living with diabetes. I just had to hang on. I would just have to hang on to that hope and so it was quite positive information. I didn't really believe her; I just found the whole thing quite scary but after about two years of having no health problems at all, I kind of realised it was stupid to live as though I was going to die."

Marc spoke of how he considered himself to be *lucky* because he had not experienced ill health following his diagnosis and therefore was not reliant on effective HIV treatments becoming readily available in the near future. The CD4 count Marc refers to is an HIV medical indicator of health which came into operation from 1992 onwards. For people diagnosed with HIV in the early 1980s, therefore, it should be acknowledged that this health indicator was not yet operative; consequently, medical practitioners were reliant upon HIV patients to self-report on matters of health and illness. Marc's main anxieties of living with HIV predominantly focussed on his financial status and the fear of becoming ill in the future. He told me:

"I worry about HIV sometimes but I try very hard not to, I try not to wallow. I don't really allow myself to wallow in HIV as a victim… The only worry is side effects of the treatments and I am shitting my pants, you know, will I look ugly or will I be able to walk. You know the usual stuff... My financial situation is my biggest concern and my ability to work with HIV should I become ill. I have been lucky so far, as I have not had any health problems as yet."

PABLO

Pablo was 20 years old at the time of diagnosis in 1990 and had been experiencing a sore throat and swollen glands under his arms. He did not believe it was anything too serious and went along to his GP and was tested for HIV and Glandular Fever. His HIV test came back positive. Pablo tells us:

"I will be honest, I suppose before there was any sort of medication around, my outlook wasn't that rosy. I didn't think I would live very long. If you had been interviewing me say five years ago, I would have said to you that I would probably not be around now in this particular year. I would have been dead by now. If it wasn't for the research and the medical experts and the medication that we are getting today, I don't know where I would be."

Pablo told me that his health has always been reasonably well maintained and he has shown no signs of symptoms associated with HIV. His fear of becoming ill was a major concern for him in the earlier years; he tells us:

"I was terrible really... if I was getting a blemish on my arm or a really bad sore throat or if I starting coughing or my chest hurt I would start panicking. I mean I used to automatically phone the hospital and say 'Look, I have such and such wrong with me'. I could always go and see my consultant and it was such a relief when you could just go to the hospital and find out it was just a general infection. The relief is just unbelievable. You know you have to be prepared for this because obviously one day I will become ill... one day I am not going to be as healthy as I am now. I am quite lucky because I am one of the healthiest people within my hospital. My CD4 count is 800 and my viral load is undetectable now. I mean I drink like a bloody trooper and I smoke."

Pablo recounted how a positive mental attitude helped him stay optimistic and since he was experiencing good health, he had few concerns about the lack of effective treatment being available during this time. Again, Pablo's health was monitored with the CD4 medical indicator of health and so fears and anxieties were diminished. Nevertheless, for Pablo the uncertainty and fear of becoming ill was always a principal concern at the back of his mind.

LISETTE

Lisette was 39 years old at the time of diagnosis in 1990 and was experiencing ill health whilst travelling in the USA. After a six week wait, her HIV test came back positive. She returned to the UK and went to visit her local GP and was referred to the local GUM clinic [see glossary]. Lisette armed herself with as much information on HIV as there was at the time. She described her initial thoughts:

"… It became fairly clear that anything they knew about HIV was about men and not women. So here was I armed with all this information that may or may not be relevant to me and I thought that was a real drawback… I couldn't make a decision because the information was only based on men; the decision I would take is that I wouldn't make the decision. You know, if you are asking me to take this drug, for instance, because you have got these results, but you can't show me that those results are to do with women, then I would just dismiss it entirely… because I wasn't constantly going to hospitals or clinics and getting pills and I wasn't being ill, it was like, well what can I do? In reality all you can do is get on with your life… I think a lot of my decisions are based on intuition. Rightly or wrongly, I have always had a gut feeling about the drugs. I couldn't help it. I always had this gut feeling that they couldn't be quite right. They haven't come up with a 'wonder drug'… I certainly was very suspicious of the drug companies and their motives. I am still suspicious of drug companies and their motives… I've seen them work on people; I can't deny that but I don't believe they are long-term… I can't really believe deep down that all that toxic stuff is going to do me any good."

Lisette's scepticism of HIV drugs in the early days in conjunction with long periods of good health led her not to take any treatments in relation to her HIV-positive status. Any fears and anxieties centred on the lack of effective treatment being available were minimal due to her own lack of symptoms relating to HIV. Having said this, Lisette did recollect periods of anxiety and uncertainty in relation to her health status and potential ill health, she recalled:

"I had periods of good health, you know, where nothing happened if you like… but does this mean that I'm nearer the other end of it: is something gonna happen? There's definitely that feeling of uncertainty with you and there is little point resisting it… I think I remember quite clearly saying to myself that if I could just get to the point where HIV isn't the first thing that I think of or the last thing that I think of when I go to bed, it will be a great day."

Lisette recounted that in the early days she would say things like 'I will never take this or that treatment' but in reality she believes it would have been a very different story if she had encountered prolonged periods of ill health. She told me that it would have been hard for her to 'have been sick over a long period of time and not tried an available treatment'. So, for Lisette her scepticism was allowed to flourish due to prolonged periods of good health prior to 1996 and the advent of HAART.

LARRY

Larry was 46 years old at the time of diagnosis in 1992 and had been experiencing ill health and believed he had Glandular fever. He decided to take an HIV test at his local GUM clinic and it came back positive. When I asked if he was aware of any treatments for HIV at this time, he recounted:

"To my knowledge there was AZT on its own, which in my opinion, killed many people because they got the dosages wrong... I dreaded actually the thought that one day I'd probably need to start taking anti-HIV drugs. The thought terrified me, mainly because of the side effects... I went over seven years before I actually started taking any treatments other than Septrin and supplements I bought for myself."

Larry told me that physiologically his health was reasonably good following diagnosis. Initially, he did not experience any symptoms associated with HIV. However, for six years, Larry went into a serious depression because of his HIV-positive status and completely cut himself off from his network of friends. He believed he was 'disgusting' and 'dirty' and was going to die. He described his emotional and psychological health as suffering enormously due to his personal anxieties and fears around living with HIV; he completely withdrew from his social lifestyle. When asked about his thoughts on taking medical treatment, he recalled:

"I dreaded the thought of taking anti-HIV drugs because in the old days, once you'd started on something like AZT, it was an AIDS diagnosis and it's almost like being diagnosed all over again... and that was a time when you did die, in the old days. I resisted drugs by initially denying that I was becoming ill. I'd actually been so ill for about one year to eighteen months that my partner was more aware of it than I was. I was in bed most of the time because I hadn't got the energy to do anything. I thought I was coping but my body wasn't coping any more and emotionally my health was poor."

The anxieties and fears recounted by Larry were not exclusively centred on the lack of effective treatment available during earlier times. His fear of taking AZT or other HIV drugs were centred on being re-diagnosed with an AIDS-related illness condition. He admitted to avoiding treatment issues by denying he was experiencing ill health until after 1996 and the advent of HAART.

TONY

Tony was 32 years old at the time of diagnosis in 1994 and had been experiencing periods of ill health from 1991. For three years Tony believed he was in denial about his HIV-positive status because of the prejudice and stigma associated with living with HIV and AIDS. He told me:

"I wasn't very well and I'd gone to London with my partner. I was very skinny... it was very scary seeing people who were ill and ended up looking so gaunt... you would get the finger pointed at you. When I was diagnosed I was put on AZT... they were horrible the drugs, I hid them and used to take them in the toilet with alcohol... I was looking forward to having more energy if I took them but eventually I stopped taking them."

Tony describes his knowledge of anti-HIV drug treatments as very limited. He did not recall being aware of the advent of HAART in 1996 or of any hopes or fears around effective drug treatments. His main anxieties for many years focussed on his body image and people within the gay community pointing fingers at him. Tony spoke of concerns and anxieties centred on where he was going to live and his financial status rather than fears of becoming ill and taking HIV treatment. Prolonged experiences, however, of severe fatigue and lethargy did affect his outlook on life and he felt that ambitions and hopes had been limited by his HIV-positive status.

What we have gleaned from our story-tellers who experienced ill health at the time of diagnosis is that almost all actively chose to resist drug treatment for a variety of reasons: only Tony embarked on AZT for a short period of time. This is extremely interesting and leads us to the next section which reveals personal narratives of experiences, perceptions and resistance to AZT as a monotherapy for HIV to which we will now turn.

A forgotten generation: Long-term survivors' experiences of HIV and AIDS

Fears, hopes and anxieties of AZT: perceptions and experiences

Out of the twenty eight women and men who told us their stories, twenty three story-tellers made mention of AZT as a monotherapy for HIV. Here we attempt to understand how our long-term survivors experienced and perceived every day life and maintained good health prior to the advent of more effective treatment becoming available. What were the dominant fears, hopes, anxieties and unpredictable uncertainties that came into play when living with HIV prior to the advent of HAART? What were the perceptions and experiences of AZT as a monotherapy? How were matters of health and illness negotiated before the advent of HAART? Let us now turn to the personal accounts of experiences and perceptions of living with HIV pre-1996.

Refusing AZT

PAUL

Paul was 21 years old when he was diagnosed with HTLVIII in 1985, as part of the mass screening process for people living with Haemophilia. He was tested without his consent and was not experiencing ill health at the time of his diagnosis. One concern Paul revealed to me was that he hoped that he would stay alive long enough until there was a cure for HIV. When I asked him about medical treatment prior to 1996, he told me:

"In the early days there was only AZT. I knew a lot of people on AZT and as a monotherapy it was a really high dose. People were really ill with the drugs and that scared me. As far as medicines are concerned, I have a deep fear of actually going on any HIV drugs because I know there are side effects which are extremely damaging… what I would also say is that I always had a very deep mistrust of the pharmaceutical and medical industries, basically because of my treatment on the NHS. My personal feelings regarding the pharmaceuticals were one of mistrust and one of cynicism… this is to do with my HIV and Hepatitis viruses, as this was down to the medical treatment and the NHS for supplying them. Of course I am very cynical about doctors and I am very cynical about medical companies. I didn't feel I trusted any of them, or the Government. I still hold them as part and parcel of the same mechanism really… as I have become more involved with HIV knowledge and treatments over the years, these feelings are changing. Going to conferences and getting involved in the medical side of HIV is very interesting… and yes, I have got a lot more time for drug companies now although I still don't trust them because they are profit-making organisations. And my attitude to doctors has changed over the years, as well as my attitude to my health care workers and those in charge of my health care… but there is still resentment."

Paul spoke of his relative good health for many years after his diagnosis; he did not consider HIV treatment until he became very ill after 1996 and the advent of HAART. Paul's active involvement in the HIV field armed him with knowledge as it unfolded; his scepticism, he recalled, 'put me off going on HIV medication until I was really quite ill." His concerns and anxieties were based on the fear of becoming ill and having to take medical treatment. He was 'scared of what might happen' but at the end of the day he realised that if he did not take medical treatment he might die.

ELISABETH

Elisabeth was 31 years old when she was diagnosed with HIV in 1985. She had a small lump on her breast and decided to voluntarily take an HIV test as she was a practising IV drug user. She was not showing any symptoms of having HIV and when the test came back as positive she was shocked. She recalled that there was very little information on HIV at this time. When I asked her about treatments prior to 1996, she told me:

"Let me get this straight. I got so used to the fact that there were no medicines and so I was used to finding out alternative therapies for myself… I mean the AZT screwed everyone because it seemed that people were just dying that quickly, more quickly when they were on AZT and what was happening was that they were giving people doses that were too high. All we could see as bystanders was that it was killing people. We were all very suspicious of this new medicine… No, I just wasn't going to take it."

Elisabeth spoke of her cynicism of the pharmaceutical industry and her fears around taking new drugs associated with the management of HIV. She frequently went for tests for her viral load and CD4 count which was the only indicator and measurement of health within an HIV context, as we have seen above. She told me:

"My T-cell count went down from around 600 to 60 and my doctor told me I was going to die if I didn't consider taking treatment. I thought 'I've heard all this before' and so I took three month's leave from my work and went on an anti Candida diet and did crystal healing. I did this and my T-cell count dropped to 40 and so eventually I gave in but I was very mistrusting of it... you know I think these tests are a double-edged sword. I have had 10 T-cells, Judy, and I felt great... and you know I have had 700 T-cells and felt like shit. It is the doctors' only measure of health that they have. I have a healthy cynicism and a healthy scepticism I think. The way we have been brought up is to believe what the doctors tell you, so it has been difficult for me to question doctors. But I certainly don't listen to a word they say any more."

Until Elisabeth considered her health to be at risk, she refused treatments until after 1996 and categorically would not 'entertain the monotherapy of AZT' prior to the advent of HAART. Elisabeth recalled her anxieties and fears when she became ill. She felt she was unable to experience illness 'normally' in that sneezes, coughs or colds would immediately be thought of as the onset of AIDS. She told me:

"Every ailment would be immediately linked to my HIV and it made me afraid to get sick, I suppose. I was pretty lucky really in that I never really got sick and if I had a headache then yeah I certainly didn't tell anyone... HIV was a secondary illness as far as I was concerned because I wasn't sick and the heroin took up so much of my life that most of my decisions were based around that rather than HIV."

PETER

Peter was 33 years old at the time of diagnosis in 1987. He tested voluntarily and had previously taken part in an AIDS-related trial at his local sexual health clinic in 1985. He did not wish to know his HIV-status at the time of the trial in 1985 and after 18 months decided he wanted to know the result. The result was positive. When I asked him about memories of HIV medical treatment that was available during the time of his diagnosis he told me:

"As far as I can remember there was only AZT available during 1987 or a little after this time. I was certainly offered AZT, not there and then following my positive diagnosis but not too long after and I resisted it.... I resisted because it was said not to be a cure, and it was really put to me as something that *seemed* to be helpful... but there wasn't really that much known about it; some people who were on it were claiming to feel worse, and some people still died in spite of taking it. And when I was offered it, I asked the doctor 'why do you want me to take this?' And the reply I got was 'it may help kill off some of the virus and help you put on a bit of weight.'... I felt quite angry about this because I knew that AZT did not kill off the virus, it slowed down its replication... and you wouldn't take such a toxic drug in the hope of putting on a bit of weight. As a result of this appalling incident I left the hospital which I had been going to for some years. I changed to another hospital and saw a doctor there who I knew from his voluntary work at the Terrence Higgins Trust. He offered to run my bloods to see what was going on, as far as they could then of course! The other hospital had failed to do this. The doctor later said that I could take AZT but he didn't see any particular need for me to do this at the time. I decided not to take them and I went for at least 15 years living with HIV without taking any medical treatment whatsoever."

Peter recalled enjoying long periods of good health prior to his decision to start HIV combination therapy after 1996; he continued with his voluntary work in the HIV field. He frequently went for medical health checks in relation to his viral load and CD4 count and learned more about HIV and AIDS as information developed. He found his voluntary work to be a source of comfort and therapy; many anxieties and worries he encountered during his work mirrored his own to some extent.

Experiencing AZT

SPIKE

Spike was diagnosed with HTLVIII between 1981 and 1983 during the mass screening of people living with Haemophilia; he was a child when he learned of his HIV diagnosis. From the age of 18 until 21 years, his T-cell count was only 10, which is extremely low. He spoke about 'waiting for something to happen' and having thoughts centred on preparing a Will and making plans for what he wanted to do with his personal belongings. Because of his young age, Spike's memories of anxieties and concerns on HIV treatments prior to 1996 are fragmented and vague, he told me:

"I may have been on the Concorde trial I think, which would have been when I was reasonably young... I may have been taking tablets. Yes, I remember I know I had AZT before I started my combination treatment and that would have been around the time of the Concorde trial or just after in the late 1980s. I also had Didanosine (ddI) when I first went to university so I would have been 17 or 18 when they gave me these tablets... I sort of never took them though because I knew they had no efficacy and at that age I was more interested in getting wasted really rather than being adherent to pills… but I have never become resistant to AZT."

Because Spike lives with Haemophilia as well as HIV, he spoke of his personal experiences of how the two illness conditions impacted on his lifestyle. Spike recalled that he wanted to do more things in life; this was as a result of living with Haemophilia and constantly being told what he could and could not do because of potential bleeds. He said:

"When I was a younger kid up until I was an older teenager, Haemophilia was not a problem, it was more a pain in the arse because I'd get regular bleeds and stuff, but it has never really limited me. I have always tried to do more because it made me want to do more things which perhaps I shouldn't do… I used to play football and last year I did a sky dive. I was repeatedly told by the Haemophilia Society that it wasn't advisable… It was psychologically important for me to do things like this. I have good friends… they are always sort of active and I've just joined in with everything they've done… but as I was getting older, especially these days, I still get lots of bleeds but it's more of a pain having HIV and Hepatitis C… The HIV and HCV are a lot more than a pain because I know that is what will kill me eventually not the Haemophilia, as I'm quite stable at the moment… Even though my T-cells are really low and bad I have never really been ill or anything and I have always been asymptomatic, so I probably wouldn't have known I was HIV if I wasn't told. The quality of life is very important to me and how I live my life. Morals and principles around how I live my life is important and how I interact and react with family and friends is the most important thing for me. I believe this comes through my experiences of living with HIV, I suppose… I have no materialistic desires. I don't want to work and run myself into the ground, to have a fast car or be able to go on three holidays a year. I'd rather be poorer and have the people around me that I want to have around me and lead a life where I can keep myself happy… the most important things to me are keeping myself fit and reading and stuff. I don't care how much money I have… I think that before HAART I was probably not rebellious because I had the same values and morals but I was more fatalistic, whereas now I have more stability in my life… I was more fatalistic before because I thought I was going to die."

It is interesting that Spike and others speak of having very low CD4 counts during periods of their life, yet they feel quite healthy and well. For some of our story-tellers it is quite often the reverse; when medical indicators suggest good health as a result of a high CD4 count some long-term survivors have felt ill and particularly unwell during these times. The medical indicator of the CD count therefore does not always reflect the way the person might be experiencing health or ill health. This is an important point to raise, as personal experiences of health or illness do not always correlate with medical indicators of health. Spike recounted 'my CD4 count was 10 when I was between 18 to 21 years old… it was the same for many years… I was always waiting for something to happen'. Despite having such a low CD4 count, he did not experience HIV-related symptoms associated and maintained good health during this period.

GLYNN

Glynn was diagnosed with HTLVIII back in 1983 as part of the mass screening process for people living with Haemophilia; he was 17 or 18 years old at the time. He is one of three remaining survivors out of 65 people who were diagnosed at the same time. When I asked about medical treatment for HIV he recounted:

"For HIV? Well, I got ill… it was Christmas 1990 and I had Thrush and that's when they put me on the AZT for a couple of years… I was taking them four or five times a day and I did this for 2 or 3 years. I was also taking Septrin and Fluconazole. I had to take a couple of Fluconazole a day, four Septrin a day… I got Thrush; I was hardly on my last legs or anything but it was pretty unpleasant. It was all in my throat so I was on those for about 3 years and then when the Doctor changed at the Haemophilia Society, they couldn't believe that I was just on AZT on its own. They examined my blood and could not believe why I was still taking these tablets. My blood was all right and I was told not to take them anymore. So I haven't."

Glynn described his initial experiences of taking the AZT when I asked if he considered his medication to be effective. He tells us:

"To begin with they made me feel tired and sick but gradually that went and I got used to it and it was all right. I mean it didn't affect me; I wasn't very good at taking them when I should have done, I must admit… I ended up chucking them all down my throat at 9 o'clock at night… in the end I used to get occasional night sweats and things like that. Whether the tablets have done me any good or not I don't know… the first few months I felt pretty rough from the side effects."

Glynn told me that this was the only time he had taken HIV treatment. He remembered his fears concerning the uncertainty of how the disease might progress, the potential threat of becoming ill again and, ultimately imminent death. He stated:

"I thought, 'God this is taking over my life!'... I felt down, you know, and thought am I going to get more ill and am I going to die? I suppose when you are feeling ill or you are suffering from something it brings it out even more, whereas if you haven't been ill or ill for a while, you don't think about it so often."

This echoed many of the voices I heard that spoke of how HIV impacted on everyday life dependent upon whether a person was ill or enjoying prolonged periods of good health during earlier times. Glynn reported how one of the doctors informed him that there was no advantage to taking AZT and building up a resistance to the drug when it was not needed. Glynn stopped taking the monotherapy and did not pursue other HIV treatments after the advent of HAART in 1996.

MARTIN

Martin was diagnosed in 1985 at the age of 21; he voluntarily tested for HIV following widespread coverage within the tabloid newspapers linking HIV with people living with Haemophilia and contaminated blood products. At the time of diagnosis, Martin recalled his memories of the treatments in earlier times. He told me:

"In the early days there was always the thought of how you are going to die. Then AZT came out and, as it was the first drug, it was a bit of a safety net. I was fine at that moment but if I got ill there is AZT and perhaps after that there might be something else around the corner. Then I was put on AZT for a while and that was a blow. You know, my God, I am on the safety net now and there is nothing else... My T-cell count had fallen and that is when my doctor suggested going on AZT. I think it wasn't long after the Concorde Trial had finished that I went on the treatment... I was on AZT about three years and some time later when I discussed with others that I had been taking this monotherapy for three years they were astounded. I should have only been on it for six months because after that it is doing you no good at all... I was reading a book by a guy called Peter Duesberg and I am not saying he was totally right or absolutely wrong but he said a few things that made me think... this drug had made me feel ill and that wasn't a good sign...I developed a wart on my big toe, a big horrible thing and it just wouldn't go. It would start bleeding and then it spread to the next toe. The hospital said I would have to live with it, it will never go and it is part of my HIV. I stopped taking the AZT because I had had enough of feeling shit and I felt I wasn't get the support from the hospital as to why I was still taking

AZT. I stopped taking the drug and I felt better and the warts disappeared. I made this decision myself to stop taking the drug."

Martin experienced good health apart from the notable side effects of taking AZT. He told me how he resisted taking other treatments afterwards. Despite his CD4 count dropping and his doctor advising him to take AZT, Martin stated he was fit and felt healthy at that moment in time. He recalled that his CD4 count had never dropped below 280 and believed that the 'hit them early, hit them hard' philosophy of prescribing AZT in earlier years was the only reason he was prescribed monotherapy. His fears and anxieties about the uncertainty of becoming ill were minimal due to him experiencing prolonged good health.

COLIN

Colin was diagnosed in 1985 at the age of 25 years when he tested voluntarily after establishing a new relationship. He remembered that his awareness of HIV treatments at this time was limited. Colin recalled that he had experienced quite a few years of good health before he was later diagnosed with AIDS in 1995. At the time of his AIDS diagnosis there was no effective combination treatment available. When I asked him about HIV treatments he had taken before his AIDS diagnosis he told me:

"I had sporadically taken what was available even back in 1989. I had taken AZT very briefly; I was on the Concorde trial and tried AZT. It actually gave me such horrible side effects; I gave it up after six weeks."

Soon after Colin stopped taking AZT, his partner sadly died. He recalled being absolutely determined to survive and spoke of how his positive mental attitude was all important to him and how he did not 'operate like a person' who thought he was going to die. He stated:

"I was determined to use everything I could. So, I went back on the AZT about 1990 and came off it again about a year later because I had read enough by that time to decide, and I still think I was right, that AZT by itself was probably doing people more harm than good and so I didn't then take HIV therapy again until combination therapy when protease inhibitors became available."

Colin's decision to stop taking AZT was partially based on his keen awareness of knowledge around HIV and his determination to maintain a positive mental attitude. He read research from places such as the Bristol

Cancer Institute about characteristics of long-term survival amid people living with cancer diagnoses and alternative therapies to minimise the impact of the illness condition. He later became involved in workshops centred on HIV and AIDS which became extremely important for maintaining a positive mental attitude to his own HIV condition. Any fears and anxieties in earlier times were overridden by his commitment to care for his dying partner and then later by his hope and determination to survive.

TOM

Tom was 39 years old at the time of his diagnosis in 1986. He voluntarily tested after he discovered an ex-lover had been diagnosed with Kaposi Sarcoma. He tested positive and later devoted his working life to the field of HIV. When I asked him about his knowledge and experiences of HIV treatments prior to 1996 he told me:

"Well, from 1990 to 1993 I was on AZT as it was recommended that I go on these because my T-cells had dropped from 750 to something like 350. At the same time, I was aware of the many friends around me who were ill at the time; I was aware that the dosages of AZT were significantly attributable to how ill people were and this was 1500 mg per day. I decided to postpone taking them because I was travelling to San Francisco and I thought I would find out stuff there. There was a project called Inform and they produced information on a trial that had been done over there. The cohort consisted of about 500 people in San Francisco and it was probably made up of gay men, I would think. The 500 people had CD4 counts of between 300-500 and they took 100mg five times a day and it showed a huge increase in efficacy. So when I came back to the UK I said 'yes I will go with the AZT' and I was heavily pressurised into stating why I only wanted 100mg five times a day instead of what the doctor wanted to prescribe for me. He started to write up a prescription for 250 mg and I said 'No, I want 100mg five times a day'. The doctor did not think the pharmacy would have the tablets in this form, so I told him that they would have to get some. In fact, they did have them and they worked really well for a short time and then my CD4 count started to drop again."

Because of his early involvement within the HIV field, Tom's fears and anxieties diminished as he accumulated knowledge centred on issues pertaining to HIV and AIDS. However, Tom later experienced a black out and a brain seizure at a time when his workload was extremely stressful. He spoke about loss of memory, loss of speech and being incontinent for a short period of time. Following this bout of illness, after 1996 and the advent of HAART, he went on to take his first combination therapy.

RICK

Rick was initially diagnosed in 1987 at the age of 18 using a false name. He re-retested again in 1990 at the age of 21, knowing that the result would be the same. At the time of our interview, Rick was experiencing ill health and severe side effects of his combination therapy associated with his HIV condition. He recalled in the early days that he was healthy when it was suggested that he should consider taking the monotherapy AZT. He told me:

"AZT had been out quite a long time in America and it had been out a few years in England. My doctor told me it was about time I started taking medication. It was monotherapy, AZT, and I think I was still working then. It didn't affect me because it was just three times a day. AZT has never affected me apart from maybe the first week I experienced a slight bit of nausea and headache but it has never harmed me ever."

Prior to Rick telling me this, earlier in our interview he told me that AZT had made him anaemic and as a result he was having many blood transfusions. Anaemia is a known side effect of AZT and this was possibly the case. Rick, however, was encountering many adverse side effects from combination therapy at the time of our interview and was, in fact, waiting for *salvage therapy* due to his resistance to licensed antiretroviral medications that were available at the time (see Glossary). Rick, as mentioned in Chapter three, died a few years later after his long, brave battle.

JOHN

John was diagnosed in 1989 after testing voluntarily at the age of 35. In 1987 he voluntarily took a test which came back negative. He recalled that he was not surprised by the positive result two years later. He remembered wondering if he would ever see the age of 40 following diagnosis. Death itself did not cause anxiety or worry but the threat of illness and being ill was problematic. Being unable to look after himself with a chronic illness condition was his primary concern. When I asked him about treatments prior to 1996 and the advent of HAART he told me:

A forgotten generation: Long-term survivors' experiences of HIV and AIDS

"Well, very early on I did a trial; I couldn't tell you what it was now... there were a couple of trials actually, and then was it AZT? Yes, there was a period when AZT was the thing to take, so I was on AZT for a while. Then it was concluded that AZT actually wasn't particularly beneficial so I came off that and didn't take any medication for a while."

John continued to work and he experienced long periods of good health in relation to his HIV status. Whilst he was given a medical 'death sentence' at the time of his diagnosis, his anxieties and fears did not centre on dying but on becoming ill. The uncertainty of chronic illness and the unpredictability of disease progression was a primary concern for John; he felt that there was nothing he could do to prepare himself for the likelihood of prolonged ill health. He reinforces what he told us earlier in Chapter two:

"...I didn't know what would happen, indeed what will happen if and when I become unable to look after myself for whatever reason?... it is not very predictable and is different for everybody. With AIDS, you know, some people at this stage die of pneumonia, some people go blind, some get dementia... you can't even prepare yourself in any way because it happens in different ways to different people... the uncertainty is the worst thing."

John's memory of taking AZT in earlier years is vague and he did not recount any adverse side effects. As his health was good he did not take any further HIV medication until many years later when he was diagnosed with cancer, totally unrelated to his HIV condition. He told me:

"... because I was having chemotherapy I was put on combination therapy because chemotherapy depresses the immune system... I had six months of chemotherapy and some radiotherapy and carried on taking the drugs for, I don't know, two or three years and then I came off them. It was the doctor's advice... I had no symptoms and my T-cell count was high and my viral load was low enough so he suggested I came off the treatment."

John believed that he had been very lucky in that he had never experienced any side effects from any of the medication he had taken, not even with chemotherapy. He had no interruptions in his work pattern and he soon resumed a healthy status.

RICHARD

Richard was diagnosed in 1990 at the age of 21 after testing voluntarily. He was working in London at the time of diagnosis, away from his home town. Soon afterwards, Richard resigned from his post and moved back home to be nearer to his family for care and support in the event of chronic illness, as he believed death was imminent. He acquired suitable accommodation and promptly secured new employment in a similar position to that in London. Two weeks into his new employment, Richard started attending hospital appointments and his employment was terminated soon after. When I asked him about his awareness of treatments prior to 1996, he told me:

"There was only AZT around when I was diagnosed and the medics were not really very sure about this treatment. What I did know about AZT is that they gave it out in quite large doses of 1000mg a day and a lot of people who were taking AZT were becoming anaemic and there were other risks too. I was put on AZT immediately… It was dangerous. I am sure I used to get bits wrong with me."

Richard later refused to continue with AZT treatment as a monotherapy because of the side effects he was experiencing and based on what others had told him. He recounted:

"I can remember point blank stating that I would not continue to take AZT because I had noticed in other people that it caused major mood swings, nasty moods and strange feelings. I didn't know what was going on. It also gave me incredible diarrhoea. I could not believe what came out of me; it was not nice. I was 21 and I shat my pants on the bus."

Richard spoke of fears and anxieties about prolonged periods of ill health and side effects of the monotherapy. His concerns also centred on the stigma attached to HIV and his loss of employment. He spent a long time believing that people had the right to know of his HIV-positive status. He believed that control had been taken out of his life and was now in the hands of others. Richard experienced short periods of ill health prior to the advent of HAART in 1996 and enjoyed periods of good health prior to taking combination therapy when this became widely available.

Positive experiences of taking AZT

MINNIE

Minnie was diagnosed with HTLVIII at the age of 21 back in 1981 after being tested involuntarily. As a blood donor with a rare blood group, he discovered his positive status after receiving a letter from his Regional Blood Transfusion Unit. Minnie experienced prolonged good health in relation to his HIV-positive status for over fifteen years. When asked about his awareness of medical treatments prior to the advent of HAART, he told me:

"I went back to work and carried on with my life and learned about the disease as knowledge unfolded. Lots of my contemporaries were being diagnosed and they were dying… it got to the mid 80s and we were all being given AZT because that was the only treatment. I don't know why but I didn't believe that this drug was the answer. Why are these people swallowing all these drugs when they are not ill? That was my idea… I knew my body well enough to know when it would be right to go and do something about it."

Minnie recalled being in good health from 1981 until early 1996 when he started to experience a high temperature and had developed a rash which started to spread from his waist downwards. He was hospitalised for almost three months. He was given an AIDS diagnosis, his CD4 count was zero and he was experiencing opportunistic infections associated with HIV. Minnie was prescribed AZT, he told me:

"They put me on monotherapy with AZT because I had never had it before and they had now discovered that 250mg per day was quite sufficient as opposed to 1000mg three times a day or whatever they dished out in the mid 1980s like sweets… and that on its own worked for me for nine months and brought my CD4 count up to 34 from nothing. It stayed around 34 for a year but AZT was only used for nine months and then I embarked upon combination therapy as it had only just become available in 1996… had it not been for me surviving nine months on AZT I don't know… the AZT worked."

Minnie referred to himself as a person living with AIDS from 1996 onwards. He did not recall any specifically related fears or anxieties in earlier times due to his HIV-positive condition because of his persistent good health for many years. Minnie was aware at the time of his severe illness that HAART was soon to be introduced in the UK. Minnie lives with other illness conditions unrelated to HIV or AIDS.

TYLER

Tyler was diagnosed with HTLVIII in 1984 following a routine check up. He was 38 years old at the time and tested voluntarily. At the time of diagnosis he was aware that there was no treatment available and prior to diagnosis he had experienced repetitive bouts of chest infections. He recalled taking treatment prior to 1996 and the advent of HAART. He stated:

"I'm still alive and, well, I put it mainly down to AZT a bit. I think that kept me going when times were really bad, whereas some of my friends didn't take it... I don't know between 1989 and 1991 I guess... I assume that this is why I lost so many of my friends because they weren't on it. I was on the experimental trial on Concorde... so I was lucky, you see, because I was on it when others weren't. So I am convinced that's why I am still alive. Otherwise I would have gone with all the others obviously, especially bearing in mind the bad chests when many of my friends didn't have bad chests but they still died with pneumonia; I mean most of them went with pneumonia and one or two with a brain tumour... I was just asked if I wanted to go on it [the Concorde trial] and became a regular at the clinic because they were keeping a check on me every month... my CD4 count was checked and they monitored any damage to the liver and kidneys and so on... from then on I was in good hands and they kept a very close watch on everything since then."

Tyler recalled experiencing periods of ill health with chest infections; he did, however, also experience periods of good health. His primary concern, following his HIV diagnosis, focussed on being told he had only months to live. As time passed by, he found himself living in extreme poverty. All aspects of his life changed after diagnosis; his life was consumed with anxieties and uncertainties around life expectancy and imminent death. His awareness of medical treatments prior to 1996 was vague and he told me 'I am losing my memory a bit now, which is also part of the HIV; I don't care what anybody says... I forget what I am doing most days.' His general opinion of AZT, nevertheless, was a positive one and a drug that he believed saved his life in the early days.

A forgotten generation: Long-term survivors' experiences of HIV and AIDS

NEIL

Neil was tested involuntarily and diagnosed with HTLVIII in 1985 at the age of 24, whilst having routine blood tests for an illness he had experienced since childhood. He was working at the time and stayed in employment for many years until he became ill in 1995, ten years following his diagnosis. He told me:

"I have kept well, I mean in a sense that I have not had any major illnesses at all with hardly any time off work… I was doing very well at work, things were good at home and I just started to get tired all the time… I found it hard to get up in a morning even if I had time off work I would just sleep and always felt tired. I'd had a cough which lasted a year and I'd feel cold all the time… that went on for about a year. I'd been losing weight too… I also had a second bout of Shingles… I had oral thrush which is why I had been having problems eating… I was tested for my CD4 count… it came back as 20 which I didn't know what this meant…. The doctor said that this is very low and I would probably deteriorate over the next two years and get really ill and may be I have four years at best… I did take six weeks off work… I was diagnosed with bacterial pneumonia. I took antibiotics and recovered pretty quickly from that."

Neil was aware that HAART was on the cusp of being introduced as a more effective treatment for HIV and AIDS. When I asked him about medical treatment for HIV he recounted:

"I had the bacterial pneumonia and they treated that which cleared up quickly and then they told me that I was at the stage where I need to consider taking AZT. They started the treatment of AZT … I think there was another drug too but I have forgotten what it was now… so they changed the drugs in the following year. I came off AZT and had no problems with it that I can recall."

Like Minnie, Neil experienced prolonged periods of good health from diagnosis up until early 1996 when HAART was about to be widely distributed as a more effective treatment for people living with HIV and AIDS. His recollection of taking AZT was unproblematic; he only took AZT for less than 12 months prior to embarking upon his first combination therapy. We will explore Neil's experiences in more depth in Chapter six.

WOODY

Woody was diagnosed in 1992 after voluntarily testing for HIV at the age of 35. He was working at the time and when tested presented a CD4 count of 250; he was prescribed AZT treatment immediately. His consultant believed that Woody had been living with HIV for a considerable amount of time and his condition was therefore advanced. Woody told me that he was not experiencing any symptoms associated with HIV at the time of diagnosis and did not feel unwell. He recalled:

"I went straight on to treatment with AZT because my CD4 count was 250. I didn't have any side effects from taking the drug... I wasn't ill... I think there were noticeable side effects that were caused by the AZT but I can't remember... I went on AZT and then AZT with something else... I think it was ddC. I don't think I suffered with side effects from AZT but when HAART became more widely available I changed my treatments and stopped with AZT."

The particular medical treatment Woody had trouble remembering was not ddC (Zalcitabine or Hivid) as this was not yet available; it was Didanosine (ddI) as this was licensed in 1994. Woody was prescribed AZT in 1992 and was not experiencing ill health. His fears and anxieties during these times, he stated, were centred on becoming ill and the psychological impact of being diagnosed with HIV. He spoke of apathy, depression, loss of sexual appetite and financial uncertainty for the future. He did reveal that his medical practitioner was very explicit when prescribing the AZT and allayed fears and anxieties, to some extent, about taking this drug. We will explore Woody's experiences further in Chapter six.

We have come to the close of this chapter and I invite you to think about what you have learned and how this might have affected or impacted on your own thoughts and feelings. To give a sense of when the first drug treatments became available for people living with HIV or an AIDS diagnosis: the failed chemotherapy drug AZT was licensed in 1987 as a monotherapy, and later in 1994 Lamivudine (3TC) and Didanosine (ddI) were introduced. As many story-tellers were diagnosed in the early 1980s before scientific and biomedical advancements had been established, this potentially presents its own fears and trepidation. Many voices spoke of fear, anxiety and the uncertainty of 'waiting for something to happen.'

Throughout this chapter we have unravelled how long-term survivors coped with living with HIV on a day-to-day basis. A number of story-tellers participated in the Concorde trial for AZT monotherapy and one refused to participate on the basis of not knowing whether he would be taking AZT or a placebo. Many story-tellers perceived AZT as a drug that was offered in too large a dose, which subsequently went on to kill those who were taking the drug. This has been well documented and established over time. Some story-tellers firmly believe that their refusal to take AZT in earlier times had saved their lives; others who had taken AZT, like Minnie and Tyler, believed that AZT prolonged their lives until the advent of HAART in 1996.

We further witnessed how some story-tellers had taken AZT over a long period of time, which was not considered advantageous as after nine months or so, the drug was ineffective. There are crucial differences in medical practices amid medical practitioners about how low CD4 counts should be before patients required monotherapy; equally, the dosage and the length of time patients should be taking AZT was inconsistent amid medics. We learned how, in earlier times, new doctors entering the medical field of HIV had limited knowledge of HIV matters and relationships were problematic. A great number of long-term survivors had experienced long periods of good health after diagnosis, but as many story-tellers implied: do periods of good health mean that soon I am going to become ill? Many spoke of the fear and anxiety of becoming ill during periods of good health and experiencing financial hardship associated with illness. Another interesting feature is how story-tellers perceived their own health status when they received a good or poor CD4 count during medical HIV health checks. At times when CD4 counts were particularly high, the patient did not necessarily feel particularly well and vice versa. This begs the question: are CD4 counts a good indicator of health?

Retaining a positive mental attitude and getting on with everyday life was, for many, the only way to maintain a healthy approach to life. Being in good health produced less fear about the lack of effective drugs being widely available but did present unease in terms of when good health would end and illness would begin.

What can be gleaned here is that few story-tellers had many fears and anxiety about the lack of effective HIV medicines being available. What becomes evident is how uncertainty and fear associated with having to take combination therapies in the future were more profound due to the possibilities of severe side effects. Was this largely the result of the huge loss of lives and the problems associated with AZT?

The profound uncertainties of living with HIV or AIDS at a time where there was limited scientific knowledge or effective treatment have to be appreciated. How might you maintain good health in the context of HIV? How would you manage your fears of becoming ill? What might be your hopes and aspirations? How would you have negotiated treatment options? For example: knowing that AZT, a failed chemotherapy drug, was the only option open to you if you presented HIV-related symptoms, what would you do? Fear and anxiety about AZT and the possibility that this drug might kill you was very real during earlier times. How might you have reacted in this context? Ask yourself if your opinions or feelings have altered since reading and actively engaging in this chapter? Who can you relate to and empathize with? Once again, take time to reflect on your thoughts and beliefs before moving on.

A forgotten generation: Long-term survivors' experiences of HIV and AIDS

CHAPTER FIVE

Positively living as sexual beings: intimate relationships

∞

"In the beginning was sex and sex will be in the end... I maintain... that sex as a feature of... society was always central and remains such."
Goldenweiser

"It is an infantile superstition of the human spirit that virginity would be thought a virtue and not a barrier that separates ignorance from knowledge."
Voltaire

Introduction

As we know from the mid 1980s onwards the increased recognition of HIV and AIDS as a public health issue led to a widespread phenomenon of HIV-related stigma, prejudice and discrimination at many levels and at varying degrees. We have seen in the media construction of HIV and AIDS how people living with an HIV-positive diagnosis were, from the onset, chiefly blamed for contracting this disease either because of their 'permissive' sexual practices and/or 'undesirable' behaviours and 'immoral' attitudes. Dominant and repressive ideologies filter through our social and cultural environment and impregnate our social values and shared beliefs which impact on our lived experiences; these have become further contaminated by the fear of the spread of HIV and AIDS. We have also witnessed how moral panic [re]produced moral dilemmas which subsequently led to legal reform (the criminalisation of HIV) as well as scientific and medical intervention in our [sexual] lives.

This chapter possibly presents the most challenging predicaments for readers to critically reflect upon. Nevertheless, I ask that we think more deeply and openly about divergent practices of sex and sexual expression as a defining feature of our own sexualities and sexual identities. We often tend to categorise certain sexual behaviours into sexual identities: this has presented an enormous problem when dealing with matters of HIV prevention and the promotion of sexual health. For example: why is there a tendency to classify anal sex as a sexual practice belonging only to gay men when clearly this is not so? Often when a person self-identifies as gay, many people immediately think of the sexual practices this person might engage in. Yet if a person identifies as heterosexual, our thoughts about what types of sexual behaviour they might practice is not immediate in our minds. If a woman self-identifies as a lesbian, people often think 'is she the male or the female in the relationship?' Why does this happen do you think?

We should never take for granted our sexuality and its relationship to self-identity, as this does not always truly reflect wide-ranging sexual practices and variations of sexual morality from both within and outside of different sexual communities. For example, we would not have a need to construct the category of 'men-who-have-sex-with-men' (MSM) if sexual practices reflected homogenous sexual identities; clearly there are men who do not self-identify as 'gay' yet engage in same-sex sexual practices from time to time in their sexual lives. Similarly, there are many heterosexual couples who engage in anal sex, 'swinging', 'wife swapping' and 'dogging' practices which might involve more than two people engaging in intimate sexual behaviour. How do we categorise these practices? Then, of course, there is the complex category of bisexuality.

Current disputes over sexual values, erotic conduct and debates about what constitutes 'good' and 'bad' sexual practices, especially within an HIV framework, often become the vehicle for transferring social anxieties towards people living with an HIV-positive diagnosis; these can be internalised in ways that might be destructive to a person's social well-being and self-esteem. This chapter explores the personal perceptions and experiences of all our story-tellers which depict their sexual and intimate lives following diagnosis. HIV and AIDS enter into sexual relationships in many different ways and living with an HIV-positive diagnosis has had a profound impact on the long-term experiences of sexual intimacies both within and outside of partnering relationships. Because of the very nature of the subject matter, this chapter is extensive.

Asking human beings to talk about intimate sexual practices is not an easy undertaking, particularly within the context of HIV and AIDS. The women and men in this study were extraordinarily open and honest and spoke frankly about their sexual relationships. I therefore seize this opportunity to sincerely thank each and every person for their truthfulness and candour.

A forgotten generation: Long-term survivors' experiences of HIV and AIDS

Thank you for allowing us to gain valuable insight into your personal experiences as sexual beings.

Preserving enduring relationships: conflicts, anxieties and intimate practices

Out of twenty eight long-term survivors who shared their personal experiences of living with HIV with me, three story-tellers were in the same relationship from the time of diagnosis to the time when our interview took place during 2002. There were, of course, other story-tellers who remained in the same relationship following diagnosis but sadly their positive partners had later died from AIDS-related complications. We must acknowledge that negotiating sexual intimacies within these established relationships are on-going, involve an assortment of anxieties and concerns and are certainly not straightforward. It is to these we now turn.

NEIL

Neil, a self-identified gay man, was 41 years old at the time of our interview and living with his long-term male partner in a sero-discordant relationship. Diagnosed in 1985, Neil has been in the same relationship since his HIV-positive diagnosis and his partner has been his main source of support. When asked how living with HIV has affected intimate relationships with others, Neil recounts:

"I think what is in the back of my mind does tend to be physical contact… you know it can only be transmitted in certain ways but I kind of have the feeling of being positive and someone else being negative and that makes some sort of physical difference. It can make me wary about touching people… even now, I mean, if I go swimming I do tend to think… are there any cuts or nicks. I know that this is not a route of transmission but it just makes me wary… it does make you feel like a leper [*long pause*] and it does knock your confidence."

Neil spoke of his extremely strong and close relationship with his partner. He told me from around 1995 he has not engaged in sex with his partner because of problems he was experiencing with erections. He tells us:

"I just started to go off sex, since not being able to get erections, so that certainly affected our relationship. Although it was discussed with the doctors at the time, it has only been in the last year or so that they have sort of recognised this as a problem that affects lots of people with HIV. So now there are things we can do about it. But for a long period there was nothing... it didn't seem that there was any way in which we could improve the situation, so I just stopped having sex for several years... In a funny way, it has kind of made our relationship stronger, but I mean actually what we do now is we live together but we actually have sexual relations with other people... we sleep together but we don't have sex together, we have sex with other people. I have only really been able to do that for just about the last year and because of Viagra."

I asked Neil if this arrangement was likely to be permanent and he told me:

"It looks like it, but things might change. I mean that is OK if it's like that and it might change which again would be OK. It is where we are now with the relationship and we are both happy about this... We have been together twenty years this year and the thing that keeps us together is that we have a very strong family life... My parents, my nephew and my brother and my partner's family all come from the same area and we have a strong family life... I mean there are lots of in-fighting but it's a very strong relationship."

Neil spoke about how he meets other HIV-positive people for casual sex using the internet and gay chat rooms. He told me that in his profile he discloses his HIV-positive status to others to avoid sexual rejection. He tells us:

"I say that I am positive and I just go into positive chat rooms... at first I just tended to meet other positive people to have sex and I assumed that that was fine and that was how it was going to be... but there are a number of people who are positive who don't say they are and they approach me. If someone has got 'positive' in their profile then I don't tend to bring it up, as it were, because it is just assumed. But if it is not in someone's profile, before I do actually meet anyone, it is a comfortable way for me to say that I am HIV-positive. It is slightly distant but honest... and a fair number of people say 'well I am too' even though they haven't stated it... and there are one or two people who aren't positive who I have seen and that's a bit strange actually... because there is intimate contact and I am positive and they are not... I feel a bit strange about it, you know, in terms of feelings of responsibility and being conscious enough to know what you are doing and not going to that sort of stage where you get so 'in to it' you lose your senses and let your body take over... especially as I have a lot of pre-cum as well, so I am conscious of that... I mean I become very conscious of becoming very intimate, sort of personal, physical, sexual things that for me starts to wreck my whole confidence... in the sexual act."

Neil continued to talk about how his erection problem has impacted on the way he has sex and how it changes things for him. He believes it is something he is now coming to terms with:

"It's part of the change, including my appearance change, you know... I do have a very clear sense of Neil in 2002 to Neil in 1994/1995... it's almost like two different people... part of me does look back and wish things hadn't changed as much as they have. Hindsight is a great thing - I wish I knew then what I know now and I think that there would be certain things I would have done differently."

Neil spoke at length about his physical appearance, lack of confidence and body image in relation to his HIV-positive status and medication; this is something that we will be exploring further in chapter six.

DAVID

David, a self-identified gay man, was 64 years old at the time of our interview and living with his long-term male partner in a sero-discordant relationship. Diagnosed in 1990, David has been in the same relationship since his diagnosis and his partner is 10 years younger. He considers himself and his partner as *'very lucky people'*. When I asked if he had ever encountered problems with sexual relationships in relation to his HIV-positive status he told me:

"Yes, the one and only one that matters. My partner and I very, very rarely have sex now and I feel very bad about it because he is ten years younger than me and I can remember how horny I was at his age. He is not such a sexually rampant kind of male that it matters much to him, but I just do feel that I am not giving him what he probably needs. In terms of everything else about our relationship, I give him totally everything he needs and if you are talking about sex, where does it begin and end? The fact that we sleep together, cuddle each other and kiss each other every day; and he comes home and we hug and kiss, is that sexual? I don't know! I mean here are we just talking about the point where males ejaculate? Is that sex? Because that is the thing that is in our relationship but, yes, it is very much a man-to-man loving relationship, so in those terms it is sexual... when I go to see the consultant he asks me how I am and I say I am tired, so is it age or is it HIV? That is always a question I ask, so I can blame both really. That's my excuse, my let out!"

In terms of his personal relationship with his partner, David, believes on balance that HIV has made them stronger together because they both have got the confidence in knowing if HIV could not separate them then nothing else will.

RACHEL

Rachel, a self-identified heterosexual woman, was 37 years old at the time of our interview and was living with her husband in a sero-concordant relationship. Diagnosed in 1993, Rachel spoke of relief that she and her husband were both HIV-positive. When I asked if her sexual relationship had been affected by HIV, she told me:

"It wasn't no! What we worried about was if one of us was, if we turned out to be discordant. We did worry about that I have to say. For both of us, in a sense, it was a tremendous relief that we were both HIV-positive because we didn't know how we would handle it... because quite honestly we have tried condoms and they are bloody awful... well, I was quite worried about whether our relationship would survive; not because we didn't love each other but because of whether there would be some kind of inhibition because of the fear of the negative partner being infected by the positive partner... that would have been devastating and very, very difficult for us to handle. I am glad that we weren't put in a position to have to handle it, quite honestly."

Rachel did tell me of her initial devastation at the thought of not being able to have children with her husband. However, following her husband's encouraging response to medical treatment and medical advancements in knowledge pertaining to HIV and reproduction, Rachel recounts:

"... then we could start planning and start looking ahead... we could start thinking about the possibility of a future, the possibility of having children even and seeing them grow up and what we want to do with them... we really thought that the diagnosis meant no family because we couldn't, in all fairness, think it was sensible to look into having a family if we weren't going to be there to look after them. I mean, if you reckon on only having a ten-year life span, then it is not fair to have a child... we had such long talks with various people, particularly the women's health advisor, which we probably spent a good two hours talking to her... we had decided that if the transmission rate of risk could be reduced to well below 10 per cent, it was a risk we were prepared to look at... and this was also grounded in knowing that somebody was going to be around to look after the child in case of our premature deaths... we needed to know that we were going to be there and that our child was, relatively speaking, going to be safe."

Rachel has two daughters who are HIV-negative and considers that HIV has not unduly hindered her sexual life apart from episodes of HIV-related ill health.

Sex outside of relationships: conflicts, anxieties and intimate practices

The next set of narratives of personal stories focus on sexual experiences of our story-tellers who were not in relationships at the time of interviews during 2002. We explore how sexual intimacies were negotiated, established and practiced over time. Dominant themes concerning anxieties and tensions around disclosure, fear of rejection and the burden of responsibility in knowing one's HIV-positive status are revealed here.

MINNIE

Minnie, a self-identified gay man, was 42 years old at the time of our interview, lived alone and was not in an established relationship. At the time of diagnosis in 1981, he was in a sero-discordant intimate relationship which later ended but not as a result of any HIV issues. Minnie described his current sexual lifestyle as celibate. He told me:

"Coming to terms with a celibate lifestyle is about enjoying it. I like my own company, I like living alone with the dog and pleasing myself and doing what I want to do... I was very extrovert and 'out' early on as a gay teenager. I have always been a gay man. I have spent half of my life living with this virus. I was very open, 'out' and I went clubbing and was, you know, very promiscuous. I spent some years on and off as an escort, as a rent boy to start with and then progressed. I did rather well out of it and progressed into doing escort work and I didn't give it up. I couldn't give it up until I was 19 and then I went back and had a dabble even later than that... it was good money and I was good at it. I was a pretty boy in those days [*laughing*]."

Minnie preferred to socialise in a predominantly heterosexual community 'as a gay man', because he thought 'it was healthier'. He had not personally experienced any problems associated with homophobia in pubs he used to frequent and enjoyed the same things other people enjoyed in this community. He recounted:

"The pub I drank in was notoriously rough and I had some pretty good friends behind me... more to the point I liked the same things that they liked. They couldn't understand why a *poofter* could possibly want to watch the boxing, for example... they then decided to have a 'gay night' the first Monday of every month upstairs in the pub. I didn't want to go upstairs and spend the evening with two fat dykes in the corner and an orange, you know, and some old queen that comes out of the closet once a month. I wanted to stay downstairs with everybody else... the straight men I used to pull in that pub was unbelievable."

Minnie spoke of how he had always practised safer sex since his diagnosis back in 1981. He did not place himself in any complicated situations where his HIV might pose a problem. He would categorically refuse to have sex unless protected sex had been negotiated. He did not disclose his HIV-positive status to potential sexual partners, but would refuse to engage in sex if the sexual partner wanted sex without a condom. Minnie saw this as a protective measure for himself. When he started to lose his libido, sex became less and less important:

"I lost my libido and that was either drug-related or not. Sometimes it reared its ugly head but that's easily sorted out with a bloke anyway... you can have a wank, the odd wank and sometimes I would even give that up half way through. I used to think 'I will do it next week' [*laughing*]. I can't be bothered. I don't want the hassle of somebody's baggage which normally I associate with being 'gay'. I can't cohabit with a partner. HIV has not really impacted on my sexual lifestyle. I protected myself as far as anyone else was concerned. I didn't disclose my status and I didn't have unprotected sex. And other people should be doing the same."

GLYNN

Glynn, a self-identified heterosexual man, was 37 years old at the time of our interview, lived alone and was not in a relationship. Diagnosed in 1983 as part of the mass screening process for people living with Haemophilia, Glynn was only 16 or 17 when he discovered he was HIV-positive. When I asked him if he had encountered any problems in relation to HIV and sexual relationships he told me:

"I don't know because I don't know where I would be if I didn't have it. I don't think it has changed my life in any way, except yes, I was married and I am not married now. I don't think this really had anything to do with HIV although children were brought up and obviously that may have had an effect on it. I think it did really to some degree. I have got a daughter now anyway, but she wasn't planned or anything... and she is fine... I think the breakdown of my marriage was to a certain degree because of children. I mean I just knocked it on the head and thought I would never have children and that was that! Although, when I was married we did go and find out about, I mean... we did think about 'sperm washing' but we didn't do that. Then we were going to get sperm donations but we didn't do that either... I mean we separated anyway [*long pause*] and HIV, to a certain degree, probably had something to do with it but it wasn't the only cause."

I asked Glynn if he could recall at the onset of diagnosis whether HIV impacted on sexual relationships. He recounts:

"Yeah, it did put you off I suppose! I thought, well what is the point? Although I did have relationships and if anything sexual was going to happen then I would wear a condom or I would tell them anyway... if I was going to sleep with someone I would tell them... some of the relationships lasted and some of them didn't and some of them didn't go any further because of the fact that I told them I had HIV. It was clear rejection and I mean it pissed me off to begin with and then it didn't... I mean I wasn't seeing a different girl every night or anything like that! But I think it was on two or three occasions that as soon as they found out that was it! I mean you have to say something anyway because it is obvious that there is something wrong with my leg... they can see me limp, and if they ask you about it, what do you say? 'Oh, I broke it in a parachute jump' or what? You know, it is ridiculous isn't it, so you say I have got Haemophilia and then they ask 'what is that then?' and perhaps they then click on and say 'oh right!' and so sometimes you carry on and tell them about HIV and other times you don't. If they need to know you tell them."

In the above quote, Glynn refers to having 'something wrong with his leg'. Because he experiences severe bleeds from time to time as a result of Haemophilia, he has a serious problem with one of his legs and walks with a distinct gait. At times he has extreme difficulty with mobility; this is something he cannot hide, and therefore he feels it is sometimes necessary to disclose his Haemophilia condition. The public exposure made by the mass media linking Haemophilia and HIV has complicated matters for people living with Haemophilia in terms of disclosing their HIV status to others. I asked Glynn to tell me more about having a family and his daughter:

"I love children and would love to have more children. My daughter is two and a half now but I mean she wasn't planned and luckily enough she didn't become infected and neither did her Mum, so I got away with it. I mean that is probably mainly because my viral load is down, so if that hadn't have happened then I wouldn't be a Dad. My ex-partner and I have split up and my daughter will soon have a step-brother because my ex-wife has got another boyfriend and is pregnant... but I mean I can't see me adding to my daughter's family because of the HIV and the fact that I am not in a relationship now. I suppose my age is also a factor, as I am getting on now. I would like to have more children but there are risks."

Glynn spoke of coming to terms with the idea that he would not have any more children because of his age, the risk factors involved in HIV transmission and the fact he was not in a long-term relationship. His passion and desire for more children, however, was immense.

TYLER

Tyler, a self-identified gay man, was 54 years old at the time of our interview, lived alone and was not in a relationship. He was also single at the time of diagnosis in 1984. Tyler spoke of having been involved in three relationships since his HIV-positive diagnosis. When I asked him to what extent HIV might have impacted on his sexual relationships and sexual lifestyle, he told me:

"I haven't gone around spreading it. That is probably another reason why I am alive; I only have the one strain of virus in me... I was extremely distressed after my diagnosis and I didn't want to spread it around... it makes you feel it is the end of your life. I don't care what people say, sex is important. Obviously the older you get the less important it is; so I am at that lucky age now where I don't even notice people in that way, which is a bonus. Because if I was still noticing people that way and wanting to do it, it would be a big issue but I don't want to spread anything or have any accidents. It doesn't enter my head now but in the early days, yes, it was a big issue. I have had only three relationships but it was all above board and it was not a problem. The relationships I have had have not been ones I have sought. They happened by accident."

Tyler recalled how being HIV-positive had physically stopped him engaging in sex and how he felt that this had virtually ended his sexual life. He did, however, tell me how lucky he was to find his last sexual male partner, who tragically died after only 15 months of living together. The short time they spent together was a wonderful experience for Tyler and is a memory he will cherish forever. He told me:

"It was a wonderful 15 months... he brought a lot into my life and I was buzzing all the time; he was so lively and full of mischief. There was quite an age difference between us and he was HIV-negative but that didn't matter. I was aware of him obviously wanting different things to me and we were quite happy with that and he never really left here except for the fatal weekend."

Tyler told me how sex was no longer an issue for him and he was quite happy to 'withdraw from it all', as it did not enter into his head. He considered his health to be poor and his doctor had recently told him he was going to die soon. As a consequence, he was taking each day as it came.

PAUL

Paul, a self-identified heterosexual man, was 38 at the time of our interview, lived alone and was not in a relationship. At the time of diagnosis after mass screening for contaminated blood products in 1985, Paul was in a long-term relationship with his girlfriend. The relationship ended after a while and Paul believes this was largely because of his HIV-positive status. He told me:

"... We stopped having sex. And then we started having sex again with a condom. I don't know! I really had so much going on inside my head I just couldn't have sex basically. It just became a really big issue... Sex is part of my life and then all of a sudden it became not a part of my life. Not only that but it became a big issue in my life... I didn't have sex because I saw it as a responsibility. I can have sex with somebody and I can give them AIDS. It was such a big issue that I didn't feel it was worthwhile me ever having sex with anyone again. I didn't ever want to put anybody at risk. That level of responsibility was overwhelming and I didn't have any support at this stage. So, quite obviously our relationship soon split up. I didn't have a sexual relationship for a number of years after this. I didn't have any relationships with any women at all. Looking back, I just thought this is crap. Anyone I got close to I would just shun away. I bet some women thought I was a freak. I enjoy women's company and I used to enjoy going out for a drink but if anything happened that looked like signs of romance, I used to go very cold. I made excuses to leave. This is quite unnatural for a young man like me... I didn't want to get into a situation where I had to sleep with a woman… I didn't want to have sex anymore because I didn't want anyone to catch HIV. So I thought I am not going to have sex anymore and I didn't."

Paul spoke about his anxieties and fears around disclosing his HIV-positive status whilst negotiating sexual relationships. He recounted:

"It was like when do I tell a woman if I was going to have sex? OK, so you tell somebody that you are HIV-positive because this is the proper thing to do. If you inform them, and they are informed and they still make the decision to have sex with you, then the issue of responsibility has eased. It hasn't completely gone but it has eased. But you cannot tell that person you are HIV-positive unless you completely trust them. You can't utterly and completely trust them until you are in a relationship with them… no, it is a strange situation all round. There were a couple of women I had sex with and I purposely told them that I had been exposed to Hepatitis through my blood products. That was my 'ace' card! I have been exposed to Hepatitis B because of my Haemophilia. A lot of people don't bat an eyelid, as they don't really know what this means. I guess some women are probably quite happy if the bloke makes the decision to use a condom. So, there are issues there but I could never get into a relationship. Only occasional casual sex. I never talked to anybody about my HIV. They were lean years on the sex front."

Paul recalled that as he got older he started to realise he had lost his life since his diagnosis. He did eventually meet a woman who he felt comfortable around and subsequently told her about his HIV-positive status. He told me that she was fine about things for a while. When their relationship ended, he also felt safe about having disclosed his HIV-positive status, as his ex-girlfriend did not know any of his friends. He could still maintain his HIV 'secret' from the heart of his social circle. Paul went on to have a six-month relationship with another woman he had told about his HIV-positive status; they did not have sex. He stated:

"We never had sex. We never had oral sex. We never touched each other's genitalia or anything. It was a relationship in that we went out together and kissed and cuddled. We slept in the same bed with each other. It was a very weird relationship and she didn't want it to go any further because of my HIV… I didn't talk about it at the time. It wasn't something I was comfortable with. It completely and utterly screwed up my sex life. I thought it was right to tell people and not have sex with them. You had to tell them. I couldn't tell them about the risks first without telling them about myself. The bottom line was that I felt that it was difficult to tell anybody because of trust. There were lots of people I could have had sex with, one-night stands... those I would never see again. But I couldn't. I could not face it."

The moral dilemmas of disclosing one's HIV-positive status, as Paul reveals here, were shared by almost all our story-tellers who spoke of concerns in relation to the tensions and complexities of disclosing to potential sexual partners. Who do I tell? Who will they tell? When should I tell? The cultural expectation that HIV-positive people should always disclose their positive status to potential sexual partners is somewhat unrealistic, impractical and unreasonable. Knowing you are HIV-positive carries with it: an unnecessary burden of responsibility; a potential risk of sexual rejection; possible isolation, and a real fear of people telling others. Why should HIV-positive people disclose their status to others? Each person's sexual health is their own responsibility and is not the responsibility of other people. The practice of safer sex is there for all.

ELISABETH

Elisabeth, a self-identified heterosexual woman, was 48 years old at the time of our interview, lived alone and was not in a relationship. At the time of diagnosis in 1985, she was in a sero-discordant relationship, which later ended but not as a result of her HIV-positive status. Elisabeth lived with an HIV-positive diagnosis for 8 years before she decided to stop using heroin and move 'in different circles'. When I asked her to what extent had HIV impacted on sexual relationships over time, she told me:

"I suppose I was lucky in that I was already in a relationship when I was first diagnosed, so you know, sex was just something I carried on having. I remember when we split up, the next person I had sex with was also positive, so that wasn't an issue either; I got very used to it. And then the next relationship was with a guy who was not positive and he didn't even know I was an addict, so that was just so prolonged. I had never gone out with somebody for so long without sleeping with them and it was because I was too scared to tell him. I didn't want to have sex with him because I knew it just wasn't going to be a one-night stand... I have had one-night stands and not told them because I just never saw them again. I was comfortable with not disclosing because I used condoms... The one thing I had to be very sure about was that I wasn't going to see a guy again. It is very, very hard to know where a relationship is going... There were lots of guys I fancied and I can remember thinking 'no I can't have sex with this guy' because I am HIV-positive and he couldn't cope with it. So, I guess with the sex thing it has stopped me doing a lot of things because of this...

If I wanted to have sex with a guy I would get very scared of telling them and thinking about what their reaction would be. I guess it was silly really because I'd never had a bad reaction really, but you never know how people are going to react."

Elisabeth told me of her overwhelming desire at times to just tell people about her HIV-positive status for the 'shock element'. She did, however, speak of her anxieties and tensions when disclosing at times, particularly within friendship networks. She was always conscious of the 'what ifs' especially in terms of telling someone who then told others around her.

TOM

Tom, a self-identified gay man, was 55 years old at the time of our interview, lived alone and was not in a relationship. At the time of his diagnosis in 1986, Tom was in a sero-discordant long-term relationship with his male partner. He described his partner as a wonderful and incredibly supportive man. His partner tested several times after Tom's diagnosis and was HIV-negative; for Tom this was a 'huge relief'. When the relationship came to an end, they remained as close friends. When I asked Tom how HIV might have affected his sexual relationships and sexual lifestyle, he told me:

"I am not by nature a very sexual person largely because I lack the motivation and the energy to go out and look for it. But on the occasions when I have, it always seemed that I initiated safer sex... for five or six years of my life after the break-up with my partner, my sexuality consisted of anonymous bath room sex in Amsterdam and San Francisco with totally anonymous strangers and I wanted it that way. I didn't want to speak and spoil the image that I had; spoil the fantasy that was in my head... but where it involved some kind of verbal communication, I always made a point of telling people about my status. And it generally brought on a huge sense of 'Phew! Glad you said! Glad you brought condoms up' kind of thing."

Back in 1992, Tom recalled one incident at a Leather Club one Sunday evening in the city where he lived. He told me:

"I saw this youngish, blonde guy in his early twenties, obviously cruising with his eyes and he just didn't really 'do' anything for me... anyway he followed me outside of the club and we stood on the street corner chatting. I was doing everything I could to deter him and he asked if he could come back to mine. I said OK and told him of my status, thinking 'that will get rid of him' but it didn't. So, he came back, we had coffee and sure enough, you know... we finished off having sex and I insisted we used a condom and he was like 'erm, well yeah ok'... anyway to cut a long story short I didn't have another date with him after that; but the next time I saw him out, he came over to me and said what a learning experience it had been for him; he liked the reality of being fucked by somebody who was positive, even using a condom... and the experience had really got home to him and he went for a test a week later... it turned out he wasn't positive anyway but he did say that if he'd have gone with somebody who hadn't have insisted on using a condom or hadn't disclosed his status, he would still have had this blasé attitude about HIV."

Tom told me of how being HIV-positive presented certain limits regarding sexual relationships with other gay men in terms of sexual practices. He recounts:

"I did feel I had got the ability to be lethal... you know the guilt thing although I am not sure that guilt is the right word. But I had the potential to do somebody else harm; and, having been through the emotional turmoil, I obviously wouldn't want anybody else to go through the same thing. I would do everything in my power to make sure that this didn't happen... I discovered that nipples were quite erotic and got round to having my nipples pierced and things like that... anything but using your dick... it's a learning thing. I do think it's a great myth both within the gay community and outside of it that all gay men are interested in is fucking each other... the vast majority of gay men that I know aren't really into penetrative sex... So, unless I have been away on holiday, I have never been a particularly sexual person... I am too tired and not bothered to get up and go out... I am not driven by a need to have sex, but it doesn't stop me missing it if you know what I mean... Again, there is a myth that positive people are all promiscuous. I know some people who have only had sex with three men in their life and they are still positive... you can describe it as 'the luck of the draw'... HIV gave sex a whole new dimension."

Tom recalled how he was non-sexual for a year because he was terrified of infecting somebody. It was not until he started to think about sex being a two-way thing, that the burden of responsibility for negotiating safer sex was lifted from his own shoulders. He told me about a five year relationship he had with one sexual male partner:

"... I had a great relationship which was 99 per cent sexual and I learned an awful lot more about myself and that's probably why I feel frustrated now that I am not using it. I just discovered the wonderfulness of long-term sexual activity and how many orgasms it was possible to have in various parts of my body before I ejaculated… I am one of those guys that once I have ejaculated, I go to sleep. So, I would try and draw it out, draw it out, draw it out – it was just wonderful. I could probably have seven or eight amazing orgasms before I ejaculated; I learned so much about my body and so much about having a relationship with somebody… where you try things to see what response it has on the other person. You can build up a sexual repertoire and I really enjoyed that. I would like to find at least one more person that I could do that with again… it seems such a waste having discovered it and it not being used."

Tom was extremely candid and open about his sexuality and sexual practices and spoke of how on the basis of his tallness and bodily image, gay men often assumed that he wanted to be 'active' in any sexual encounter. He told me:

"Because you don't have any hair and you look kind of 'butch', gay men assumed I wanted to be active… I was actually first fucked in my bisexual period and found it extremely uncomfortable and so it didn't happen to me for quite a long time afterwards. Eventually I got to physically enjoy it but I had this huge psychological problem that being fucked was not a thing that men do. I would be angst-ridden for days afterwards thinking 'why the hell did you let that happen'… I worked through this and became happy with all that kind of thing and then b-o-o-m what happened? I am HIV-positive. So getting back to 'bare-backing', I verbalised to somebody recently that the kind of thing I missed was when you are being fucked by somebody without a condom; the particular sensation you get when they ejaculate is really magical. I didn't have much opportunity to experience it but I still miss it. I couldn't say that I miss anything else or that I don't do anything because of HIV. That is it really!"

Tom's willingness and enthusiasm to go out is diminishing; he puts that down to his age and the fact that he 'can't be arsed'. However he believes it would be good to share his life with a 'significant other' if the opportunity arose.

CLAIR

Clair, a self-identified heterosexual woman, was 40 years old at the time of our interview, lived alone and was not in a relationship. At the time of diagnosis in 1987, she was married and her husband later died from an HIV-related illness after contracting HIV from contaminated blood products. When I asked Clair to what extent HIV had impacted on sexual relationships, she told me:

"I am not in a relationship now and I do wonder whether deep down HIV affects me in terms of relationships... I don't think it does! Well, it's more like where do you go? It never gets to the stage where I have to make decisions... well it hasn't recently. It was a few years ago now the last time I got involved with someone and that was absolutely no problem whatsoever. I just don't get to meet anybody and I just think 'what's wrong?' [laughing] What is wrong? You know, I just laugh but I think it doesn't help when you spend a lot of time in an HIV ward and spend a lot of time with gay men... Every now and again I have to remind myself that 'oh yes, this is me'... but you don't really know what you take in and I don't really know what might be stopping me. I might be protecting myself... it's only because I don't seem to meet men I like, or the ones I have liked have not been interested; so it's just not happening at the moment."

Clair was in a relationship with her husband for 15 years until his death. Some while later, she met a man and formed an intimate relationship until they both went their separate ways. For the past few years, she told me that she had not been involved in an intimate relationship and tells us:

"I really know the importance of love and sharing in a partnership and having someone to come home to. This affects me more. I mean the HIV is nothing in comparison to not having someone to love... but you know there is nothing you can do. I mean I don't want to be desperate but I am aware of it and I just think that I could do with a friend to go to the pub and do things like that. I certainly don't have any problems with establishing a relationship. I know somebody who refuses to ever have sex again but that's just nonsense! I would have to know someone, the person would have to know and it would have to come out... but that's just another new area again. The moral responsibility and that sort of thing... but I just know that it's such an open part of my life. You can't keep that from anyone... I never have one-night stands; I am not interested in that. It's just not me really! And that's nothing to do with HIV that is to do with me."

Clair stated she did not have a problem with issues of disclosure and would not allow this to be a problem if the right situation arose. She spoke of a woman she knew who was HIV-positive and in a sero-discordant relationship with a man. She recalled:

"I know this woman who just freaked out because the condom split or something and she was going crazy. I just thought 'what on earth'; the guy realised with terror that he might get HIV and I thought 'what is the problem?' This is something I have questioned time and time again because of my own situation with my husband. Just how transmittable is this disease particularly woman-to-man?"

Clair believed HIV had changed and broadened her mind and she had encountered some wonderful experiences. She found it difficult to articulate how HIV had impacted on sexual relationships, as it was hard for her to imagine the type of life she would have led without being HIV-positive.

CHRISTOPHER

Christopher, a self-identified gay man, was 51 years old at the time of our interview, lived alone and was not in a relationship. At the time of diagnosis in 1988, he was living in a sero-discordant long-term partnership which lasted for 26 years. Twelve months before the break-up of the relationship, Christopher told me of how his male partner had undergone a 'massive personality change' and had started physically and mentally abusing him. His partner was ashamed of Christopher's HIV-positive status and did not want others to know. When I asked if HIV had affected his sexual lifestyle he told me:

"HIV is a big thing for me as far as the sex side of things is concerned. I couldn't knowingly pass it on to anybody so therefore there are times when it will restrict me from certain sexual practices. For many years, I wouldn't have sex with anybody because I was very unsure... you know, in the late 1980s, people were very unsure how it was transmitted. So, it was easier to abstain or just have mutual masturbation and that is all I ever did with my partner after diagnosis. I was diagnosed in 1988 and I split up with him in 1997."

I asked Christopher if he would like to tell me more about how HIV restricted certain sexual practices. He recounted:

A forgotten generation: Long-term survivors' experiences of HIV and AIDS

"Well! Although I have been a passive male, I do know that the risk factors are much lower for transmission… but I always use a condom for penetrative sex… I am always passive. I practice very safe sex. Since I have been on my own, I have not had what I would call a true loving relationship. I have had sex with other people but I've not had a loving relationship. So, I don't think of HIV as a burden as such, but I just feel that the sort of person I am it does restrict me… because I would be absolutely terrified of infecting somebody. I take the responsibility very seriously."

Christopher clearly takes the role of responsibility seriously and is always aware of his HIV-positive status. I asked him whether he felt the need to take sole responsibility for the practice of safer sex during sexual encounters. He stated:

"Absolutely not, no! Since my diagnosis, I have had unprotected sex however that has been the choice of the other person. I will not be forced to be 'outed' about my HIV-positive status. So, if I say to somebody 'I am not having penetrative sex with you without a condom' and they then say 'No I want it without a condom' and you then say 'no, I am not having it that way' and they continue to want to have sex 'bareback' and all the rest what do you do? I would say 'there is a high risk for both of us and we don't know each other'. If that person is willing to take the risk and just do it, it is their responsibility. This has only happened I think twice since my diagnosis, and the first time I felt very guilty until I got my head around it. I then thought 'Oh no! I gave that person every opportunity'. Also the risk factor of him contracting HIV was fairly low, as I was passive and there was no bleeding; so there was nothing where he could have got fluids from me… the risk was very low for him but I think that I cannot carry the guilt. I used to, but I can't now. After learning more about it, and listening to others and discussing this with others, I give myself permission to lead my life to the full. I can't be responsible for every individual who comes into contact with me. I wouldn't knowingly harm anybody or pass the virus on anyway."

When Christopher refers to being 'outed' he is relating to being put in a potentially harmful situation where a possible sexual partner might wonder why he is insistent on using a condom; this might lead to the sexual partner asking Christopher about his HIV status. It is Christopher's choice to disclose his status to others; he should not be put at risk or be expected to say "I am not prepared to have unprotected sex with you because I am HIV-positive." Christopher went further and said:

"I would love to tell more people but it is my choice. The people I have regular sex with, I always have sex with a condom, always. One person did ask me if I would have unprotected sex with him and I said 'no'. He then went off and had unprotected sex with a friend of mine. I then had to say to this friend of mine that he should go to the clinic as they had both been very irresponsible."

Christopher told me that after the break-up of his long-term partnership, his partner told his family about Christopher being HIV-positive status. Christopher felt this was his partner's way of justifying the break-up by saying, 'I am splitting up with Christopher after all this time because he is HIV-positive and I can't stand the thought of him being ill; I wouldn't want that burden and I don't want to carry him should he be ill.' Not surprisingly, Christopher was angry about being outed in this way. He has, however, since learned to like himself and love himself with the help of an HIV support group. He is a completely different person compared to fourteen years ago when he was diagnosed HIV-positive.

JOHN

John, a self-identified gay man, was 48 years old at the time of our interview, lived alone and was not in a relationship. At the time of diagnosis in 1989, he was single and living in the South of England. When I asked John whether sexual relationships had been affected by HIV he told me:

"On a scale of one to ten, when it comes to me seeing new men it hovers around 8 or 9 I suppose… because it is all this stuff about who do you tell? This is still something that I have not got a formula for… I suppose when it comes to casual sex I don't worry about it too much… I assume that people are doing what they are comfortable with; I only do what I am comfortable with. So, I don't personally feel any obligation to protect other people. In fact, early on, I had some very intense discussions with a couple of friends I was quite close to. They took the line that it was my responsibility to safeguard other people and we very quickly didn't stay friends any more. One was a man and the other was a woman and, whilst I have no direct evidence, I believe they were both quite sexually promiscuous and probably afraid. But they took that line and I didn't agree with it and … well, we very quickly stopped being friends. On some occasions when I have been in groups of gay men talking about these issues, everybody in those groups maintain they always disclose their status and wouldn't put anybody else at risk. I just don't believe it! When I am in a situation where I am with somebody who I think I might possibly develop a relationship with, it becomes a much more difficult issue. Do I tell them straight away, or later, or what? In fact, last night I met somebody for the first time who had just come out of a 10 year relationship. We got on very well! Erm, I don't know what or when I am going to say anything to him. I think I will probably see him again but I don't know."

John recalled a violent incident he witnessed when he was with two other men in a sexual encounter. He could not remember whether he had been diagnosed himself at this time or not. He told me:

"We'd meet other guys and we would all arrange to go back to various people's flats and we got there and the guy whose flat it was said 'before we do anything else, I just want to tell you both I am positive'. The third person just started beating him up... and drew blood. We got this guy out of the flat and I stayed the night because the positive guy was very upset. This is the only occasion I have come across any HIV-related prejudice of this type."

John was totally shocked by this incident. He hopes as time elapses HIV will become less of a stigma and less of a problem; so that HIV-positive people, like himself, will not have so many 'hang ups' about keeping HIV a secret. He tells us:

"Because HIV is predominantly sexually transmitted this is the problem... it isn't talked about. I remember when I was a little boy it wasn't nice to have cancer and it wasn't talked about... My thing about cancer is linked to Kathleen Ferrier, who became a very famous opera singer. She collapsed on stage in Covent Garden because she had cancer of the cervix. At that time, this illness was connected to or perceived to be the cause of being sexually promiscuous. It was only about 3 months ago I discovered that it is actually a virus that causes it. You know, this wasn't talked about, and so she just got ill and went off and quietly died somewhere. This all came out later... so, yes I think there is a perception that it is because people are drug users and sexually promiscuous. And, probably it is the case that lots of people who are HIV-positive are but certainly some people aren't. I knew someone who was infected with blood products because he was a Haemophiliac, and he was happily married. He became very ill, which was unpleasant for him and the whole family. He had two daughters and they were somewhere in their teens. It was very unpleasant for them because obviously part of the stigma associated with HIV was transferred on to the family."

PERRY

Perry, a self-identified gay man, was 40 years old at the time of our interview, lived alone and was not in a relationship. At the time of diagnosis in 1990, Perry was single and had recently given up his working career. When I asked him how aspects of his life had changed since his HIV-positive diagnosis, he told me: 'Well I have no sex life. I don't really have one now.'

Perry was not the only story-teller who failed to resume his sexual lifestyle following diagnosis. For Perry, however, it had become difficult for him to separate his HIV and his mental health condition for which he takes medical treatment. He told me of how his anti-psychotic drug treatments makes him lethargic and therefore cannot tell whether being HIV-positive has affected his sexual lifestyle.

LISETTE

Lisette, a self-identified heterosexual woman, was 51 years old at the time of our interview, lived alone and was not in a relationship. At the time of diagnosis, she was not in a relationship. When I asked to what extent HIV had impacted on her sexual lifestyle and sexual relationships, she told me:

"I don't really know because I haven't had any relationships since I've had HIV. No, I'm telling a lie. I did have one little fling but he was a positive guy so the issue didn't really arise… but it's kind of hard to know if I haven't had a relationship because of HIV. I've just never met anybody. That's really the answer. I think had I met someone I would have dealt with whatever I had to deal with… but I guess you could also say that it may be! It's not easy to go out and meet anybody, but I don't really know. I honestly think that had the right person come along I would have tried to deal with whatever… but they just never have."

MARC

Marc, a self-identified gay bordering on bisexual man, was 38 years old at the time of our interview, lived alone and was not in a relationship. At the time of diagnosis in 1990 he was single. I asked him if he believed HIV had impacted on his sexual lifestyle or sexual relationships and he told me:

"No, I normally tell people I am positive before they come back if it's, you know, casual sex. I try and get the information out quite quickly and I don't know how many people I have had sex with in the last ten years, but let's say at lot! In ten years I would probably estimate about four people, when I told them I was HIV-positive, kind of freaked out. Maybe four out of about a thousand really; I am not sure if it was that many but a lot. It is such a small percentage... you see I found that being honest and straightforward with people normally got a good reaction, but this is in the gay community... I was so glad that I told them. There was a guy I brought back who said 'tie me up and shag me' and you know I was wearing a condom. And afterwards he said 'oh are you HIV-positive?' and stupidly I forgot to say before we had sex. So I told him 'yes' and he kind of completely freaked out. I thought you stupid fool – you say to a stranger 'tie me up and shag me' and then you worry that they are HIV-positive. Anyway I was wearing a condom and so he didn't even see that he was not at risk. I just thought 'you stupid idiot'. Obviously people don't have enough information but it didn't make me feel bad about myself."

Marc went on to say that being HIV-positive had perhaps impeded his voyage of discovery into heterosexual land. He recounted:

"Because of my HIV I have been a bit hesitant because I would want to tell someone I was HIV-positive before I had sex with them. But on the gay scene, I know how guys would, well from my own experience, how they were going to react... but I think on the heterosexual scene I don't have many personal experiences and, I don't want to sound sexist, but my impression is that it is more of an issue for straight women than it is for gay men... I just imagine it... I mean guys are just dogs... I gave up men and I just think men find it easier to be sexual objects than women... I mean I had a relationship with a woman for a few months in 1998 and just from that experience I can see that women behave differently to men. Is that fair? They do in many instances. I think it is fair... because I want to be fair... I think women do more in their head compared to men. I have just become really bored with men and I would like to have a relationship with a woman. I don't really understand how women think... but I have started engaging with women in a way that might you know lead to a relationship."

WOODY

Woody, a self-identified gay man, was 45 at the time of our interview, lived alone and was not in a relationship. At the time of diagnosis in 1992, he had recently established a relationship with a new male partner. His partner was HIV-negative and the relationship ended soon after, although Woody does not believe HIV was anything to do with the break-up. When I asked to what extent HIV had impacted on sexual relationships and sexual lifestyle, he told me:

"Well… there was a loss of sexual appetite, not wanting sex… I suddenly became a different person and everything that I used to do, like going out and meeting people, I looked at everything from the point of view of a person with HIV. I thought out what I could do and what it meant and what I couldn't do. I thought about if I met somebody I wanted to have a relationship with, how that would differ being a person with HIV…"

Woody spoke about the break-up of his relationship with his partner soon after his HIV-positive diagnosis. He recalled:

"He was very supportive… we stopped seeing each other shortly after that but why is too difficult to go into… it might have been in my mind. He might have thought that I wasn't such a good long-term prospect and I might have thought the relationship wasn't such a good long-term proposition as it might have been. I really don't know. I don't think it was love's lost dream, but I was absolutely destroyed because I was HIV-positive and he was negative. At least if he was positive he didn't tell me either then or since."

In his early twenties, Woody had previously lived in America and London and been part of a large gay community. During his mid-30s, he returned to his home town, settled into a new house in a quiet rural area and thus believed he was moving into a new phase of his life. He did, however, mention depression being a major factor affecting his sexual lifestyle. He told me:

"I was more depressed about being HIV-positive than anything else. I wasn't desperately worried about infecting people because it was fairly well established that safer sex using a condom every time you had sex was fairly safe. If you wanted oral sex, it was generally accepted that oral sex without condoms was OK because of the acid that was in your stomach and your digestive system. I mean oral sex wasn't a big concern for me anyway… I was just so depressed and that affected my desire to go off and have sex… I never got back to the things that I was doing before I was diagnosed. I was in a six-month period of shock and so I never got back to being as involved socially or sexually as I was just before the diagnosis… The year after, I met somebody else who lived abroad and I used to see him one weekend in every three or four. He used to come to England one weekend in every three or four. I saw him for about 8 months and then we stopped seeing each other. HIV has slowed me down and made me think about going out and meeting a lot of people. After I finished seeing this guy there is just a big gap of basically nothing."

Woody spoke about his age being an important factor in his diminished sexual appetite. Overall, Woody believes that HIV has had a large impact on his sexual lifestyle and relationships in conjunction with the ageing process.

JAY

Jay, a self-identified gay man, was 35 at the time of our interview, lived alone and was not in a relationship. At the time of diagnosis in 1992, Jay was in a sero-concordant relationship with his male partner. This relationship ended as a result of Jay's partner being physically violent; it was not as a result of HIV. When I asked Jay how HIV had impacted on his lifestyle and sexual relationships, he told me:

"Well I suppose it has made me appreciate other people. You know like before I used to go out, you pick up a bit of trade, you go home, you have sex and you disappear in the morning. Now it's got to be a bit more and then obviously you being the person with HIV, you have to be protective of others in a sexual way. No more unsafe sex… I think it is up to me to make sure condoms are worn and things like that because it would be unfair to infect anybody else. I wouldn't have sex with a person if they refused to use a condom."

Jay did not have any problems in terms of his sexuality or his HIV-positive status; he considered himself as 'strange'. He did not always disclose his status during casual sex encounters because he always used a condom. He spoke of issues around disclosure:

"I don't go out of my way to tell anyone but I mean if someone asked me then obviously I would tell them… I mean if you want to have a relationship with someone then obviously you'd have to play all your cards on the table and be totally honest and up-front from the beginning… but if you are going out on the town and if you just want to pick up a quick shag, that sounds horrible doesn't it?… well you know everyone does it! You know if it's a quick shag, wear a condom. Nine times out of ten the other person wants to wear condoms anyway. So, there has never been a problem. If you are going into a relationship and it's somebody different, then you sort of do all the going out for cups of coffee and dinner and things before it leads up to anything else; then I'd make sure they knew so they had a chance to stop it, in case they didn't want to be put in that position of being with someone who is positive."

Jay spoke freely about his sexuality and believed that his sex drive had increased since his HIV-positive diagnosis. He told me how he had always wanted lots of sex beforehand, but his sexual drive was even greater now. He described himself as a 'deviant' and said 'I am a slag when it comes to sex'. HIV had not inhibited his sexual lifestyle, apart from always having to use condoms. Indeed, said Jay, he was probably more sexually adventurous now and likely to try new things than previously.

SANDRA

Sandra, a self-identified heterosexual woman, was 37 years old at the time of our interview, lived alone and was not in a relationship. At the time of diagnosis in 1994, she was in a sero-discordant relationship with her long-term partner and they got married following the death of their five-month old son due to an AIDS-related condition. Her marital relationship became deeply affected by her HIV-positive diagnosis and ended in divorce four years later. She recounts:

"I became afraid of any sexual contact in case I infected my husband. I felt guilty enough that I had passed it on to my child; I just could not cope with the idea of the possibility that I could infect my husband, because I loved him, I still do love him... so I decided the best thing for me, well for him and me, was for me to leave... I have had a lot of psychological help over the past three years, but most of the help hasn't centred on the HIV. You know, I had issues in childhood, child abuse and I have dealt with all of that...HIV was just another thing to mess up my life and I am sick of it... I just thought I could kill myself and I tried and failed and I thought 'bloody hell, I can't even kill myself. I am stupid'... after three years of therapy, I started to love myself after I had dealt with all the other garbage in my life. I now need to accept that HIV is here to stay and accept this. I will exclusively date positive men because I don't want it to be an issue."

Sandra spoke of initially losing all interest in sex which was a contributing factor between her and her husband growing apart. She was fearful of infecting him and was unable to relax. She told me:

"Logic tells me people should be responsible for their own sexual health but it is because I know what the consequences of being infected are, so I wouldn't want that on anyone else. You cannot totally relax with people when they are not in a similar situation as yourself, and that is why I made this mental decision to exclusively date positive men; and that only leaves you with a very small sort of pool that you can date from. I could never envisage being in a sexual relationship with a negative person. It is too much hassle and is not worth it. You know, if things did work out and it could be wonderful for a few years, there is always this thought that one day they are going to sue you or something and I can't be dealing with all that rubbish. It isn't a balanced relationship. It would always feel as though I wasn't quite good enough for them and I couldn't live like that; I would rather not have another relationship."

Sandra told me of her hopes to one day meet an HIV-positive man who would accept her as she is; someone who she could be comfortable with. She looks forward to the day when she can 'just be herself' and not have to live in fear and isolation with her 'guarded secret'.

Sex within relationships: conflicts, anxieties and intimate practices

The last set of narratives focus on the personal experiences of our story-tellers who were in a long-term relationship at the time of our interview during 2002. We explore how sexual intimacies have been negotiated, established and practiced over time following diagnosis. Many personal accounts expose similar tensions around issues of disclosure, a noticeable lack of sexual libido, fear of sexual rejection and overbearing fears of the possibility of infecting sexual partners. Again, we must acknowledge how these personal experiences remain on-going throughout the sexual lives of our story-tellers.

SPIKE

Spike, a self-identified heterosexual man, was 27 at the time of our interview, lived alone and was in a sero-discordant relationship with his girlfriend. At the time of diagnosis between 1981 and 1983, Spike was only a young child when he was involved in the mass screening process for people living with Haemophilia; he is the youngest member of this study. When I asked him to what extent HIV had impacted on sexual relationships he recalled:

"I have never been fobbed off! As far as I could tell anyway, I've not. I'm lucky I suppose, because I have always had good people around me and that includes partners. So, no it's never affected any sex relationships. Obviously it changes perhaps sexual relationships to some extent because I am always taking precautions and I have always made sure I wasn't in a position to infect anyone else. Obviously you can't guarantee that, but I've always tried to make sure that whatever has happened there would be nothing that could possibly infect someone else."

I asked Spike about whether or not he wanted to have children in the future and he told me:

"Yes, I do want a family. I mean this is something me and my partner have talked about; we have actually found some information out and worked out the risks and how we'd go about it if we wanted children. Probably not at the moment, but in a few years time, we would seriously consider having the sperm washing done. If we want kids then we will have them… if we have a boy and he has Haemophilia then that's fair enough, but I think it is less likely because my partner is not a carrier."

JO

Jo, a self-identified gay man, was 53 years old at the time of our interview, lived alone and was in a sero-discordant relationship with his long-term male partner. At the time of diagnosis in 1982, Jo was single. Jo's partner lives in the same building complex and they have an open relationship. When I asked to what extent has sexual relationships been affected by his HIV-positive status, he told me:

"Yes, I think sexual relationships have been affected. There are times when my libido is sort of low anyway, so at that point it's not a problem. I tend to go out less and less to clubs, pubs and bars… I suppose that is because of the notion of having to negotiate, you know in terms of sex, we've got to continue to negotiate sex… you know 'I'm HIV-positive, how do you feel about that?' It's difficult! It's not straightforward. Occasionally I have had people say 'Look I can't hack it' or 'I'm not interested' but not a lot. I have not put myself in a bad position but it is an area that is difficult."

Jo mentioned how he did not want to knowingly infect someone else, which played on his mind from time to time; this he believed potentially diminished his sexual desires. There were also times when he thought:

"Oh God! Fuck safe sex, let's go bareback – and then I would think 'No, I can't!' It is really difficult… Whether my lack of sexual desire is to do with the HIV drugs or whether it is to do with age or whether it is to do with the virus, I don't know... I was able to get Viagra because I went to a clinic for sexual dysfunction and amazingly I fit into whatever strange categories the NHS have. If you are colour-blind you fit into a category because it is a gene fault within your genetic make-up. It is bizarre! HIV has impacted on my sexual lifestyle because I was always promiscuous; one of the most amazing things about having a lasting relationship in one's later stage of life is we are very open. We have an open relationship and he has a relationship with someone else. That is fine! It has been something that has been on-going because there are aspects of his sexuality that I can't satisfy and don't want to satisfy, so you know, that is fine. He has a good sex life and mine has got smaller and smaller... my sort of sense of sexual self. It has its positive sides and negative sides, but I don't think I could ever be celibate."

MARTIN

Martin, a self-identified heterosexual man, was 38 years old at the time of our interview and lived with his wife and their son. At the time of diagnosis in 1985 he was not in a relationship. When I asked him what factors affected sexual relationships after being diagnosed HIV-positive he stated:

"I found it a lot harder to interact with girls and I never saw a future with a wife and family and it was always a secret. I started seeing a girl... my first love, almost... I don't know why I am talking about this... I suppose it wasn't a great relationship... I didn't tell her straight away. I found that if I were to meet a girl I couldn't tell them my status straight away because I could see no way of building a relationship. I thought that they would just walk away, so the only way I coped with this was to get to know them first and let them get to know me and then tell them. Hopefully they would see me and not those three letters [HIV]. The sexual side of the relationship was cool, we always practised safe sex and I told her eventually after six months. Obviously, she was very shocked and upset but we carried on going out and then some six months later she said, 'I can't cope with this anymore so I will have a test and if I am negative I am going to end the relationship and if I am positive we can carry on.' Luckily, she was negative and so she walked. I would have felt bloody awful if she was positive. We were not compatible as two people."

Martin spoke of how one of his friends was always telling him how he should disclose his status to girls before he had sex with them. After work on an evening, Martin would go to the pub and he became familiar with one or two barmaids who would come back to his flat. He had been drinking most of the evening and therefore was incapable of sexual intimacy on most occasions. He recalled:

"I just wasn't physically capable of doing anything but I was jumping in and out of these relationships and my friend was always saying 'you have got to tell the girls'... and that really pissed me off because I knew of my own responsibility with the HIV but he was a bit of a Casanova. I felt that it was unfair because he was going out with lots of different girls and having sexual relationships and he wouldn't wear condoms because he didn't like the feel of them. When I mentioned to him that heterosexuals can get HIV as well and he should go for a test, he said 'No, I can't have the test. I couldn't cope with the fact that I might be positive.' So he felt that not knowing his status made it OK for him to go out and have lots of different sexual relationships; whereas because I knew my status I had a responsibility. His argument was flawed and unfair. His sex drive was always in overdrive, and he was always examining his equipment. He just considered those sexually transmitted diseases such as Syphilis as one thing and HIV as another."

Martin recalled how when he was sober he could not establish any sexual relationship; after a few drinks his view changed as his inhibitions were reduced with alcohol. Long-term relationships though were 'out of the question' because of the tensions and anxieties around disclosure; the potentiality of sexual rejection was a real fear. Martin needed to get to know a person first to be able to gauge their reaction; and so sexual relationships were complicated by issues of trust. Martin's wife was present during our interview and she told me how Martin broached the subject of him being HIV-positive. She recounted:

"We kept going out and we were having sex and he would be all over me like a rash. The next day though he would be really cool. This was part of the attraction but there was always something huge there lurking. As I worked in the same organisation I managed to read through Martin's personnel file and I always knew he was a Haemophiliac. I remember that his brother had died of AIDS, and I remember thinking 'I wonder if he is HIV-positive'. I thought 'no he is not' because he is very fit and well. Martin was very different from anybody else I had been out with because he was so remote. I found it to be a huge challenge. He wasn't acting as predictably as men do and I really liked him. We would go out on a date, have a drink, we would have sex and then he would be really off with me. I couldn't work it out. This went on for about six months and I thought 'Fuck it! I am not having this.' I asked him what was going on and that I couldn't cope with the mood swings and that we should call it a day. And then he told me. It was such a relief because I was convinced he was gay. I said to him, 'Is that it? Is that the problem? Is that all the shit I have had to put up with just because you are HIV positive?"

Martin spoke of the stigma associated with HIV and why he was unable to say anything to her at that time. He spoke of his deep-rooted guilt and his unhappiness. He was still grieving over the loss of his younger brother who died of AIDS. Martin told me of how he had been unable to speak about HIV with his brother at a family wedding. His brother had wanted so much to talk to him and Martin was too vulnerable to do so. His brother later died in hospital. Martin became very disturbed by these memories and asked why he was still alive when his brother was not. We took a break from the interview until Martin regained control of his emotions.

COLIN

Colin, a self-identified gay man, was 42 years old at the time of our interview; he was cohabiting with his male partner between their two homes and in a sero-discordant long-term relationship. At the time of diagnosis in 1985, Colin was in an established relationship with a different male partner who died four and half years later of AIDS. Colin cared for his dying partner until his death. When I asked Colin if HIV had affected his sexual lifestyle and sexual relationships over time, he told me:

"Yes, yes of course! I think it is really difficult and I don't gloss over it all. I told some gay guys and they said, 'Oh, what's the problem! I'll put a condom on every time, there's no problem with that.' Dah-di-dah. And then you talk to other rebels, you know, people who essentially keep it a secret. I think it is really problematic. I have had enormous problems. I will be honest… there are people who say 'I always disclose' and they are either people who are a lot stronger than me, or they are just lying to themselves because I find it difficult. I have suffered quite a number of sexual rejections when I have disclosed. But you have to, unless it is casual sex; unless you are not going to see that person again. If you are going to see them again then you have to tell them. I don't generally. I think some people just do come right out with it from the word go. I don't. With my current partner I didn't. I told him after the third time we'd met and he said he would have to go away and think about it and he might not come back. He did come back… it comes down to whether people like you enough to want to make a go of it. I still have problems with it and I don't think I'll ever not have problems with it… because I think people are scared of AIDS and HIV; they're scared of it and that can manifest itself as prejudice or it can manifest itself as very rational. If I was negative, I am not sure I could have a sexual relationship with a positive person unless I was really into them. So it is difficult really."

Colin then spoke of the use of condoms during sex; he was mulling over the idea of whether one realistically or rigidly adheres to using condoms in every sexual encounter or do you take risks? He stated:

"Do you take negotiated risks or not? Do you seek out positive people to have sex with? We have a kind of open(ish) relationship where we both have shags on the side and although this causes its own problems, I also think it's sort of good and has brought a bit of air into the relationship. My partner goes out where he doesn't have to worry about it and I go out sometimes with other positive guys where I don't have to worry about it. Our relationship is sero-discordant, which has definitely affected our sexual relationship. I think it has tended to make me the passive partner which is not necessarily what it used to be. You can enjoy it but… Yes, sod it I will talk about this! It's very personal and every long-term sero-discordant relationship decides what is safe enough to include for the two of you. What is safe enough for us is that I am on combination therapy and my viral load has been under 50 for four years. It is very unlikely that I could even try and infect somebody with HIV, you know, from what I have read. I don't think there has ever been a case of transmission where someone has a viral load under 1500. Also, if I am the passive partner then I am much less likely to pass it on to him. So, what we have sort of stumbled into is that if he shags me he doesn't use a condom, whereas when I shag him I very much do. I think that this means inevitably I tend to take the bottom rather than the top, which is ok, I don't mind. I think he minds it more than I do. I think he would like it the other way round. So, this is one of the ways it has distorted our relationship. It might have been very different if we had both been negative or positive. It would have been very different if we had both been positive, I can tell you that!"

Colin stated how they both struggle with these tensions all the time. They have been together almost 10 years; the sex as in any long-term relationship, says Colin, tends to 'tail off a bit' but it has not vanished. Both Colin and his partner are still clearly attracted to each other; however HIV has brought with it many difficulties which have impacted on the quality of their sexual relationship over time. Colin recalled some of his earlier memories of sexual rejection on the grounds of his HIV-positive status. He tells us:

"Yes, sexual rejection… which I have clearly experienced to the extent of actually literally getting chucked out of somebody's bed at 2 am in the morning... I will tell you about that! A very nice guy, he seemed very intelligent and well-informed and he told me he had been in a relationship with somebody who had died of AIDS. At 2 am in the morning he wakes me up "I am sorry you are going to have to go!" I said 'A-ha' and the guy said: "I don't think I can stand having a relationship with another positive guy, in fact, I don't even really want you here." And that was it, you know, his psychological reasons... I mean he was pretty clear about why but prejudice is always based on fear anyway. I am very careful about who I come out to. I have experienced direct rejection because I have disclosed my status. And yes, rejection is part of the scene and you get used to people turning you down because you are too old, or too fat and as you get older it becomes the rule rather than the exception."

RICK

Rick, a self-identified gay man, was 32 years old at the time of our interview, lived alone and was in a sero-concordant relationship with his male partner. At the time of diagnosis in 1987, Rick was in a different long-term relationship with his partner who later died of AIDS. Rick cared for his partner until his death. When I asked him how HIV had impacted on his sexual lifestyle and sexual relationships over time, he stated:

"In between partners I might have seen a man or two. I have to sit down with them first 'cos I am not like other people; the first thing I say, even if all I want to do is give them a kiss is 'do you realise I am HIV-positive?' Most people turn round and say they are fine with that. I am fine with it too. A couple of people have said there were not fine with it. Even my current partner was strange. I talked to him for a long time but it turned out that he had two strains of HIV and had unprotected sex when he was drunk."

Rick told me because of the problems associated with his medication and ill health his libido was dramatically reduced and sex was not the first thing on his mind right now. Throughout our interview he made many references about the HIV press and HIV newsletters in relation to safer sex messages. I believe it is worthy of mention as Rick had strong views about the way in which HIV was recently being advertised as a 'background illness.' As a person who had lived long-term with HIV, he told me:

"I read adverts in the gay press and in Newsletters *'HIV-positive no problem! HIV-negative no problem!'* It is given as a background illness but why are they putting these adverts in the HIV press? Young boys and young girls are not bothering about it because the press is saying that HIV can be a background illness for 20 or 30 years now, just like diabetes or a heart condition... so people, especially young gay lads are going out drinking, taking speed, some take GHB (GammaHydroxybutrate – a modern rave-party scene drug) and are not giving a damn about AIDS because they read in the magazines that it is no longer a problem. If some of them had to go through what me and my partners have gone through, and if they catch it they will do eventually, then they wouldn't be so carefree... when you take the HIV drugs there are side effects. OK there are messages saying 'protect yourself' but in a way it is also saying 'you are still gonna live to a ripe old age' and these papers like Positive Nation shouldn't be putting these articles in because the young people are still going out, getting drunk and taking drugs and having unprotected sex. These adverts are in the HIV clinics, in the HIV press, in gay magazines. It is wrong, totally wrong."

Rick made mention of this on more than one occasion during both interviews; he felt very strongly about the way in which HIV was portrayed as a background illness that brought with it few problems because of medical advancements in HIV treatment. Rick told me of his younger years:

"Look, when I was younger, I mean you could have called me a 'slut' in the beginning when I lived in London. A lot of men and women who went to College did that sort of thing. You know, I slept around with loads of men and I didn't have proper partners; you would get drunk, because you were young and carefree... young people are still doing this today but what about HIV?... Now, sex is not on my mind at all. I am too tired and lethargic for every day things, let alone sex. No, sex is not an issue for me now."

Rick was only 32 years old when he told me this but at times he said he felt like a very old man. He was quite ill at the time of our interview and was in the throes of changing his HIV medication due to resistance issues and allergies to certain established HIV drugs available. Rick had no regrets in his life.

PETER

Peter, a self-identified gay man, was 48 years old at the time of our interview, lived alone, and was in a sero-concordant relationship with his male partner. In 1985 when Peter learned he was HIV-positive, he was single. During our conversation when we spoke about intimate relationships, Peter became very emotional and was reduced to tears on several occasions. I would like to thank Peter for his bravery and perseverance in continuing with the interview. I asked him to tell me about HIV and its impact on his sexual lifestyle and sexual relationships, he recounted:

"It is very difficult because I have a partner... I am like a mother to him and very supportive and he is unable to be supportive to me. He has a degree of learning difficulty and so although he is in his early thirties, very often he can be somewhere between five and fifteen. I find it rewarding when I am able to help him and when I see positive development in his life and well-being; this gives me a lot of pleasure. But when I am feeling unwell and when he says inappropriate things about how he will cope when I am dead and how my friends are going to have such a job clearing up my flat because I have got it full of loads of stuff... he says that it will take them ages to sort out when I am dead... [*Peter is crying now*]

Peter told me of the difficulty in coping with this but spoke of his deep love for his partner. Some friends have told Peter to tell his partner to 'fuck off' but Peter said he could not do that to someone he loved. He continued:

"It's a very difficult relationship because he is like a teenager in many respects and I am like a Mother to him. I say Mother rather than Father because I almost hear my mother speaking through me to him... but I mean it's me doing my best to look after my partner and there are moments of great beauty. I am also very self-critical and I beat myself up quite a bit sometimes... sometimes he says things and it is so amusing and funny and I think 'oh I am so glad you are my partner'. I love him very much and can't imagine being without him... he says he is HIV positive but I am not sure. Our relationship isn't sexual anyway. I am not sexual. I have sexual dysfunction which I have had for some time. I don't know whether it is HIV-related or not... About four years ago I was experiencing problems with ejaculation rather than erection. I wasn't ejaculating until I lost my erection and sometimes there would be blood in the ejaculate. I had various tests with nothing conclusive. I felt, once again, that my HIV specialist wasn't particularly interested in the problem, you know 'yes, some people with HIV do have sexual dysfunction problems but they are usually mental more than anything else' type-of-thing. I didn't accept this."

Peter stated that his sexual dysfunction was not, in his opinion, a mental issue. He had not, in the past, experienced problems with sexual performance after his HIV diagnosis, in fact quite the reverse. Before he was with his present partner, Peter had used his HIV-positive status as a 'pick up' line. He told me:

"People actually respected my openness and honesty in a 'cruise situation' because I informed people that I had HIV; they felt more comfortable about coming back with me and having some kind of sexual encounter because they knew that safer sex was not going to be a worry issue. I mean there are some gay men that could hardly believe it... this was in the Eighties. I was scoring more than most and it was so funny. I didn't expect that. In some respects to actually be up-front and open at the onset means that all the negotiation problems are sorted out at the beginning of the encounter... it had endless value! Because my desire was to try to help people, to live as positively as I could as a gay man in London, and not put up with the intolerance of society. It was almost a crusade to educate people; and I mean if gay men in a cruise bar can't talk about safer sex and about enjoying sex then where can they do it? So, most of the time I scored and I am no oil painting... but it was my openness and honesty that did it. There were occasions when it didn't happen but nevertheless very often it involved meaningful conversations with other people; some of whom said I was the first person that they had met who had told them they were HIV-positive. Nobody had told them before and so they had the opportunity of asking me questions. So, I mean there was some real quality stuff going on there and so, for me, my sexual dysfunction is not a mental thing that affected me sexually at all."

Following a battery of tests, the medical profession have dismissed Peter's sexual dysfunction as a 'mental issue' common amongst people living with HIV. For four years, Peter has not been sexual; this no longer bothers him because his partner is not sexual. He described his sexuality as *'disinterested'* and said that *'once it is used up, it's gone. Finished.'* We were both laughing at this point.

PABLO

Pablo, a self-identified gay man, was 32 at the time of our interview, lived alone and was in a long-term sero-discordant relationship with his male partner for five years. At the time of diagnosis in 1990, Pablo was in relationship with his female partner who was also HIV-positive. The relationship broke up shortly after his diagnosis; his ex-partner died of AIDS within two years at the age of 22 years. When I asked if HIV had impacted on sexual relationships and intimate practices, Pablo recalled:

"I told my current partner straight away and that was pretty hard for me because over the past years when I have told people they have run a mile.

A forgotten generation: Long-term survivors' experiences of HIV and AIDS

There is always that thought of when do you tell somebody? Do you tell them straight away? Do you wait and see how the relationship goes before you tell them? Then there is the problem of, you know, you tell the man straight away and then you sleep together. Later you have a big fall out and then the next day the whole of the village or town knows. This is so scary… I don't know how to explain it. When you tell someone you are always thinking 'what the hell are they going to be like? Are they going to scream and shout at you?"

Pablo told me of an incident he experienced when on a blind date which was set up by one of his friends. Pablo was told that the guy on the date would be 'cool' and not have a problem with his HIV-positive status. He recounted:

"We met in a pub and we got chatting and he was telling me about his life and his family; and I was sort of talking about me and saying what I had been up to over the years, and then all of a sudden, out of the blue, I just said, 'before we go any further I need to tell you I am HIV-positive'. His face twisted with a look of horror and disgust. You know, he was sat there talking to me. I hadn't even touched the guy or even kissed the guy. He jumped up out of his chair and literally ran out of the pub and I never saw him after that. My first reaction was that I felt dirty and ashamed of myself. I later thought about it and decided that it was not really my problem but his and he will have to deal with it."

Pablo went on to discuss his relationship with his current partner. He told me:

"My partner has been brilliant. I am very lucky. He has been my log really. I have always had quite rocky relationships with people who have said they can handle the HIV, and then two or three months down the line they say they have changed their minds and cannot handle it. Rather than talking about it and trying to sort things out, they have just run away from the relationship. People are scared. I am lucky now I have my partner… we actually met through a chat line and were on the phone for about two and half hours chatting. We decided to meet and hit it off. I remember saying to him, 'look you have told me a lot about yourself, it's my turn now.' I had said a lot over the phone but there are certain things you cannot say over the phone. I just said 'Look, I want to tell you I am HIV-positive' and he said 'Fine, that's not a problem'. I asked if he meant it because of the others in the past running a mile. He said he wasn't going to do that. And five years later we are still together and we talk about things all the time."

Before he was with his partner Pablo recalled how he felt strange in a potentially sexual situation. He told me:

"If somebody came up to me to sort of try to come onto me, I used to say I was with somebody even though I wasn't. I was terrified to actually meet up with them or go home with them and end up in bed. Honest to God, I would be petrified of not being able to perform and not being able to do anything. I would just probably freeze. Me and my partner were fine when we first met. Sexually it was OK but even now sometimes it's not... It doesn't bother me. Sex doesn't bother me at all. We are not really bothered about sex. We have had conversations about it and I have said that I don't really want to have sex because I would be scared of infecting him even though we always practice safer sex. But, it is always at the back of your mind... I suppose as I have got older as well, it's really hard to explain, I wouldn't want to put anybody's life in jeopardy... I mean sex doesn't bother me at all. My sex drive has diminished."

Pablo reported how he did not have problems achieving erections but when it came down to actually engaging in sex he could not go through the motions. He found this really *weird* and did visit his consultant about this. Pablo also stated that actually discussing these issues with other HIV-positive men in HIV groups had helped him enormously:

"I have spoken to a lot of people about this... those in long-term relationships just don't seem to have sex anymore. It was a relief to actually know it was not just me but others as well. I suppose HIV really does affect you sexually because you wonder if you should actually be doing this and that and the other. It plays on your mind all the time. You can end up just going mad and not having any sex life whatsoever. We are quite happy together. Sex happens once every blue moon to be honest. I thought at first it was because he was scared of me infecting him but he is just not bothered about sex. He is 47 now and you can put some of it down to age."

RICHARD

Richard, a self-identified gay man, was 32 at the time of our interview, lived alone and was in a sero-discordant relationship with his long-term male partner of 10 years. At the time of diagnosis in 1990, Richard was not in a relationship. When I asked to what extent had HIV impacted on his sexual lifestyle and sexual relationships, he recounted:

A forgotten generation: Long-term survivors' experiences of HIV and AIDS

"The day I found out my diagnosis, the innocence had gone... at first I felt guilty and dirty. I thought everybody had a right to know... partners who you are having sex with where there is no risk taking place... nowadays it is different... forcing people to disclose is wrong unless there is a significant risk of transmission; obviously there is a responsibility involved but it is also necessary for positive people to have protection and safety, and confidentiality is absolutely essential."

Richard spoke of how certain sexual intimacies were no longer attainable because of HIV, as he always engaged in safer sex practices particularly within casual sex encounters. However, Richard's sexual lifestyle and sexual relationships were not deeply affected by his HIV unless he was experiencing illness. He perceived that perhaps his relationship with his long-term partner, on occasion, was affected because of his HIV-positive status; however this had never actually been voiced by his partner and so was only in his mind.

LARRY

Larry, a self-identified gay man, was 56 years old at the time of our interview, lived alone and was in a sero-discordant relationship with his male partner. At the time of diagnosis in 1992, Larry was divorced from his wife and was single. When I asked Larry to tell me how sexual relationships had been affected following his HIV-positive diagnosis, he told me:

"Once I realised I was HIV-positive I made a conscious decision to not have sex. I could have decided to have 'safe sex' but I decided not to have sex because it worried me that I could pass it on. There is no such thing as 'safe sex', there's 'safer sex'... so there is still a tiny percentage where you might accidentally but not mean to infect someone else. I wasn't prepared to put myself in that position... you are responsible for yourself and for your own actions. I don't blame anyone. I don't even blame myself. Blame doesn't help any one. Awareness helps. Being aware. Blame is the worst thing anyone can do to themselves; whether it is blaming other people or blaming themselves. It is completely non-productive."

Larry went on to speak about his relationship with his current partner:

"I have a relationship with my partner who is 35 years younger than me, or something like that. I love him to bits but I won't have sex with him and now he's only 21 and he finds that extremely, extremely difficult. I am aware that every healthy twenty one year old does need sex and a lot of it. Well, I'm afraid I don't have sex with him. I don't think it is purely physical; I think most of it is psychological. I'm too worried about infecting him and one thing I have always said to him is, 'I can't promise that you'll never become HIV-positive but I can promise you that you'll never become HIV-positive because of me.' That is how I have put it to him and that is how much I love him."

Living with an HIV-positive diagnosis had completely and absolutely affected Larry's sexual lifestyle; he had stopped engaging in sex. He told me that the longer it has gone on, the less it bothers him. He recalled how in the early days his body still wanted 'it' and it was on his mind; he used to masturbate on his own to pictures or images on the Internet but as the years have rolled by, he no longer lives for sex at all. He described his current situation as:

"Wonderful. It has released me. I think this is one of the reasons I have managed to move forward because I haven't got this sexual force holding me back. It's left me, you see… now it's one of our most primeval drives isn't it, like eating and sleeping. We need sex. I don't know! I have probably educated my body to not wanting it. I am able to get on with other things… it is not an issue for me but it is an issue for my partner. I am finding it almost impossible to deal with, at the moment, because I realise I am going to have to give him – this sounds awful doesn't it – permission to go off and do something about it. I realise I am going to have to allow him to go and have sex elsewhere and that's worrying me silly. I might lose him because if, once he gets into bed with someone, he might fall in love with them. It worries me but I have got to do it. This is the biggest thing on my mind at the moment, his needs. Not my needs, but his… He has said to me, 'am I shared?' and I know what he means: can I go with someone else? Twice I have said 'yes' and I have got to mean it, and really he shouldn't be waiting. He shouldn't have to wait for me to say 'yes'. I cannot really give him permission; it is his life isn't it?"

Larry never believed he would be in a relationship with someone of his partner's age; he thought it might be more ideal with someone of his own age. Larry also had concerns about his partner's sexual safety:

"He does need sex regularly and what worries me is if he goes off and has sex elsewhere and comes back and sleeps in my bed. I mean we do kiss and we do cuddle… and if he's gone with someone who has a sexually transmitted disease, or got scabies or whatever, I'm a little worried about that. I can't be with him all the time."

A forgotten generation: Long-term survivors' experiences of HIV and AIDS

At this stage, our interview stopped for a short while so that Larry could compose himself. He was becoming distressed and this situation was clearly problematic for him. Larry finished our conversation relating to intimate relationships by stating that his sexual lifestyle had been severely affected, was on-going and probably always would be.

TONY

Tony, a self-identified gay man, was 40 years old at the time of our interview and lived with his male partner in a newly established sero-concordant relationship. At the time of diagnosis in 1994, Tony was not in a relationship. When I asked to what extent HIV had impacted on sexual relationships and his sexual lifestyle, he told me:

"Yes it has impacted on sex, I guess. Yes and no really! I like being penetrated. I am not into penetration. I go through phases… I am more into masturbation. I have always been like that. Once I am comfortable with a person I always tell them because I feel it is important to do so. Well, sometimes it would be a one-night stand and I have made everything so obvious but haven't disclosed, so I suppose no I don't always disclose my status… Sex is crap. It is a personal thing and for me sex is crap. I mean with my partner, because he is HIV-positive, he feels it is easier to have sex now. He is comfortable with what we do. I don't think I have never had sex or not done different sexual things because I am positive."

Tony spoke of being lethargic and lacking sexual energy. Masturbation was something he preferred. His health status was an issue at this time and so he perceived sex to be a waste of valuable energy. As he stated on a few occasions, sex, for him, was crap.

In closing, we have exposed how our story-tellers have personally experienced sexual and intimate relationships after discovering their HIV-positive status. We have learned how long-term intimacies have been renegotiated and managed in sero-concordant and sero-discordant relationships, as well as in casual sexual encounters. Some long-term survivors have revealed how tensions and issues around touch and physical contact with sexual partners have been problematic in terms of guilt and the potential of causing harm to others. Many story-tellers have experienced a considerable loss in sexual libido and have encountered sexual dysfunction as a result of either being HIV-positive, getting older or the possible side effects of combination therapy. A few long-term survivors made a decision to stop engaging in sex at the onset of diagnosis but later renewed their interest in sex as a result of 'coming to terms' with their status. The loss of confidence and psychological problems associated with HIV have impacted on: the ability to retain erections; sexual desire, and sexual behaviour; feelings of being dirty, 'contagious', and feelings of shame have been voiced during earlier years.

A prominent theme revealed throughout these personal experiences is tensions and confusions around disclosure. Who should I tell? When should I tell a potential sexual partner? Who will they tell? It is not a realistic expectation that HIV-positive women and men should disclose their status to potential partners within particular sexual contexts. The risk of sexual rejection and being exposed by those you tell may lead to social isolation which is potentially harmful with powerful consequences; the burden of responsibility does not lie with HIV-positive people. Many story-tellers have recounted how they have insisted on practising safer sex during sexual encounters and therefore had no desire to disclose their HIV status. For a few, HIV has not affected sexual behaviour to a large extent, whist, for others, HIV has undoubtedly limited certain sexual practices, particularly 'bare-backing' [having sex without a condom]. Without doubt, all our story-tellers have been extremely open and candid in terms of their personal experiences of intimate sexual practices which should be highly commended.

Again, I ask you, the reader, to critically reflect on how these personal experiences have impacted upon your own feelings and opinions. How might you describe your own sexual behaviour? What types of sexual practices do you engage in? Can you relate to the problems and dilemmas exposed in these stories? Are there any experiences you cannot fully engage with? Please think about why this might be. Do you know your own HIV status? How might you react if you were in a sexual encounter with someone who disclosed their HIV-positive status? How would you negotiate sex if you were HIV-positive? Who would you tell if you were HIV-positive? I am sure that there are personal accounts outside of your own experiences so I ask that you consider these in terms of how they might make you feel.

CHAPTER SIX

Experiencing HAART: managing combination therapy

∞

"Patients may recover in spite of drugs or because of them."
J.H. Gaddum

"Poisons and medicine are oftentimes the same substance given with different intents."
Peter Mere Latham

Introduction

Knowing you are living with a chronic illness condition and knowing there is effective medical treatment for the management of your chronic illness is, to some extent, reassuring. For all of our HIV-positive story-tellers, medical diagnoses occurred years before effective medicine was accessible. From late 1996 onwards, the rapid expansion and advances in effective HIV medical treatment has significantly assisted in the successful management of HIV as a chronic illness condition. There is undoubtedly a powerful connection between the advancements of scientific and medical developments and the continued changes, revisions and transformations in health care provision for the treatment and management of HIV and AIDS across the globe. In the era of Highly Active Antiretroviral Therapy (hereinafter referred to as HAART), for those willing and able to access combination therapies, the cause for celebration is beyond doubt for an abundance of reasons. Certainly, people living with HIV in the UK can now expect to encounter prolonged periods of good health with the absence of HIV-related symptoms and look forward to a longer life expectancy. Yet how does such optimism for the future impact on people who have lived long-term with HIV?

As previously witnessed, prior to the advent of HAART there were few effective HIV treatment options available: to remind ourselves these were the failed chemotherapy drug Zidovudine (ZDV, commonly known as AZT) licensed in 1987 and Lamivudine (3TC) and Didanosine (ddI) which were introduced in 1994. Pre-1996 was a bleak and challenging time for people trying to manage life with an HIV-positive diagnosis. Yet in spite of medical optimism with the new combination therapies, these transformations produced many psychological and social challenges for people who had already lived long-term with an HIV-positive or AIDS diagnosis.

As well as facing the possibility of severe and adverse side effects as recipients of new combination therapies, many long-term survivors had to contend with the changing uncertainty of the likelihood of premature death in conjunction with uncertainty around episodes of chronic illness and disease progression. At a social level, medical optimism in its advancement of effective treatment for HIV has now impacted on social welfare changes in the UK; the potentiality of returning back to the workplace has become a social reality. Over time medical advancements have generated societal and attitudinal changes in relation to how we publicly perceived HIV as a chronic illness condition as opposed to a fatal disease.

As we have learned so far, living with HIV and AIDS in earlier times, raised an assortment of concerns and presented profound uncertainties in terms of longevity, maintaining health and encountering periods of chronic illness in every day life when medical treatments were less effective. In chapter one, we explored the concept of health as a state of *being* that is subject to wide-ranging individual, social and cultural interpretations. Certainly, ideas about health are created by the relationship between individual perceptions and dominant social influences [including medical practices] within different social and cultural environments. We have acknowledged how notions of health can differ between individuals and across diverse social groups within our social world. We also accept that other governing factors help shape how we view health which may depend on our age, gender, ethnicity and social class which requires particular attention. How do we attain good health in the context of HIV? Is effective medicine the only answer?

This chapter explores how periods of health and illness have been experienced by our story-tellers after effective combination therapies (HAART) became widely available in the UK. We attempt to gain insight into the variations of what a healthy state is for a person living with an HIV-positive diagnosis from both a medical and individual perspective. It is important to recognise how we effectively connect our psychological needs with biological and medical requirements. How did our long-term survivors cope with the daily challenges of taking complex HIV combination therapies? How did story-tellers consider the efficacy of new treatments? What were the implications in terms of severe side effects? One puzzling element about long-term survival is how we begin to understand why some story-tellers who have never taken HIV medication continue to maintain a healthy state and good quality of life whilst others do not. Mystery is a big part of our lived realities.

Out of twenty eight women and men living long-term with an HIV-positive diagnosis, who shared with us their personal experiences, ten were medically defined as being 'asymptomatic' at the time of our interview. The term *asymptomatic* refers to individuals who have tested positive for HIV but show no clinical symptoms of the illness condition. Seven story-tellers were not taking any HIV-related medication at the time of our interview and five out of seven had *never* taken HIV medication since diagnosis. Despite the absence of clinical symptoms, three of our story-tellers were taking HIV combination therapy at the time of our interview. The remaining eighteen long-term survivors were medically defined as '*symptomatic*' (experiencing clinical symptoms associated with HIV) and were taking combination therapy for HIV; with the exception of Tyler and Rick who were both waiting for *salvage therapy* (see Glossary) due to problems associated with previous combination therapies.

We begin our journey by exploring the experiences and perceptions of seven of our story-tellers who were asymptomatic and not taking combination therapy at the time of our interview. We then move on to reveal how three asymptomatic long-term survivors personally experienced taking combination therapies for HIV. From here we focus on how our story-tellers who are medically defined as *symptomatic* experienced health, illness and combination therapy as part of every day life. We expose how severe side effects of combination therapies have been experienced and managed from 1996 onwards. As with the previous chapter, the personal experiences of all our long-term survivors are featured here whether or not they were taking combination therapy at the time of our conversation.

On being asymptomatic and living without HAART: health and HIV

GLYNN

Glynn was diagnosed with HTLVIII in 1983 aged about 17 or 18 years old after voluntarily testing as part of a mass screening process at his Haemophilia centre. Out of 65 other people who were diagnosed at the same time as himself, he is one of three survivors. He has previously taken AZT during 1990 for two or three years in conjunction with Septrin and Fluconazole for a thrush-related condition. This is the only medical treatment he has taken. When I asked him about how he medically monitors his health, he told me:

"I go and see my consultant for my Haemophilia about every three months and pick up Factor VIII and things like that... they do blood tests and then every six months I see the HIV specialist... I think it is every six months and they do the viral load and CD4 count... my viral load is under 40 and I think my CD4 is about 400 or 500 or something like that."

Glynn spoke of the side effects he had experienced with the AZT treatment and explained how he had to separate his Haemophilia, HIV and HCV as three illness conditions in terms of how he experiences health. In terms of HIV, Glynn confirms he is healthy, asymptomatic and perhaps ought to eat more healthily. He tells us:

"Yeah, I look at myself as a normal bloke who has just got Haemophilia, HIV and Hep C and walks with a limp. I don't see myself as HIV first or Haemophilia first or anything like that."

Glynn has some interesting perceptions and views on the medical profession and health practices in terms of how he contracted HIV and Hepatitis C which we will explore in chapter seven. He remains optimistic in his outlook on life and considers himself to be in good health. He does admit, however, to sometimes experiencing bouts of depression and anxiety about the possibility of future illness and not being able to do what he wants to do. Relating to HIV, he said: *"having it always there in the back of your mind that may be one day I am going to die before I should do."*

MARTIN

Martin was 21 at the time of diagnosis back in 1985 after voluntarily testing following mass media coverage which linked HIV to people living with Haemophilia and contaminated blood products. Like Glynn he had previously taken AZT for approximately three years and was not taking combination therapy at the time of our interview. Martin actively chose to stop taking the drug AZT after feeling that he was not being given appropriate support from his medical consultants as to why he should continue this treatment. When I asked him how he perceives living with Haemophilia in contrast to HIV he told me:

"I feel that I am very lucky. A lot of my peer group, Haemophilia wise, are badly disabled with twisted joints in legs and arms... but for some reason I have coped very well. I have had very few debilitating bleeds... I see them both as being totally different. The Haemophilia affects me from a physical side but not all the time. I do get bad bleeds but, as I said, I am quite lucky within my peer group... The HIV affects me mentally and not physically... you know I think about it a lot. Every day I guess."

Martin considers himself as quite physically fit and cycles every day. When asked about his perceptions of HAART and the possibility of taking HIV medical treatment in the future, he tells us:

"I don't know a lot about HAART and I don't know about the survival rates. I have heard of people that have had to keep changing their combination... I would say that if things started to go wrong or if things took a turn for the worst, then I have got a few more years perhaps than I would have had if HAART wasn't there... I would see starting taking treatment again as being definitely a sign when things had taken a turn for the worst... I would see that as the beginning of the end... the only reason I would go on HAART is if things were really bad."

CLAIR

Clair was diagnosed with HIV in 1987 at the age of 25 whilst trying for children under medical supervision with her late husband's Haemophilia consultant (see Chapter two). Her husband was diagnosed in 1985 with HIV following mass screening of people living with Haemophilia; he died several years later from an AIDS-related illness. From 1985 onwards, Clair was tested regularly for HIV and received negative results until September 1987. She has never taken HIV treatment and revealed:

"There has been nothing wrong with me... I think they [medical professionals] might call me 'not dead yet'... you just have to get on with your life, leave it and it just goes away... as I say, I haven't had [medical] tests since 7 years ago and then I stopped going for tests. I used to have regular CD4 count blood tests and I have never had a viral load test because I thought what is the point? You are living off numbers; people I used to meet like would say "ooh! What is your T-cell count?"

Clair explained she had never had a viral load test (see glossary) because at the time she ceased attending HIV medical health checks, these tests were not yet available. She took the decision that perhaps these tests were counter productive, she tells us:

"It was a decision I took not to have blood tests... what went through my mind was 'will I be able to live with the results or will I be left wondering what these tests really mean?' The answer is there again: just forget it and get on with life. I believe the whole process of having regular blood tests taken is not good. What if one day your tests were bad? Would this be a dangerous thing in itself? What is causing this? For all I know, Judy, I could have no T-cells but the point is I am alive and healthy. People actually come up to me and say that this is crazy... you know HIV-positive people can see how well I am and say to me 'you don't have medical tests? So how do you know you are well then?' I am like [laughing] well I can cartwheel and even stand on my head. I regularly do Yoga and I am healthy."

Clair's conscious decision of opting out of medical checks that monitor HIV health is rather unique yet very much requires our attention; the point she pertinently makes requires considerable reflection. How should we understand the variations of what is a 'healthy state' for a person living with an HIV? Are blood tests enough? Should we not consider our own indicators of health? Individual perspectives on maintaining health, when living with an illness condition, are important yet are often overshadowed by medical practices.

Within an HIV context, it is a social expectation and obligation to turn to the medical profession to monitor health and the likelihood of potential illness in terms of blood tests which present the CD4 count and viral load. Yet how we assess our own health in terms of our own bodies is significant to us all. Many story-tellers have revealed how when they received a low or high CD4 count following blood tests this did not correspond with how they felt in terms of their own health. In chapter four, Elisabeth told us how, on one occasion, she was feeling very well yet her blood results revealed an extremely low CD4 count; similarly, on another occasion, her results showed a remarkably high CD4 count of over 700 but she felt 'like shit'. Individual perceptions and personal experiences of ill health or being healthy should be recognised as important markers of health and illness.

JOHN

At the age of 35, John voluntarily took an HIV test and tested positive back in 1989. John was involved in an early clinical trial in which he took the monotherapy AZT for a short while until it was medically considered not to be beneficial. At the time of our interview, John was not taking combination therapy. He had, however, taken HAART during the time when he was diagnosed with testicular cancer which was totally unrelated to HIV. He did not recount any adverse side effects from the HIV drug treatment or indeed the chemotherapy. He tells us:

"I was put on combination therapy because chemotherapy depresses the immune system...I took it for, I don't know, two or three years and then came off it... Because the treatment had finished, the doctor advised me that the latest research opinion was better to delay treatment for as long as possible... I had no symptoms and my T-cell count was high and my viral load was low so I came off it. I have been very lucky and never had any side effects from the medication. In fact when I had the chemotherapy I had it on a Friday afternoon, so I left work early, spent Saturday in bed and went back to work on Monday. I didn't have any time off work."

John continues to attend his health clinic every 3 or 4 months for HIV medical checks and reports that his T-cell count is about 600 and his viral load is extremely low. He considers himself to be in good health and remains optimistic about not having to take combination therapy for some considerable time.

LISETTE

After voluntarily testing for HIV whilst travelling in the USA in 1990, Lisette learned of her HIV-positive diagnosis at the age of 39. She held a deep-rooted scepticism of HIV drugs because most research and clinical trials had been primarily based around men. With prolonged periods of good health and in conjunction with her 'suspicions of the drug companies and their motives', Lisette made a conscious decision not to take HAART based on her own intuition. When asked about her health, she recounts:

"My health! I think that I probably tolerate quite a lot of things because of my HIV condition, erm... like fatigue and things like Thrush and Herpes. They are the same things that I have been dealing with since I was diagnosed and I think it is a case of you get on and live with it...Rightly or wrongly I always had this gut feeling about the drugs, I couldn't help it. I always felt that they couldn't be quite right... I have seen them work on people, I cannot deny that... but I have certainly never ruled out taking them if I was really sick."

Lisette was 51 at the time of our interview, asymptomatic and was consciously avoiding taking combination therapy for numerous reasons.

One example she spoke of was her experiences of the menopause and living with HIV. She recalls:

"I've also had to try and deal with the menopause and HIV and it is just another one of those 'here you go take this drug but we have no idea what it will do to your HIV' You see, had I have been taking anti-HIV drugs the medics certainly have no idea what HRT and anti-HIV drugs will do together… this is a decision that I feel is taken out of your hands because I am not prepared to take those kind of risks."

Lisette identifies herself as a family member attempting to cope with an HIV-positive diagnosis and all that goes with it. She now sees herself as a Granny and a Mummy, but in the early days:

"When I was first diagnosed you kind of lose sight of who you are; you are just HIV, you're a walking little T-cell count out of control. But at the end of the day, if it isn't going to kill you and you have to go through being in hospital eventually to die, then what else can you do but resume, if you like, the life that you had before."

MARC

Marc tested positive in April 1990 at the age of 26 after voluntarily testing following a period of ill health. He was aware of clinical trials at this stage for AZT and knew people who were participating in such trials. As many reported rather bad side effects because of high doses, he decided to avoid AZT as a monotherapy. He has remained asymptomatic and enjoys periods of good health and had never taken HAART at the time of our interview. When asked about his health, he recounts:

"I'm pretty healthy. I haven't had any medical treatment at all. If I need to I will take them but otherwise I won't… I expect I probably will have to take these drugs at some point… I am just waiting until the side effects management can be at its very best. I am kind of holding out until the pill intake reduces and the side effects are less."

DAVID

David was 52 years old at the time of diagnosis in 1990 when he tested voluntarily following a change of his GP. David is the oldest member in this study and has never taken combination therapy for HIV; he also lives with

Hepatitis C (HCV). When I asked him for his views on medical treatment since the advent of HAART, he recounted:

"I made a positive decision not to have anything until I have tried all the alternative options. The only treatment I have had has been Interferon for Hepatitis because I felt I had to have a healthy liver in case I had to go on combination therapy… that date can't be far away now because I have been offered treatment now for at least eight years and I have always declined."

David spoke of his extremely healthy eating regime which consists of a vegetarian diet of organic food wherever possible. He also takes many vitamin supplements and seriously pays tribute to one particular supplement:

"I am a great advocate of Spirulina, which is the bottom of the food chain, because it is not animal or vegetable, it is an algae which grows in water…I take all sorts of other vitamin supplements and I see the HIV nutritionist."

David revealed that he attends regular HIV medical health checks every three months as well as taking acupuncture and other complementary therapies. He told me:

"In the past six months my T4 cell count has dropped from 600 to 340 and this is during the period when the acupuncture ceased and when my mother died… the other issue during this time is that I had run out of my herbal remedies… the viral load has gone up to about 3,000 copies from about 1,000 and my T4 cell count is dropping rapidly… the consultant said that this might be an immediate effect rather than a long-term effect due to these circumstances and offered another blood test in two weeks to see if this was a one-off."

David remains sceptical about the new combination therapies and recounts:

"If I do take combination therapy it would be really the last resort and I will be expecting that I am taking a poison; that is the way I see it, so I am very very reluctant to start."

The abovementioned personal experiences of our story-tellers bring to light how periods of good health in conjunction with being asymptomatic have led to conscious decisions not to embark upon new combination therapies for HIV. We have also exposed how a few of our story-tellers embrace a deep-rooted scepticism towards the pharmaceutical industry and are somewhat cynical of medical health indicators and the long-term effectiveness of combination therapies. For many, the onset of taking HIV combination therapies is perceived as the last resort.

On being asymptomatic and taking HAART: health and HIV

CHRISTOPHER

Christopher was diagnosed with HIV in 1988 at the age of 36 whilst in hospital with an arthritic condition. He was tested involuntarily and is medically defined as asymptomatic. Christopher has experienced two strokes which are unrelated to his HIV condition; at the time of interview he was taking *Combivir* and *Indinavir* for HIV and aspirin as a preventative measure for future strokes. He has not changed his combination therapy; however he has stopped taking some drugs which were originally combined in 1997. He has experienced no adverse side effects. When I asked him what factors influenced him to start taking HAART, he recalled:

"It was 1997 when I started taking medication... I had been with my partner for 26 years; the last 12 months he had a massive personality change and he started to physically abuse me, mentally abuse me and I was going through an awful lot of stress and my CD4 count dropped to 60. On the advice of my hospital consultant I went on to medication for preventative reasons. I have not been ill with HIV since my diagnosis fourteen years ago... I have not experienced any side effects... except for awful wind [laughing] windy bottom... After two weeks of taking the combination therapy they did blood tests and my CD4 count had tripled from 60 to 180. My CD4 count now is 430 which is the highest it has ever been since diagnosis."

Christopher considers himself to be healthy and has never had time away from work for HIV-related illness. He has not experienced adverse side effects and has always been compliant with his drug regime. Christopher believes being compliant with medicine is of paramount importance as a management strategy for maintaining his healthy status.

A forgotten generation: Long-term survivors' experiences of HIV and AIDS

PABLO

In 1990 Pablo was 20 years old when he discovered his HIV-positive status after voluntarily testing following a general illness. He is medically defined as asymptomatic, has an extremely high CD4 count of 800 and an undetectable viral load. He considers himself as healthy and extremely lucky. Pablo has not experienced ill health as a result of HIV. At the time of our interview, Pablo was taking Nevirapine, Lamivudine and Abacavir and had previously taken other combination therapy which had produced side effects. I asked him about the factors that influenced him to start on medication; he recounted:

"It was 1997 when I first started taking medication… a friend of mine was on combination therapy and I saw the changes in her really… I mean she had lost a lot of weight and had been quite ill and then suddenly she went on medication and it was like a miracle cure… all of a sudden she gained weight and looked so healthy… I had had numerous conversations with my consultant about pills and stuff and I thought to myself 'is it really worth me going on these tablets?'… I mean I didn't need to take them; I am quite healthy and my sort of perception was they only gave them to people who was ill…I wondered if there was any point in spending more of the Government's money on somebody that's really healthy?... I mean this was coming from my consultant who said what they try to do now is get people on treatment sooner rather than later."

Pablo told me how his HIV consultant advised him to start on combination therapy as a preventative measure. Despite reservations about taking drugs for the rest of his life Pablo agreed to embark on medical treatment for his HIV. He described how his first combination impacted on his daily life:

"The first lot of drugs dramatically changed my life as there were certain times you had to take them; you had to take some with food and others you had to take an hour before food and so on… I missed a hell of a lot out because of my lifestyle, mostly at night… you would go out and forget to take them before you went out and then you would think 'Oh! I will take them when I come home'. Then you have been out and you have probably got that pissed, to be honest, you come home and fall into bed. You get up in the morning and think 'Oh shit! I didn't take my tablets last night' and there is no way you can catch up… so if you miss them you miss them. It's not good to miss them. I think I am quite lucky now in respect that I have got a good combination therapy."

Pablo has changed medication only once and his adherence to this current medical regime has greatly improved. He puts this down to the fact that now he only has to take medication in the morning and the evening; his combination therapy does not require that these have to be taken with food. Pablo does not consider his medication as intrusive to his daily lifestyle. When recounting on his earlier combination therapy, he told me:

"I have had side effects... I was terrible. I can't remember what they called this bloody tablet [it was ddI]; it was like a big horse tablet, a big white thing and the only way you could really take it was to crush it up and have it with apple juice... the taste was disgusting and horrid... Shit! I had diarrhoea, sickness, violent headaches, and I was hallucinating quite a lot... I was very paranoid with the slightest thing somebody would say to me and I would snap. My temper was really bad and I thought I was going mental."

After Pablo changed his combination therapy he has encountered few long-lasting side effects and is happy with his current treatment. He is healthy and is reluctant to take any risk in terms of stopping treatment in spite of his on-going healthy state. He is aware of how others often take a break from HIV medication yet this is not a decision he is willing to take in maintaining and managing his own health.

JAY

In 1992, Jay aged 25, was living with his HIV-positive male partner when he discovered his HIV-positive status after voluntarily testing following a short period of ill health. He was not shocked by the result and had a very relaxed and laid-back attitude to life. Jay first started taking HIV medication back in 1998 and these consisted of: Combivir and Nevirapine and Septrin twice daily. His combination therapy had since changed at the time of our interview to: Stavudine, ddI and Nelfinavir alongside the continuation of Septrin. Jay was medically defined as asymptomatic but spoke of the factors that made him decide to embark upon medical treatment. He tells us:

"Let's see... it was probably 1998, four years after I was diagnosed. I did quite need them. Basically I was in a relationship with a guy and he was a terrible person. He was a liar, a cheat and used to beat the crap out of me. I just got to the stage where I felt so bad; I didn't know whether I was coming or going. I went to the doctors because basically I was quite ill... I'd lost quite a bit of weight and my face was gaunt and it was all due to this guy beating me up as well I suppose... My CD4 count was just so low and my viral load was so high that the doctors told me that I needed to go on medication. They gave me it and I started taking it and it brought me straight back to normal; I was fine again."

Jay had to change his combination therapy after four years due to medical opinion that it was no longer effective. Jay puts this down to his failure to adhere to the treatment because of his violent relationship and his forgetting to regularly take medication every day. He recalled:

"I messed up on the first medication... to be quite honest I don't think I can stick to a regime where you have to take them with food and special diets. I mean I eat when I'm hungry and not at set times... I don't think I could actually stick to a regime that takes a load of messing about. It's messing about as far as I'm concerned. It is life-saving as far as others are concerned I know this... but since changing to the second lot I have never missed, well probably one or two, but I have taken these since April 2002. You know, I have never experienced bad side effects and it's just like putting the kettle on in a morning as soon as you get out of bed, it's just normal."

The above narratives reflect the personal experiences of three story-tellers who were medically defined as asymptomatic and taking HIV combination therapy as a preventative measure. Matters of being compliant and problems associated with adhering to medical regimes have been raised; experiences of side effects have revealed that some combination therapies had been problematic. All our story-tellers who were medically defined as asymptomatic were experiencing good health.

On being symptomatic: HIV, HAART and health

This next section explores the personal experiences of eighteen long-term survivors who were medically defined as symptomatic and were recipients of combination therapy during the time when our interviews took place in 2002.

Experiencing HAART with no side effects

Only three story-tellers reported that they did not experience any adverse side effects whilst taking combination therapy during our conversation. We shall explore these stories first.

PAUL

Paul was involuntarily tested at his local Haemophilia centre at the age of 21 back in 1985 after a routine visit and as part of a mass screening process for people living with Haemophilia. He was diagnosed with HTLVIII, the precursor to HIV. Paul enjoyed many periods of physical good health following his diagnosis (psychological issues excluded) and did not consider taking HIV treatment until he became very ill after the advent of HAART. At the time of our interview Paul was taking Combivir and 3TC for his HIV; Nevirapine for HCV and Factor VIII for Haemophilia. His fear of embarking upon HIV medical treatment (see Chapter four) was based on his deep-rooted cynicism of the pharmaceutical industry until he became ill and his choices were diminished. He tells us:

"HAART is a very positive thing as it keeps me alive… It has made me think I am not going to die of AIDS anymore because if there is no treatment there is no hope. The drugs are intrusive in the fact that you cannot have a day without them. The emphasis on adherence is so hard. It makes you feel very guilty if you forget. It is a responsibility that I have; my daily responsibility is to make sure I take my tablets on time… it is a burden but if you think about the alternative of not taking them properly, I am going to get ill. So it is not a burden as it is keeping me alive. I think of it more in terms of a responsibility than a burden."

Paul did not report any adverse side effects from his combination therapies and has maintained good health. He did recount how having to stick to a rigid drug regime during earlier times was extremely difficult to manage. He spoke of his anguish around whether or not he had taken his daily pills at a certain time, or if he was out somewhere did he have the correct dosage with him. These issues were a constant reminder of being HIV-positive in daily life.

LARRY

Larry tested positive after voluntarily testing following the onset of illness back in 1992 at the age of 46. For six years following his diagnosis, Larry experienced long periods of good health yet psychologically he suffered enormously with prolonged bouts of depression and social exclusion. He was the only person in the study who was unable to identify the route of transmission for his HIV condition. Larry attends regular HIV medical check ups and, at the time of interview, he had only been taking combination therapy for two and half months. His treatment consisted of: Trizivir,

Acyclovir and Septrin in conjunction with complementary therapy. I asked him what factors influenced him to start medication, he recounted:

"I dreaded the thought... I was terrified because of the side effects which I was aware of from other friends which can be severe and permanent... I realised that the minute I started any kind of HIV therapy it was going to compromise future treatment...I'm afraid that I'd actually been so ill for about a year to eighteen months... I'd get up and half an hour later I would be back in bed. I hadn't got the energy to even stay up and that's terrible when I look back... The doctor put it in a good way and that was helpful... he said my body wasn't coping very well and although my test results are not very good, they're not actually very very bad but my body was having to work overtime... I thought that was a good way of putting it. I did need to go on some kind of treatment as I had systemic Thrush, which in the old days used to be an AIDS-defining illness... this was a clear sign for me that my body was telling me it wasn't coping."

Larry recalled at the onset of his ill health how he sought out treatment advice and support from organisations such as the Terrence Higgins Trust, as well as speaking with other HIV-positive individuals; as a consequence he took an active role in choosing his own drug regime of Trizivir (a combination of AZT, 3TC and Abacavir). When I asked what kind of things have changed since embarking on the combination therapy, he told me:

"Well the only way I can describe it, it's like something or someone has breathed the life back into my body again, because after about two weeks I noticed a subtle difference. I was getting up in the morning and staying up. I was able to stay up and I started doing jobs that I hadn't done for two years... like the house had got left... these tablets have actually breathed life back into my body... it's a bloody miracle! I have no side effects and the doctor tested my liver... I am actually going to discuss this again with him because I've got terrible pains down here, internally... but no side effects. It's wonderful, absolutely wonderful."

Larry's takes his medication every twelve hours and he copes well with adherence. He does not consider his medication as intrusive in daily life, as he can take his tablets with or without food. For Larry, the advent of new combination therapies has been a positive experience without adverse side effects, which was a source of great anxiety and fear for him in the past. It is worth mentioning here that HIV combination therapies had been available for over 7 years and had rapidly changed prior to Larry starting his medication.

RACHEL

Rachel was 28 when she was diagnosed as HIV-positive back in 1993. Her husband had previously tested positive and had contracted HIV in West Africa from an infected syringe that was used to treat a Malaria attack. The injection saved his life; there was no bitterness or blame apportioned for his HIV condition. Rachel expressed a sense of relief that she was not in a sero-discordant relationship at the time of diagnosis (see chapter two). After careful medical supervision, Rachel went on to have two daughters who are both HIV-negative with her husband. At the start of 2002, Rachel embarked upon triple combination therapy due to her CD4 count dropping below 200. She had taken combination therapy previously for the last three months of each pregnancy. She recalled during her two pregnancies:

"I went on a triple combination that I chose... I spent a lot of time on the internet as there hadn't been many studies of drugs in pregnancy, apart from AZT, 3TC and Nevirapine... at that time 3TC was not available, Nevirapine was but AZT plus Nevirapine wasn't a terribly good combination on its own... so I went for AZT and ddI which hadn't had any studies but appeared not to have any side effects anecdotally on the baby and I went for soft gel Saquinavir, the first protease inhibitor which wasn't actually licensed at the time but it was flown in for me."

Rachel took the decision to come off the combination therapy following the birth of each child. She spoke of being 'lousy at complying' with the taking of tablets and was only willing to start medication again when it was necessary. She recounted:

"The combination treatment when I was pregnant was a nightmare... there were five different times that I had to take pills and that really was difficult... I could never have taken these long-term, not by choice, but it was the one I chose for safety for each pregnancy... I knew that this was for a short term because I planned to stop as soon as the babies were born."

She told me of the factors that influenced her to consider combination therapy following several bouts of ill health. She stated:

"I had actually had a couple of really nasty sore throats and infections and I hadn't been able to shake them off as well as I used to... I can't say that I was ill with anything directly related with HIV but I knew I wasn't shaking off infections... that suggests to me that things are beginning to get to the stage where I need to start looking at taking treatments... there are some treatments I would wholeheartedly avoid because I have seen how it has affected my husband and how it has affected other people. So, for example, you won't catch me taking Efavirenz; not on your life."

Rachel actively chose her own combination therapy and has not experienced any side effects associated with the drug regime. She takes tablets twice a day and spoke of her continued difficulty in remembering to take them regularly. Her health has improved and she hopes to return to work in the not-too-distant future.

Experiencing HAART and adverse side effects

The final section of this chapter explores how story-tellers negotiated health in terms of managing combination therapies and the side effects associated with certain drug regimes. How do complex treatment regimes impact on daily life? As usual we start with those who were diagnosed earliest and take a detailed exploration into the factors that influenced our story-tellers to take medical treatment. We examine how earlier combination therapies and problems of adherence in conjunction with adverse side effects impacted on long-term survivors since the advent of HAART from late 1996 onwards. We conclude with the personal experiences of Tyler and Rick who were not on treatment at the time of our interview due to them awaiting 'salvage therapy'; they had run out of HIV treatment options and we will see how HIV medicines had impacted on everyday life.

MINNIE

Minnie was diagnosed with HTLVIII back in 1981 at the age of 21 after being tested involuntarily following routine screening as a blood donor of a rare blood group. He experienced prolonged bouts of good health from 1981 until 1996 when he was hospitalised for almost three months. Minnie survived on AZT for nine months before embarking on combination therapy as soon as it became available. At the time of our interview, Minnie was reliant on a wheelchair (possibly unrelated to HIV) and was taking the following medications for HIV and other conditions: Lopinavir (Kaletra boosted with Ritonavir), D4T (Stavudine), 3TC (Lamivudine), Tenofovir, Septrin, Methadone, Gabapentin, Diazepam (Valium), Diclofenac, Fluconazole and occasional short courses of Acyclovir. He also took complementary therapies such as cranio-sacral healing and reflexology. Minnie told me how he became ill in July of 1996 and was subsequently hospitalised. He recalled in detail:

"I had a high temperature and I developed a rash from the waist downwards, spreading down my legs to my ankles. I didn't know what it was, it was just incredible. I went to my GP... I think I was in his surgery at quarter past three that afternoon and by 4 o'clock I was in a ward for infectious diseases at my local hospital. I was treated for a streptococcus infection...I didn't have any CD4 cell count and there was no viral load testing available then... I'd been in bed for three days and on the fourth night I woke up and I could not feel my legs from about the shin below the knee... I had the most agonising pain. I weighed so little at this time. They hooked me up to Morphine and told me what was happening to my body... vasculitis is the body's way of destroying itself... normally the renal system is affected but I suffered the extremities, which were my feet. Peripheral Neuropathy. I could have lost fingers with gangrene but it was my feet... the tips of my toes went *ischemic* (grey/black) and I lost the tops of two toes on my right foot. They would not operate; they insisted that the toes amputate themselves because they were frightened that my foot wouldn't heal because I had no resistance, no CD4 count... they offered me steroids and I declined this treatment because steroids mask infection... I was full of infection. The streptococcus was one thing but what sparked off the vasculitis nobody ever discovered the root cause."

Minnie stayed in hospital until the beginning of October and lost many of his toes on both his left and right feet. He lived with gangrene for two years and he described the pain as difficult to control. Minnie was put on AZT as a monotherapy for nine months until HAART became available in the UK (see chapter four). His CD4 count slowly rose and he was medically advised to start taking combination therapy immediately. He told me:

"I have suffered an awful lot of side effects with the drugs I have taken... you know for me this was par for the course. I live with a disability which is degenerate myopathy of the legs but I'm still feeling physically well enough to function. I have a car...I am a person living with AIDS; I've had an AIDS-defining diagnosis since 1996 and I have had every opportunistic infection and no CD4 count. I live with a particular horrific dietary problem but there is no hard evidence linking it to HIV, only anecdotal. I guess it is like the Crick's belly anecdote way back with Indinavir where they discovered fat being produced in places where it shouldn't be. I suffered a reaction to Ritonavir and developed a resistance to it. I experienced extreme night sweats and diarrhoea is, of course, par for the course... you get used to it... I can only put it down to Ritonavir but I've got no medical evidence because my consultant's not prepared to put me through more biopsies. I have horrific bowel problems sporadically and I'm also living with spontaneous incontinence... it's on and off and I have no control over it; I don't know when it's going to happen... it's just a bloody nuisance. I get Tenor for Men."

Minnie spoke of how he accepted the side effects and the changes in his life as being part of what was 'wrong' with him. Two years prior to our interview, Minnie had nerve conduction tests and a biopsy to identify why the myopathy in his legs was rapidly progressing and if this was related to him taking d4T for his HIV. There was no empirical evidence to suggest that HIV drugs played any part in the degenerative condition of his muscles. He is now taking Ritonavir again as a pharma-kenetically boosted part of the Lopinavir drug; he firmly believes, however, that Ritonavir is causing adverse reactions to certain foods such as wheat; he stated:

"I tried omitting wheat from my diet and within two weeks for the first time since 1996 and taking combination therapy, I didn't have diarrhoea any more. I thought that can't be coincidental... so it has now progressed to omitting gluten, wheat, oats, rye, barley and malted grain... I have to be careful with stabilisers, emulsifiers or any food that may be of a wheat derivative because I have an instant reaction to it... Again, I can only put it down to Ritonavir but I've no medical evidence to support this."

Minnie firmly emphasised how he liked to take control over his various drug treatments and the various strategies for managing his HIV condition. He listens to his own body and is able to function to the best of his ability on a daily basis.

SPIKE

Spike is the youngest person in this study at 27 years old and was a child when he was diagnosed with HTLVIII around 1981 – 1983 as part of the mass screening process for people living with Haemophilia. From 1997 onwards, Spike started combination therapy, and at the time of our interview, his medication consisted of: Nelfinavir, Combivir, Septrin and Factor VIII for Haemophilia. He occasionally uses aromatherapy massage as a complementary therapy. He considered himself as extremely healthy despite having a low CD4 count. On being healthy and HIV-positive he tells us:

"It is hard to categorise really... if the medical indicators of health with the T-cell count and viral load tests are true, then I have lived with an AIDS diagnosis for the best part of the last ten years or more... because my T-cell count is still under 200... but I don't think I should have this sort of label over me. It was nice to have a gauge, a predictor of how you are doing and stuff, but my count has never been more than 400 since I was a teenager… it would go down from 200 to 170 to 150 to 120 and it is has been under 10 before now. My viral load has been undetectable since I started HAART… everything is medicalised but their [the medics] definition is quite unrealistic in terms of my own health. I am healthy with a low T-cell count. Obviously since HAART I have got more stability in my life in relation to long-term plans. I try to keep fit and have gone back into education… It took me two years after I started HAART to think I am now in a position where I can move on; I can do other things… before I was more spontaneous in life."

I asked Spike about his combination therapy and how intrusive his medication might be on a daily basis. He told me his current regime was pretty good. He takes his tablets in the morning when he awakes and later before he goes to bed. He did mention that in the past he had been hospitalised because of the side effects of his previous medication. He recalled:

"I have always taken Protease Inhibitors and my first combination started in January; it was Ritonavir… I tried to keep taking the medication for ages, sometimes up to six weeks, but then I would actually come off it… I was just throwing up as soon as I was taking the tablets and experienced really bad nausea. The second combination was Indinavir, another Protease Inhibitor… that was OK for a while as it kept my viral load down… then I was having *haematuria* (presence of blood in urine)… I was pissing blood and I had to drink up to 15 litres of water a day to try and keep my system flushed… I was pissing clots in the end and I was hospitalised and taken off the drugs. They put me on Nelfinavir which was meant to be taken three times a day, but I just took it twice daily and it worked. I have been fine ever since, so I have been lucky. I know lots of people who have become resistant to most drugs and are knocking on the door of salvage treatment now, so I consider myself lucky."

Spike regularly attends a health clinic for medical monitors and blood tests for his HIV and Haemophilia and sees his current medical treatment as giving him a new lease of life.

JO

Jo was diagnosed in 1982 with HTLVIII after voluntarily testing following a short bout of illness at the age of 33. He enjoyed prolonged periods of good health following his diagnosis until he started to experience severe fatigue years later. He regularly attends a health clinic and is on his third combination therapy. At the time of our interview Jo was taking: Saquinavir, Ritonavir, Tenofovir, Abacavir and occasionally used osteopathy as a complementary therapy. He was currently experiencing good health after previously falling ill with extreme fatigue after taking a voluntary 'drug holiday' for 18 months. When I asked him about his experiences of taking combination therapy he told me:

"The problems associated with adherence are complex and difficult to manage at times. I'm lucky because at the moment I am on a number of pills that I only have to take once a day… At one point I was being given medication that was twice a day, and other medication that was three times a day… at the beginning I had to take pills five times a day because of the hours in between… you were forever having to think 'when do I take this pill?' I am fairly pragmatic and therefore fortunate to be able to deal with this, but eventually I could not cope… twice daily I can deal with but some tablets every six or eight hours I can't hack… I would rather deal with the consequences of not taking them and have done. I am on my third combination now and this works."

Interestingly, many story-tellers spoke of adherence issues and the problems associated with taking complex drug regimes at particular times; some drugs had to be taken with or without food and the medical expectation that people would change their lifestyle to suit the medicine was unrealistic. These then became really big issues and extremely difficult to manage over time. Jo spoke of anxiety when attending medical HIV health checks:

"When one goes to give blood, you have to give blood two weeks before your appointment with the doctor, so the results are there. It's highly stressful because what happens if you start to fail with your medication? What is the next generation? What happens if we've reached a point where actually there are not that many new drugs that are available? What doctors used to say was that basically you have got ten years on medication IF you can tolerate it. If you can't tolerate it then you're up shit creek anyway… The whole sort of toleration is quite difficult and gets to be a big pressure in your life… I mean there is constant uncertainty that one is always dealing with, but then life is uncertain."

The dominant factor that influenced Jo to embark upon combination therapy was extreme lethargy and his quality of life had diminished. He explained:

"I'd reached a point where I was so lethargic... I was so fatigued I couldn't do anything that I enjoyed. So my quality of life basically for me has always been important... as long as my quality of life was good, then that was fine. If it wasn't then I wanted out... I'd reached that point and spoke to my consultant who felt that it was time that I really had to bite the bullet. I had reached a point where I no longer had an alternative... At first, the initial experience was wonderful! I mean after about probably three months I had such energy. I couldn't believe it... I was able to do anything; it was incredible and wonderful, I had such a high rush of energy. I was lucky though as I tolerated the drugs and it was a very easy combination to take so it wasn't complicated."

I asked Jo if he had encountered any side effects with any of his three combination therapies. He reported:

"After about a year I developed Peripheral Neuropathy which was associated with two of the drugs I was taking ddI and d4T... I remember one day I sort of could barely walk; I was leaning on a trolley in the supermarket. I just thought that this was it. You know one of my pleasures has always been walking. I really like walking in the Fells, walking in the Dales and in the Southern Welsh mountains, you know, it's great! So not being able to walk was absolutely awful. So they took out the ddI and the d4T and put me on Combivir, which was AZT and 3TC as one pill but after 15 weeks I couldn't hack it. I still don't know whether it was the AZT; I had such hatred against GlaxoWelcome and AZT and everything that it had done in the past. You know, whether it was psychosomatic or whatever, but I was just continually nauseous. I was back to lying down all the time. I couldn't move; I felt just awful. The consultant believed I was worse off now than I was before so I came off them. I had an 18 month drug holiday and it was fab."

After experiencing another bout of ill health around lethargy and fatigue, Jo went back on combination therapy and is now experiencing good health without any adverse side effects to this treatment. Jo further mentioned how since the advent of HAART he experienced significant confusion and uncertainty around new treatments and revival accompanying renewed health. He told me:

"I mean one of the things that has happened around HAART is that there's been this huge change in terms of, you know, for years one was expecting to be dead next month and... it's such a terrible stress and sort of strain to be dealing with this... you come to terms with the fact that you know you're not going to be alive and then suddenly you are alive and what are you going to do? I think they refer to it as the *Lazarus Complex*… it is very daunting and very difficult to manage."

For people like Jo who have lived long term with HIV and especially for those given an AIDS diagnosis a long time prior to effective treatment being available, psychosocial concerns about hope, revival of good health, identity and the problems of continued life have led to different levels of confusion and uncertainty. This kind of experience has been acknowledged by significant others and is commonly referred to as the *Lazarus Effect* or *Lazarus Syndrome*.

NEIL

Neil was 24 years old when he was diagnosed with HTLVIII back in 1985 after been involuntarily tested following a visit to his GP due to ill health. He experienced prolonged periods of good health until 1995 when he discovered he had oral thrush and was rapidly losing weight. His GP believed he ought to be medically monitored more frequently for HIV and perhaps start looking at medication in the future. Neil took six weeks away from work, during which time he was also diagnosed with bacterial pneumonia which was effectively treated. Neil returned to work and later in July 1996 he was prescribed AZT and another drug which he cannot recall. He explains to us:

"My CD4 count was 20 and my doctor said I will probably deteriorate in the next two years and get really ill… I actually did plan and change what I was doing because I believed that I was going to be dead in a few years and that was a really big moment…they started me on AZT and I think another drug… I went on the first triple therapy in Autumn of 1997 and now I am on my fourth combination therapy."

I asked Neil about his experiences of side effects with his combination therapies and how this impacted on his daily routine and his work life. He recounted:

"It was tough! I had pains in my legs, in my chest and I always felt physically sick taking the pills… I was often sick actually and I had diarrhoea… so they changed them in the following year… I came off AZT and then I had something else. I can't remember… I had to take time off work as I was ill and being sick… when I was at work I had to rush to the loo, which I really didn't like and that was tough. When people go on treatments now there is so much information about side effects and how to take the pills; back then it was all so confusing... I didn't know that I would get side effects."

Neil also recalled how his second combination therapy impacted on his daily routine. He explained:

"The second lot I started I was supposed to have them an hour before food; so when you are working and getting up, you know, an hour before breakfast, it's six o'clock in the morning... I felt physically sick with the pills and often I was sick... It was all so secretive too, as at work I would have to go and take the pills in secret somewhere. It wasn't easy at all... I felt quite down with it all but the only option was to press on and really try to keep working... it then became more increasingly difficult to work and take tablets at the same time. It was hard because I didn't really have any illness it was just the side effects, the treatment was making me ill."

Neil continued to take his combination therapy because he had become so frightened the year previously, when his consultant had told him that he was likely to die in a few years having such a low CD4 count. He believed he had to give himself a chance of survival and persevere with the effects of taking the drugs. He told me:

"I got myself a computer and there was so much information on the Net. It would have been better if I had had a computer earlier; I find out so much about other people's experiences... I mean it never occurred to me not to take the pills, I mean some people decided not to take them... you know, looking back I had some really bad side effects. I am curious now to see what would have happened if I hadn't taken the pills... then of course the doctors say the reason I am still here is because the pills are working... but sometimes I do wonder."

I asked him how successful his other combination therapies had been and he told me that his fourth combination therapy was less intrusive and had fewer side effects. He recounted:

"I still have diarrhoea and have to take anti-diarrhoea tablets every day and even taking one in the morning and one in the evening I still have off days; so I have to increase the dosage... it isn't quite completely under control. Now though I only have to take two lots of tablets twice a day, which makes life a lot easier... but for all those years beforehand, there were all sorts of complications... I had diarrhoea and then there's the neuropathy, nerve pains and chest pains and rashes. I also had two operations on my toes because it affected the skin around my toes; again, nobody knew about this for a couple of years when I went to see my doctor… but now it has been recorded as one of the side effects of one of my tablets, Indinavir."

Neil spoke at length about problems associated with *lipodystrophy* and lipdoatrophy (see Glossary) which he considered as a major side effect of his long-term medication. After three years of taking various combination therapies, Neil told me:

"Another difficulty has been the loss of fat cells in my legs and mainly in my face. Certainly after being on medication for about three years, in about 1999, a lot of people like my family and like my sister-in-laws have said to me 'what's wrong are you ill?' This is because I have lost a lot in my face and I am so thin. To be quite honest other people are saying the same and I find it easier to socialise on the Net. It is a visual thing… and it really bugs me. It does make me quite nervy about meeting new people and it makes you aware of yourself, even on the High Street. I think my doctors don't really take it on board how important it is for me… as you can see I have got sunken cheeks and sort of hollow eyes and a bit in my temples. I did actually start going to a lipodystrophy clinic, which was advertised as a specialist clinic. I was told that once you have lost the fat cells you are not going to get them back… they have suggested one or two treatments that might help but they can only offer me them on a trial basis and I thought that there's not much point starting and stopping treatment. They talked about Thalidomide and anabolic steroids but only for a limited period… apparently there is a new product that has been developed called NuFill and I am awaiting the results from these trials but this is only for the face. It is quite expensive so I can't see this being offered on the NHS… It does make me feel like a Leper at times; it makes me feel physically different from other people… Yes, it does make me very very conscious in most situations, like going to the Gym. I am trying to build up my lean body by going to the Gym and I do feel conscious there."

After taking combination therapy for over a year, Neil decided to take medical retirement from work due to the complications associated with the side effects of the treatment. He recalled:

"The side effects just weren't letting up and I thought that the time had come to consider medically retiring. I had diarrhoea and the pains in my legs were difficult to cope with and I thought that this was going to be like this for the rest of my life. At one time my doctor suggested I go part-time. The problem with that was that if I ever did retire this would affect my pension and to be quite honest the system was such that it was easier to retire medically than to reduce my hours. Financially I would actually miss out if I went part-time."

Neil went on to tell me that if there had been more information at the time of him embarking on new combination therapy, especially in relation to the side effects of specific drugs, he might not have taken some of the treatment and persevered so long with these side effects. In addition to this, Neil recalled how in 1999, three years after he started with medical treatment he developed Lymphoma. He remembered:

"Even when I was on HAART, I actually developed Lymphoma, which is an AIDS-defining illness and so this makes me question how good HAART was in a sense... This was three years ago; I had chemotherapy and I started to get well and this has now cleared up... but it shook me a bit because I thought if I was on medication why have I progressed from HIV to AIDS? The cancer treatment depresses your immune system and I already had HIV so I was not in a good position. Psychologically it did mean that I was diagnosed with AIDS so I had moved on and progressed to having an AIDS diagnosis."

Neil continues to attend medical health checks for his HIV but now negotiates his own health status from his own psychological point of view. Whilst he always considers the results from his CD4 count and viral load tests, he does believe that as long as he can stand up and do what he wants during the day, he is healthy; if his test results are at odds with how he is feeling, he will push these aside. *'One of the big changes with how I perceive how well or how ill I am is that I am more confident about judging my own health, rather than simply letting medical people judge my health.'*

ELISABETH

Elisabeth was diagnosed at the age of 31 during the Christmas of 1985 after voluntarily testing for HIV; at this time she was a practising IV-drug user which continued for eight years following diagnosis. She attends regular health checks for her HIV and described herself as relatively healthy despite having a serious liver complication. Similar to other story-tellers, Elisabeth spoke of times when her HIV results for her CD4 count were often 'at odds' with how she was experiencing health. On one occasion when her CD4 count was over 700, she felt 'shit' and conversely when it fell below 20 she felt relatively healthy. At the time of our interview she was taking the monotherapy Kaletra and had previously taken other combination therapies. I asked Elisabeth to tell me what factors triggered her decision to embark upon taking medical treatment for her HIV, she told me:

"My T-cells disappeared from about 600 to about 60... then went down to 40 so I decided to give in and I went on combination therapy but I was very mistrusting of it... I've had terrible trouble with prescribed medication with lots of side effects, rashes, you know feeling sick and even with Hepatitis, the Interferon nearly killed me... I believe it was that that nearly killed me rather than my liver."

Elisabeth spoke of relative confidence in the combination therapy over time but in many ways she firmly believed that at the onset of HAART, a number of HIV-positive people almost gave up looking after themselves and medication became the only priority. She spoke of the difficulty of striking a balance between medicine and alternative therapies, of eating well and listening to her own body. The medicalisation of HIV had impacted on individuals' perceptions and beliefs about their own health status with the CD4 indicators and viral load tests as we have learned. Elisabeth went on to explain how intrusive and confusing her previous medication had been in daily life. She recounted several past experiences:

"A lot of times if I was out and I had a tablet to take after meals or with meals I just didn't take it... You know it is so awkward and instead of organising my life around medication, I organise my medication around my life. You know my life comes first... For a lot of people medication comes first. They say 'Oh I can't do that because I've got to take my pills at this time'. I think fuck it! I had to fill in a form at the clinic on research looking at how compliant patients were with their medication... They wrote back telling me I was not very compliant and I was taking my tablets at the wrong time... I had to take them every 12 hours. I thought that's interesting! How do the pills know what time it is? And when I was in hospital when I haemorrhaged last December, this was a Sunday night. The Monday morning I had to take my pills by 9 or 10 o'clock but I couldn't because I was 'nil by mouth' and had to take food with these tablets. So one nurse was saying that I had to take the pills with just water; I said No! To take these pills without food will make me sick and it is absolutely horrendous and I'm not taking the risk. Then another nurse says to take them later. They make up their own bloody rules and I had to get that operation."

Elisabeth spoke of additional side effects with other combinations:

"I was on one combination therapy and I got Peripheral Neuropathy and so they took me off the tablet that caused this and put me on something else which made me lose my appetite and I was unable to eat... I can't even remember which medication this was. It made me quite sick. I lost loads of weight. They wanted to replace this tablet but I refused and stayed with the two tablets. That was fine. Then my liver got bad and they put me on Interferon... the side effects of the combination drugs I have taken have always been so horrendous that the doctors had to take me off them and give me new ones... now I'm allergic to quite a lot of them. I really pushed to go on to Interferon because of my Hepatitis C (HCV) and it nearly killed me... but you know at least I tried."

Elisabeth spoke of her experiences of the medical profession since her HIV-positive diagnosis which we explore in chapter seven. At the time of our interview, Elisabeth was experiencing reasonable health after a prolonged period of ill health and was awaiting a liver transplant due to problems associated with her Hepatitis which is further complicated by her HIV.

PETER

Peter was 33 when he discovered his HIV-positive status in 1987 after previously being involved in a clinical trial in 1985; he chose not to know the result during the trial but some eighteen months later he changed his mind. Peter regularly goes for HIV health checks and is currently on combination therapy (Trizivir) and Warfarin for DVT - Deep Vein Thrombosis (not related to HIV). In earlier times, he was offered AZT as a mono therapy but declined. He describes himself as reasonably healthy and spoke about the startling factors that influenced him to start HIV medication some 15 years after diagnosis in 2000. He reveals to us:

"... I gained information about HIV through my voluntary work at THT and various other publications in the Gay press. I had come to realise that it was a sensible course of action to take medication when my CD4 level had fallen no lower than about 250 and my viral load had been higher than 50,000 for more than three months. What happened was in the course of the year my viral load rose from 20,000 to 50,000 and then to another stage of 100,000 and at the end of the year to a third of a million and my CD4 count which had been steady(ish) around about the 450 mark dropped to 350 and then to 250. I knew there weren't many choices to be made so in consultation with my doctor, I went on something called the Forty Trial... a randomised trial involving three or four drugs according to what the computer threw out. I was hesitant about going on the trial at first, mainly through ignorance about trials and drugs because although I knew quite a lot about HIV, I hadn't really investigated the treatments as they were forever changing… The doctor pointed out that this particular trial was not using people as 'guinea pigs' in a sense of trying something new; it was actually taking a combination of several drugs that had already been licensed and had their value proved and I would be monitored very closely… I know one of them was Nelfinavir, one was Nevirapine and I think another ddI and the other might have been 3TC… it was a faulty trial for certain. Anyway I got all four drugs thrown at me and they reduced the viral load very rapidly, er wonderfully well, although they didn't do a great deal for my CD4 count which stayed around 250… unfortunately after some weeks I found it very difficult to eat; I had nausea and felt very unwell and basically was sent home with anti-sickness tablets. I actually felt so unwell I thought I ought to have been in hospital and quickly went to see my local Social Service department who arranged for me to go in a hospice… The next day I had blood tests which showed that these drugs were actually harming my liver and kidneys… apparently I was within an inch of needing a blood transfusion. Two of the drugs were stopped immediately… I went to see the doctor in charge of the trial, as I was told to do by the hospice, and I felt quite angry really… I thought if I had just gone home with the anti-sickness tablets, I wasn't actually due to see the consultant for five weeks, or something, you know my next trial appointment… If I had gritted my teeth and tried to grin and bear the side effects, you know, I probably would have been dead."

Peter was not happy about the consultant's reaction to the side effects or of how he was monitored during the trial. After further blood tests Peter was advised to come off the drugs completely and was to be re-assessed in the January of 2001. He recalled:

"As the drugs had initially reduced my viral load so drastically I thought I would be alright… when I did go back in the January, I had the shock of my life to discover that my viral load had soared right up again… this meant that I needed to start treatment pretty quick. Since my trial I had done more research on the Internet and had been reading NAM (National Aids Manual) publications on drug regimes and a drug called Efavirenz listed some very nasty side effects for some people. It could actually cause depression, anxiety, nightmares and if mental health problems were an issue, could make you feel suicidal. My Doctor wanted me to take this drug because my options were now limited and this drug had an excellent profile. To me, the only thing in the minds of doctors at this time was to reduce the viral load to undetectable as fast as possible and get CD4 rates as high as possible… if they can achieve these two markers then nothing else matters much…

there is perhaps the tendency not to have much consideration for the side effects and quality of life."

Peter reluctantly took Efavirenz alongside Combivir (AZT and 3TC) against his better judgement and revealed:

"The worst happened... I had nightmares and worse than that I felt suicidal on a daily basis. I could go to bed quite happily in the evening and I could wake up several hours later quite typically and feel absolutely suicidally depressed. I felt life wasn't worth living. I felt that my brain was frying and life just wasn't worth living. I went on holiday, which should have been a good time, and found myself bursting into tears in a restaurant eating a meal that I was thoroughly enjoying... there was a chemical reaction between eating food and sometimes just drinking coffee and like a wave, a horrible black vile sort of wave of depression, almost physically came over my head in the same kind of physical way that a shudder goes down your spine; I would burst into tears and it was uncontrollable... I was convinced I was going mad... that is where I was after three months of starting this drug, to June 2001 which is just over a year ago now. I saw the doctor and he decided enough was enough and took me off Efavirenz and put me on Abacavir; Abacavir and Combivir equal Trizivir and that is what I am on now."

Peter stated that he had experienced a 'tough time' over the past 12 months but felt 'a hell of a lot better' since being taken off Efavirenz. He described his own health status as relatively good.

COLIN

Colin was 25 when he has diagnosed with HIV after voluntarily testing back in July 1985 and has lived with an AIDS diagnosis since 1995. He regularly goes for HIV health checks and is 'as healthy as your average 46 year old man who doesn't take enough exercise'. Colin has previously taken 5 different combination therapies and 2 other drugs to prevent other conditions. He describes his current treatment as effective with few adverse side effects at present; he has, at times, barely escaped death as a direct consequence of his HIV. I asked Colin to tell me about his experiences of taking drug treatments and what factors influenced him to start medication, he told me:

"I got all those sort of things that people get... I got Thrush; I got recurrent stomach bugs, and not just the same ones but different ones all the bloody time... I was running to the doctors with ghastly diarrhoea... gradually this got worse and worse until one batch of really awful diarrhoea, the doctor said 'this is crypto-sporidium and that means you have got an AIDS-defining condition'... that was 1995... I was losing a lot of weight and getting sicker and sicker and getting all sorts of things... I can never remember when I was really really really ill but it was late 1995 early 1996... I had constant diarrhoea and I just couldn't eat anything. I felt tired all the time... They put me on dual medication... I was on two nucleosides, that's right."

I asked Colin if the diarrhoea was a side effect of the drugs he was taking. He recounted how ill he had become and how he knew the difference between diarrhoea with side effects and its alternative. He continues to tell us:

"No, definitely not! That is one of the things that I know the difference with the side effects of AIDS drugs and AIDS-related diarrhoea and believe you and me they are absolutely different experiences. I still get diarrhoea because of the AIDS pills but that is just a bit of a nuisance and is easily controlled. We are talking about food going straight through you and having to wear a nappy and like literally kind of not being able to be more than, you know, 200 yards from a toilet ever... just yellow water pouring from you. It is horrible. I got shingles and I've got a few KS lesions but not too badly but I still had to have radiotherapy for them. But the really awful thing that frightened me was when I got M.A.C (see glossary) which took a long time to be diagnosed. It is like TB-like bacteria and that did two things: one it started giving me terrible pain, it was awful, awful, awful pain. First in my guts and then in my back here, awful back ache... it felt like a slipped disc... all my lymph nodes were blown up to the size of tennis balls. And then at the beginning of 1996 I suddenly started getting 104 degree fevers every day and you could control it by taking really strong pain killers; it was like clock work, as soon as the fever wore off I remember getting absolutely freezing cold and would shake like a leaf. I would have to be wrapped in duvets and then half an hour later I would be pouring with sweat and burning up...eventually they had to put me on morphine because no other painkillers worked...eventually they diagnosed this M.A.C. thing and I took antibiotics and that improved my health slightly...so as soon as it became available I basically demanded combination therapy with Saquinavir but that didn't work because it was very early days and they didn't know how to dose it properly. Then the next regime didn't work because it was Indinavir based on taking it three times a day away from food... I just couldn't discipline myself to take it... so it wasn't until my third combination and that worked dramatically, almost instantly, suddenly the diarrhoea dried up and I thought that it was working but that wasn't until October 1997."

Colin had been ill throughout 1995 until early 1997. As a volunteer in the HIV field he found that his combination therapy regime was difficult to adhere to in relation to his work life. He remembered:

"So the regime... those three tablets a day regimes were completely incompatible with... I mean they could help you live but they certainly couldn't help you have a life that is how I would define it... I should say that one of the awful things that happened to me in 1996 was that I had been taking an AZT-based combo and the AZT started making me dreadfully anaemic and I had to have two blood transfusions...Now I essentially take four drugs, which is five but one of them is Ritonavir which just boosts the other PI, so it is not really a main drug or ingredient in its own right. So it is Indinavir, 3TC, ddI, Efavirenz... I have been on that ever since... I take it 97 per cent of the time; I might forget a dose once a month and it works... I have been remarkably lucky with the side effects I think."

TOM

Tom was diagnosed in February of 1986 at the age of 39 after voluntarily testing; he has been living with an AIDS-diagnosis since 1991. Tom, however, prefers to think of himself as someone living with HIV because AIDS is such a powerfully evocative word and a label that Tom decided to give back to the medics. He describes his health as relatively good at present and goes for regular HIV check ups. His current combination therapy is Lamivudine, Abacavir and Nelfinavir. Tom has previously experienced a brain seizure and severe memory loss from two embolisms found in the frontal lobe area of his brain in the 1990s; he tells us in detail of his experiences of ill health whilst continuing to work in the HIV field:

"In 1993... I was on AZT and then I went on to ddI and I had two months on ddI and I was aware something strange was happening because I was just losing my sense of empowerment... I was having to work very very hard...And then I had a total blackout at a conference...it was quite funny because I was doing things which weren't me and yet I didn't challenge them... So I went up to the hotel room and then completely was in a haze and didn't remember anything... didn't go to dinner and got up in the morning... I had no sense of time... went down to the lobby... I don't know how many hours... the doormen repeatedly kept asking me if I was OK... my support was with me and she called my partner and I remember looking at my partner and then I don't remember anything for two months... initially it was thought to be a nervous breakdown and stress-related... Finally they sent me for an MRI which showed embolisms affecting emotion and memory; I had no memory; I had no speech and I was frequently incontinent and very uncooperative when asked to do anything different from whatever it was I was doing at the time... I made this amazing recovery. It didn't seem amazing to me but to everybody else it was... the following May my consultant and psychotherapist brought it to my attention that they thought the virus was taking me towards dementia... so I had tests again and the results were horrible... I decided to resign from work and had a big bash with friends and flew off to San Francisco... and then a week after that I had a brain seizure in San Francisco and had to come home."

Tom made a good recovery from this illness event and recounted how his first combination therapy impacted on his daily life. He tells us:

"Having been literally near death's door and consciously ready to die, the first combination therapy I had worked wonders and gave me energy to go to London to access the fourth drug I needed which was important... In a day-to-day sense it is intrusive like every twelve weeks I have to go to the hospital and get my prescription, which might take up to two or three hours to make up... I have a big box in there and every couple of weeks I have to top it up... you know the worst case scenario is 36 pills over 5 times a day but it's simplified now down to twice a day... I value that... I know what it's done to me and it doesn't seem that intrusive... When I was on Indinavir you had to be careful what you ate; it's like two hours before and two hours afterwards... the good thing was it actually made me eat lunch... sometimes it was inconvenient like when you are away or going out with friends for a meal so occasionally I didn't take it but I didn't feel guilty about it and I didn't allow it to rule my life either..."

Tom considers himself fortunate as in five years since he started combination therapy he has had only one high viral load test and his CD4 count has doubled. He speaks of previously experiencing side effects with specific drugs but these were minor and he was fortunate. He recalls:

"I had PCP because of the ddI which was one very obvious effect of taking the drug... Indinavir I have a suspicion that they might have caused a kidney stone because I was passing blood... I never felt pain or anything... I just had red urine."

PERRY

Perry was diagnosed in 1990 at the age of 28 after voluntarily testing for HIV. At the time of our interview, Perry was working, regularly went for HIV health checks and was taking combination therapy: ddI, Stavudine, Abacavir and Efavirenz. In addition he was also taking anti-depressant and anti-psychotic medication for a mental health condition. When I asked him about his medication and his role in the decision-making process, he told me:

"I just take whatever they tell me to take...but I do make my own judgements of the doctor. If it's a doctor that I wouldn't trust then I would certainly see if I can change and have done before...I feel ok with treatment but I do have a few side effects. I was having bad dreams which I think were to do with the Efavirenz so I started taking them in the mornings instead of night time...I am happy with the treatment... when I was first put on medication it wasn't successful. I was on Nevirapine and Indinavir and Saquinavir and a couple of others I cannot pronounce and they didn't work... Nelfinavir was another one as well... they didn't work at all and then I was put on the regime I am on at the moment, about three and a half years ago and I have never looked back."

Perry had a low CD4 count prior to his starting combination therapy and it was the doctor's decision to start medication; Perry recalled he was quite happy with this decision as 'you don't argue because you assume they are doing the best thing at the time'. His current regime is twice daily and he finds this unproblematic.

RICHARD

Richard was a happy 21 year old man when he was diagnosed in 1990 after voluntarily testing following the discovery of a close friend who had developed AIDS. He went for regular HIV check ups, was working part-time and was on combination therapy at the time of our interview: Nelfinavir, ddI, Stavudine and chlorphenamine. He considered himself relatively healthy despite his poor diet and his difficulty in taking care of himself. Richard lived with an AIDS diagnosis for many years. He was never fully compliant with drug treatments and as he worked within the HIV field was knowledgeable on HIV issues of treatments and side effects. I asked him how successful he considered his own medical treatment since the advent of HAART and he told me:

"I'd say it has been pretty good but there are real issues for me around poverty. It sounds strange but being able to make sure that you get three square meals a day is difficult... also you have to have the ability to be assertive about dealing with the medication. People with HIV are just expected to take the medication because it is on offer and you get given a big list of instructions and you do the counselling session and they talk you through the responsibilities... they make sure that you have to eat with such-and-such a drug and get plenty of sleep... It is really hard to do this for a lot of people whether you are ill or not... even harder if you're ill and you've lived with HIV a long time... it is incredibly difficult because you have to have the motivation and high self-esteem above everything else... let me give you a few case scenarios: say if you are out with a load of friends and you have to take medication... I take over 20 tablets a day and when you pull a big handful of tablets out of your pocket it is obvious that something is wrong. The other thing is that the tablets are not very small and they do make you feel bad... the other issue is ensuring you remember your medication... It's a nightmare! Then you get the guilt because you have forgotten your tablets... research is coming out which blames middle class men for lack of adherence and for the new strains of HIV. My feeling is this is unfair as it is difficult for us all to maintain strict treatment regimes every single day... my current regime is pretty good at twice daily but I have to stop eating anything at all after 9pm, so it is quite intrusive. "

Richard took the decision to stop taking AZT in earlier times (see chapter four). I asked him to tell me of his experiences with combination therapies and side effects. He told me:

"I do feel tired... I find it difficult to cope sometimes with the effects of my illness. The taking of tablets is extremely problematic for me as well as the side effects, especially loose stools...I have become resistant to many medications and then I have to stop taking them... I do believe I have a right to choose and express my views about taking treatment and how this impacts on the quality of my life. Your quality of life has to outweigh the issues that arise from medication... I have lost a considerable amount of weight and I look dreadful."

Richard spoke later about how some medicines had changed for the better and one personal problem he had was the actual swallowing of tablets. He struggled to swallow tablets from the onset, but told me:

"Medicines are also changing and being used in different ways, for example, they have lowered the dosage and made the amounts of tablets you take smaller. The tablet sizes have been reduced in some cases, which all make life a bit easier. Also treatments are more tolerable, for example, those tablets that were powdery tablets are now in capsule form so it is easier to swallow. DDI is a good example. I used to have to take it twice a day and it was like taking two Sterident tablets; this has been reduced to one very small capsule that you have to take every 24 hours. The other thing with DDI is that it has to be taken on an empty stomach. So to have an empty stomach twice a day is very difficult. This was one of my issues with treatment early on, whereas now it is easier to adhere to the right tablets at the right time."

Richard experienced many severe bouts of oral thrush and found eating extremely difficult during prolonged periods of his life. He recounted how he had good days and bad days and said the uncertainty of living with HIV had been a large part of his every day life since diagnosis. He remained proud 'to still be here' and maintained his sense of humour and increased his willingness to constantly learn alongside his ability to listen. On living with uncertainty he recounted:

"I get really annoyed sometimes; I pick out my file of letters from the doctors and I read about things that are happening that I really don't have much control over… being in this situation means that I have to carry on and live as best I can… when I learned about the promising outlook for a healthier life with the new combination therapies, I did think 'fucking bastards'! I was getting used to living with HIV and the consequences of dying and now I am going to have to live through all this again… when I wanted effective treatment it wasn't there and now I had gotten used to my condition I was going to have to think about being healthy again and maybe even going back to work… I had mixed feelings… early on it was OK to sweep us all under the carpet and let us die quietly and now things are changing with medication. I was pretty frightened when I look back."

Richard's anger and fear concerning uncertainty pertaining to new combination therapies and the potential revival of good health have been similarly voiced by many people living long-term with HIV outside of this study. Experiences of revival accompanying renewed health in the context of more effective HIV medicines have been met by confusion and uncertainty for many people who were once reconciled to their own death (the Lazarus Syndrome). Richard did believe HAART was a life-saving advancement, in spite of his experiences of taking combination therapies, adverse side effects and difficulties he often faced with non-compliance. Nevertheless, for Richard, the effectiveness of combination therapy did raise complex issues around uncertainty as it 'constantly changed the goal posts'.

WOODY

Woody was diagnosed in 1992 at the age of 35 after testing voluntarily; at the time of his HIV test, blood results revealed that his CD4 count was 250 and he was immediately put on the drug AZT. He reported that he did not feel ill during this time. Woody attends HIV check ups and considers himself as extremely healthy. He was working at the time of our interview and was on combination therapy: Tenofovir, Epivir (Lamivudine), Abacavir, Efavirenz and Septrin. Woody has taken other combination therapies previously and considers his current treatment as effective. I asked him to tell me of his experiences of taking combination therapy and what factors influenced him to start on medication, he recalled:

"I haven't had any AIDS-related illnesses and I haven't had anything that's been a direct cause of HIV…I took a couple of different HIV treatments for a year or two when they became available… whatever they're called anti-nucleoside drugs of the first generation… then I was on Stavudine and Lamivudine… I was on those two for may be a year and my CD4 count started to go down. I think that was just before or round about the time when viral loads were introduced. Anyway the blood results weren't good and so I changed onto a completely new regime of combination therapy… this meant increasing my tablet intake from probably four or five tablets a day to nineteen pills a day… I used to take them after meals except for the ddI which I used to have to take half an hour before or two hours after and that was the soluble one… then I got the pill for which is no food two hours either side, so I found that difficult. Because when I remembered it was usually when I was hungry… I wasn't on a three times a day dose I was on twice daily so this wasn't intrusive with my work life."

Woody, like others, spoke of how sometimes if he was out in a restaurant eating with others his medication was sometimes overlooked or he had to take them later than usual. Adherence therefore is very much a problematic issue when taking medication. Lying and secrecy was a big part of living with HIV; only a couple of close friends knew of Woody's positive status, and those who knew were HIV-positive themselves. He described his medication are relatively unproblematic but has experienced a few side effects. He spoke further of his experiences of taking his medication:

"When I first started on it, it was depressing with the number of pills that I had to take and I didn't stick rigidly to what I was supposed to… I sort of didn't let them rule my life. I did experience side effects. I lost a lot of weight and I have become less sexually inclined… yeah I sort of almost am well not impotent but there's been a severe decline in desire and performance… lots of wind and sticky shit which just used to stick to everything including my bottom, my underpants, my hairs… Diarrhoea at regular intervals but not so much recently… I mean I couldn't go to work or anything because it was very unpredictable bowel movements…nasty stuff that just used to stick to everything and you couldn't wipe it clean… I had to shave the hairs off because it just used to stick to it… I used to have skid marks in my underpants which I'd never had before… oh yes! I had peripheral neuropathy in my lips… tingling lips which lasted for a couple of months and then just disappeared. Sometimes there was just the feeling of not feeling particularly good, just feeling Yuk! Over the last two years I've lost a lot of weight and people have started to comment. Off my backside; off my legs; off my arms, and a bit off my face."

Woody told me how he coped with other people's comments and observations:

"I've had various bouts of bronchitis which may or may not be related to HIV but when people mention my weight loss I suppose the main way of coping with it is putting it down to this or my age because as you get older your body shape changes and you're more prone to either put on weight or lose weight, so I am passing it off mainly as an age-related thing."

TONY

Tony was diagnosed in 1994 at the age of 32 years following a prolonged bout of ill health for almost three years. Tony believed he was in denial during this period. At the time of our interview Tony stated he was fairly healthy but lethargy and a distinct lack of energy was becoming a source of major concern. He attends regular health checks for his HIV and is on combination therapy but cannot remember the names of the tablets he is taking. He is living with an AIDS diagnosis and awaiting a new combination therapy whilst continuing with his old regime. When I asked about the factors that influenced him taking combination therapy he stated:

"The doctors advised it because my T-cell count was going down and my viral load was increasing… I had been ill previously about a year before… I had this chest infection and I got rushed into hospital but I did think I could beat it… I was very ill so they pumped this white fluid into me and I was in for a week and I did get better. The doctors decided to take me off my medication at the time and I had a whole break from it for about a year…

eventually my T-cells were getting lower and my viral load increased... I was seeing so many different doctors at this time and I got pissed off with this... every time I went for my health checks it was a different doctor and I found that when I was getting my medication it was all wrong and the amounts and stuff... I used to point out that I had too many tablets. I wanted the same doctor for continuity."

Tony stated that he found all the information on HIV medication confusing and difficult to absorb, especially in earlier times; dosages and the amount of tablets to be taken on a daily basis were constantly being changed as more treatments became available. I asked him about his medication and possible side effects. He told me:

"Well I have all the normal stuff, diarrhoea, skin problems and osteoporosis. I have now developed a problem with my eyes. I have really high cholesterol and I have high blood pressure. These are all, I am told, side effects of the various drugs I have taken over the years for my HIV... I get overwhelmed with the information and having to comply with the medication but I do try."

SANDRA

In 1994 Sandra was 29 years old when she discovered she was HIV-positive; her five month old son had been admitted to hospital and later died of an AIDS-related illness. She voluntarily tested at the hospital where the medical team were desperately trying to identify her son's illness condition. Sandra aged 37 years describes herself as reasonably healthy. She is medically retired and started attending regular HIV check ups in 1996. Sandra was on combination therapy (Nevirapine and Combivir) at the time of our interview. When I asked her about medication issues since taking combination therapy, she told me:

"I didn't start going for regular check ups until around 1996 and I found out my CD4 count had gone down and all that stuff so I decided to take whatever help was going... I started reading up on things on the Net and tried to tailor a combination therapy that would suit me... it was difficult to find something that was acceptable. You know, initially it was a case of taking twenty six tablets a day and that was a nightmare... the side effects were horrendous. I have gained a lot of weight in strange places. I look like I am seven months pregnant... it is body fat redistribution; I have got a hump on the back of my neck and that doesn't shift regardless of what I do... this is a result of those Protease Inhibitors, Saquinavir, for about two and a half years... Initially I didn't know of the side effects, it was a case of you are unwell, so take these tablets and see if you feel better... so you feel grateful just to be offered this chance of life. After a while, you think 'Wait a minute! The quality of life doesn't come into it'."

We have learned about body fat redistribution from other story-tellers and side effects such as these were largely unknown within the medical community for a number of years. Sandra continued to tell me about her second combination therapy:

"I got onto this second drug Efavirenz which had been hyped up as a good strong drug, which it is... I didn't really understand what the side effects would be, especially for somebody who is 'drug naïve' in terms of recreational drugs... I was like a zombie. I felt crazy most of the time. People who take recreational drugs kind of found it great because it puts them on a different plane but for me it was a nightmare... It was really good in terms of suppressing the virus; it killed the viral load but I was confused most of the time. My memory would lapse and you know one day I went into a filling station and filled up with petrol and got into the car and I couldn't remember how to drive the car. I just could not... I was so frightened. Apart from that there were the nightmares so I decided that even though it was fantastic for suppressing the virus, I couldn't possibly stay on it... I mean I got done for going through red lights, I got a fine and went to court and all the rest... it was a nightmare."

Sandra went on to tell me that she was now a diabetic as a result of the drugs she has previously taken; she recalls:

"There is evidence now that prolonged use of protease inhibitors can bring on diabetes and I am now diabetic... Yes and I have high cholesterol and lipids... now I am on my third combination which kind of limits my options because I have chopped and changed but it seems to agree with me... I have taken these now for six or seven months and it is workable as I take two tablets twice a day... there are minimal side effects for me and I can live with it and you kind of get into a relationship with the drugs where it is just automatic; it is just a part of life... I take my tablets after I feed my cats and then do it again in the evening, so it becomes part of your life."

Sandra initially started on combination therapy when she became unwell and exhausted. She had experienced several reoccurring chest infections and she considered her immunity to be low. Sandra then explored the Internet to find out about the various combination therapies that were available so she could 'take some control and gain empowerment over her own biomedical treatment'.

On waiting for salvage therapy

At the time of our interview, neither Tyler nor Rick were taking combination therapies as they were both waiting for new, more suitable, treatments to be made available due to resistance issues. For both men, combination therapies had been problematic in the past and salvage therapy was their only hope at this time.

TYLER

Tyler was diagnosed back in 1984 with HTLVIII at the age of 38 following a routine sexual health check after a short bout of ill health. There was little information at this time and following his HIV-positive diagnosis his life totally changed. Tyler went for regular check ups at his HIV clinic and had stopped taking medication at the time of our interview. His health was poor and he struggled with his chest and breathing from difficulties associated with asthma and emphysema; he also reported memory problems which he put down to HIV. Tyler was awaiting salvage therapy and lived each day at a time. When I asked him about his medication and experiences he told me:

"I have to live my life around HIV because it has affected me so much with energy levels and other things like my memory problems, so yeah it IS my life…I was on combination therapy which was working quite well and then I lost my mother and I lost my dad all in eighteen months…the guilt was unbearable and I had a failed suicide attempt… it seemed futile going down that road again as I didn't have the confidence to do anything successfully so I decided that the alternative was to stop the drugs. I had a word with my consultant and told him I was stopping… so I stopped for about 10 months and I started getting really bad Thrush down my throat onto my lungs… it was really painful and the doctor told me I needed to go back on combination therapy… because I couldn't stand the pain I really had no alternative but to go back on the drugs. But then like it was an about turn because then it was the drugs doing the damage and they had to take me off them… it cleared up the Thrush but I got really bad skin across the whole of my body… it was a mess and I couldn't handle it so they took me off the drugs until my skin got better… it was a matter of maintaining a quality of life… I think it was too much poison in my body over the years."

Tyler recalled some of his other personal experiences when he was taking previous medication:

"We did have a cock-up, for want of a better expression, where they gave me some, I can't remember the name of the drug now, but instead of the normal capsule I was taking once in a morning, they gave me these two huge tablets and it made me poorly… I wasn't eating and I lost a stone in two weeks and I was feeling sick so I listened to my body and stopped taking it and when it was time to go and see my consultant he told me 'how the hell have you got those because they were supposed to be pulled off the market twelve months ago because of these side effects'… I got them from the Chemist and the doctor went ballistic."

If Tyler had persisted with these tablets he might not have been here to relate his experiences. I asked him over the years how intrusive his medication had been and he told me:

"My last combination therapy was difficult… when I was on Combivir and whatever else somehow it was never a problem for me. I never ever missed a pill. But then after I took a year off my drugs it's suddenly a different ball game… when he put me back on them it was a nightmare because it was like: one at 7 o'clock on an empty stomach; one at 8 o'clock before a meal so then I had to eat at 9 o'clock whether I wanted to eat or not and I had to have a pill with that food, then I had to have a pill at 10 an hour after… I had real bad ulcers and your ulcer pill can't be taken anywhere near any of the other pills so that was 12 o'clock for the ulcer one… and then 2 o'clock for another one that couldn't be taken with HIV pills. Then you start it all over again at like 7 o'clock at night which means my dinner is at 6 o'clock… I can't change that because my body is so used to it but then I am having to force my supper down me at 9 instead of 11 to take my pills and it's horrendous… I found it very very difficult… now I am not on any combination therapy just the prophylaxis to stop pneumonia."

Tyler had built up resistance to most of the combination therapies he had previously taken and there was no suitable combination therapy available at the time of our interview; he was waiting for new treatments to emerge.

RICK

Rick was 21 years old when he tested positive for a second time back in 1990. He regularly attended HIV health-check ups, was not taking combination therapy and was awaiting salvage therapy at the time of our interview. Rick recounted how he had possibly taken up to 10 different combination therapies over the years and was unclear of all of the names. He told me of how he had previously suffered severe side effects; at the time of our interview he was experiencing severe bouts of ill health and dealing with stress due to current changes with his medical practitioners. When asked about medical treatment over the years, Rick told me:

"I have had about 10 combinations and I have been in a few trials and AZT made me anaemic so I had to have blood transfusions... some tablets made me sick, a lot of protease inhibitors don't agree with me, although they are good for my blood results... they have given me lipodystrophy, they have raised my lipids, my cholesterol and I am on other drugs to control the diarrhoea... the diarrhoea to me is the most important thing at the moment because you lose so much weight... but you know some of the combination therapies have been good for me... like I say Ritonavir and Saquinavir together got me down to six and half stones in the space of two weeks, but I had good blood results but bad side effects."

Rick also lived with congenital heart disease which was not related to HIV but his compromised immune system and subsequent poor health did not help this condition. He reported that over the last few years his medication was largely unproblematic until recently; yet he recalled as have other story-tellers about how intrusive the medication was in earlier times. He told me:

"The combination therapy when it first came out was like so intrusive... I mean when I was abroad, me and my friend had to go to the toilet to take our tablets... I had them in a bag in my pocket... also I used to visit a German family several times a year and I had to hide them and each day I had to get the right amount so that when we were out or if they were not in the house I could suddenly go to the toilet to take them... the drugs have got better now as most of them are just once or twice a day... At the moment HIV is a very large part of my life because I've got a lot of appointments, as there are a lot of different things wrong with me with all the treatments I have had."

Rick had been advised to stop his current combination therapy some six weeks before our interview. He was awaiting more suitable treatment and was experiencing problems at his HIV clinic due to members of staff leaving. Rick stated that some four weeks earlier he had embarked upon private treatment for lipodystrophy to his face; he had undergone facial injections to fill out the hollows in his face. As this type of treatment was not available on the NHS, Rick had decided to go privately as his facial features were a concern to him and a well documented side effect of the drugs he had previously taken.

As we close this chapter, it is interesting to learn how for many story-tellers who go for regular HIV health checks, the medical monitors that predict health and subsequent illness are not always congruent with how people actually feel in relation to their own health status. We are also left to wonder why some people are asymptomatic and therefore not taking medication whilst others are symptomatic. HIV certainly affects different individuals in different ways.

It has been revealed how story-tellers have had to tolerate and manage complex drug regimes in earlier days and adherence has been difficult to negotiate in every day life. Taking some tablets with food and others on an empty stomach and some two hours either way is undoubtedly intrusive in everyday life. Many story-tellers have spoken of severe side effects which include: diarrhoea, sickness, skin rashes, severe headaches, hallucinations, mood swings, suicidal tendencies and body fat redistribution (Lipodystrophy); the specific term used for fat loss and thinning of the face is Lipoatrophy which is seldom used here. Certain Protein Inhibitors have presented other illness conditions such as anaemia, diabetes, high cholesterol, osteoporosis and systemic Thrush.

For many of our story-tellers who were medically advised to embark upon HIV combination therapy at a time when they felt relatively healthy, these drug regimes simply made them ill. Many medical practitioners were unaware of the severe side effects of earlier combination therapies for many years and the personal experiences of HIV medicines have been quite astounding. It is evident that many story-tellers, over the years, have decided to judge their own health status rather than being reliant on medical judgements. Quality of life issues are of extreme importance to us all, yet appear to have been largely overlooked by the medical profession during the advent of HAART.

The expectation of medical practitioners in relation to how people living with HIV and AIDS should strictly comply with complicated drug regimes is implicit. We have uncovered how these drug regimes were simply too difficult or challenging to manage on a daily basis and were not without consequences from a health perspective. I ask you the reader to reflect and explore how these personal experiences have impacted on your own beliefs. How might you have coped with complex combination therapies? How would you have managed severe side effects? How would you

A forgotten generation: Long-term survivors' experiences of HIV and AIDS

balance the side effects of HIV drugs with quality of life issues? Can you sympathise with any of the issues raised here? What have you learned in this chapter? As usual I ask that you consider your own feelings, beliefs and attitudes and reflect on whether these remain the same or might they have changed and if so why?

A forgotten generation: Long-term survivors' experiences of HIV and AIDS

CHAPTER SEVEN

Taking control: experiencing the medical profession

∞

"The medicalisation of early diagnosis not only hampers and discourages preventative health care but it also trains the patient-to-be to function in the meantime as an acolyte to his doctor. He learns to depend on the physician in sickness and in health. He turns into a life-long patient."

Ivan Illich

Introduction

Medicine is characteristically regarded as a practice because it is what doctors and specialists *do* professionally as an occupation; this is why we talk of doctors, clinicians and specialist consultants as medical practitioners. The structure of the medical profession, both as a profession and a practice, is deep-rooted in moral rules and comprises of specialist forms of knowledge, methods and technical skills that have to be learned. When we turn to the medical profession for help, we usually enter into the 'patient role' whereby often supposed shared norms, obligations and mutual expectations are not always compatible between medical practitioners and patients. The medical profession have a presumed medical expertise and their technical and specialist training typically relies on approaching the medical consultation with the specific aim of proficient diagnosis of an illness or disease and active treatment intervention.

The patient, by contrast, approaches the medical encounter often with a more divergent or wide ranging set of goals. We, as patients, have personal and social agendas which relate to the effects of our illness on daily activities and our relationship with ourselves and our social world. Arguably, in many ways, medical training and the agenda of medical professionals might typically discourage them from seeing us as whole persons whom embody social, emotional and spiritual components as well as health-related facets to our individual lives. The professional dominance of doctors and specialists is often enhanced by their control over their interaction with patients; this is, nonetheless, continually changing with multidisciplinary approaches to health care practices and different types of relationships currently emerging which significantly shift the balance of power and mutual expectations of those involved.

Our roles as patients can be qualitatively different when we interact with health care practitioners, such as nurses, nurse consultants, health advisers, dentists, nutritionists, than say a doctor or specialist consultant. It is further recognised that relationships between doctors, specialists, consultants and clinic nurses and those of the patient can vary dramatically in accordance with where the medical encounter takes place; in other words, the institutional context or social setting is an important factor which affects how we interact and experience these relationships. Dependent on whether our medical encounter takes place at the doctor's surgery, or in a hospital, or at the patient's home or at a primary care clinic this can significantly impact on how we interact with medical practitioners. The introduction of health centres and primary care clinics in the UK means that other health care professionals, other than doctors and specialists, are now interacting more with people seeking medical care. Such changes in health care provision brings with it changes in hierarchical relationships and significantly reduces the power of medical professionals generally. Indeed, a multidisciplinary approach to health care provision means that we, as patients, may interact with a team of medical professionals during one consultation which significantly changes our roles as a patient.

Often we tend to overlook these important factors in our general encounters with medical and health care professionals. Yet it is important to tease out and recognize how we come to socially accept dominant sources of medical knowledge and how this, in turn, effects the balance of power during our medical encounter. How do we negotiate medical knowledge, power and control over our own lives within medical consultations for chronic illness? In earlier times, doctors and patients rarely spoke to each other about the consequences of illness; doctors often did not adapt their medical recommendations around a patient's lifestyle and did little to encourage a patient to express their own viewpoints on potential treatments or medical outcomes. Nowadays, especially in terms of chronic illness, we are witnessing a more open approach between patients and medical practitioners. To be sure, patients are becoming more active in decision making around treatments by assessing the risks and benefits for themselves. The rise of chronic illnesses, like HIV, have created patient-led self-help groups which has improved our awareness of medical matters and patients are now becoming the 'experts' of their own illness conditions during medical encounters.

A forgotten generation: Long-term survivors' experiences of HIV and AIDS

Changes in health care provision and widespread access to knowledge and information on health and illness matters means the patient does not always take on a passive role within medical consultations. The nature of compliance has now shifted from no longer 'abiding by the rules' of the doctor; instead we are taking a more active role in successfully managing and negotiating medical treatments to fit in with our social and personal lifestyles. We are now witnessing more mutual co-operation between medical practitioners and patients during medical consultations. For chronic illness conditions, such as HIV, the continuity of health care means that HIV specialists and patients have often developed an established relationship over a long period of time from multiple consultations. So who are the HIV experts? How do long-term survivors experience HIV medical and health care professionals?

What we have come to recognise in previous chapters is that living with HIV and AIDS presents various levels of medical uncertainty and anxiety within a health and illness context and can, therefore, be a major challenge on a day-to-day basis. Facing the unknown has been one of the most significant causes of HIV-related stress. Hope is essential for all human beings in order to create meaning in our disordered lives; it gives us an optimistic focus and allows us the prospect of a more promising future for the rest of our life span. Living with HIV and AIDS has not always offered individuals the luxury of anticipating time and presuming long life, as we have previously seen. Until the advent of more effective medical treatments, like HAART, becoming widely accessible, questionably, hope and optimism was overshadowed by ignorance, fear, uncertainty and imminent death.

In chapter six, our attention was in part drawn to how the advent of HAART from late 1996 onwards had led to more optimism in relation to living longer. Even so, prolonged periods of good health were, in many cases, compromised when HIV combination therapies became part of everyday life especially in earlier times. For those women and men who were medically defined as *asymptomatic* and not taking combination therapies, this raised questions as to why some people maintained health and a good quality of life without medicine whilst others did not. As we have witnessed, adherence and compliance issues to complex HIV combination regimens had often been difficult to negotiate and successfully manage in daily life, especially in relation to severe side effects of certain drug treatments.

From a medical perspective, it has been recognised and clinically proven that less than excellent adherence to combination therapies resulted in virus breakthroughs and the emergence of drug-resistant strains of HIV. In addition, cross-resistance amidst drugs in the protease inhibitor category can severely compromise the effectiveness of future treatments. It is fair to say that earlier combination therapies for HIV were the most complex drug regimens ever prescribed in terms of previous treatments for other chronic illness conditions. People living with HIV and AIDS who embarked on medical treatment were given the daunting responsibility to comply with their medicines regardless of quality of life issues and the impact of severe side effects. The medical profession have since had to deal with adherence issues due to the unrealistic assumption that individuals can and will comply with complex drug regimens regardless of outcome.

We cannot ignore how the balance of power within our relationships with medical and health care professionals can affect decision-making processes for the management of a chronic illness like HIV. Knowledge and power are undoubtedly interrelated. What counts as expert knowledge and how is it practiced within an HIV context? Of course, how medical health professionals and patients successfully and effectively negotiate specific information does vary according to the type of illness condition. Throughout the duration of long-term treatment plans for any chronic illness, like HIV, we often see how the balance of power changes and requires a re-negotiation of these relationships towards a more mutual participation. Many patients who have lived long-term with a chronic illness condition are likely to become increasingly more expert about their experiences of illness and thus assume a more challenging and assertive role in relation to their own health care management. How have long-term survivors of HIV experienced medical and health care practitioners over a prolonged period of time?

The dominant driving force of this chapter is to bring to light how long-term survivors' have personally experienced and managed their HIV in terms of active, passive, or mutual participation with the medical health profession concerning decisions about health and complex drug treatments since diagnosis. We explore divergent personal experiences of the medical profession which began when HIV medical knowledge was still in its infancy and explore these encounters right up until the time of our interviews in 2002. How was HIV knowledge and expertise shared between long-term survivors and medical professionals? To what extent was HIV prejudice and discrimination evident within the medical profession? It is to these matters we now turn to reveal the many ways in which the medical profession has been experienced by our long-term survivors who share with us their stories.

A forgotten generation: Long-term survivors' experiences of HIV and AIDS

Living with Haemophilia and HIV: scepticism and issues of trust

We begin with the personal experiences and perceptions of our story-tellers who live with Haemophilia and who, as a consequence, contracted HIV through contaminated blood products. Without exception, all four men conveyed a deep-rooted scepticism of the medical profession and pharmaceutical industry. We must remind ourselves that, dependent upon the severity of their Haemophilia, each person regularly interacted with the medical profession and experienced medical treatment and hospitalisation since early childhood. Equally we are reminded that Haemophilia is not a disease but a disorder of blood clotting. All four story-tellers have contracted not only HIV, but Hepatitis C Virus (hereinafter called HCV) from contaminated blood products and were, at the time of interview, awaiting further test results to learn whether or not they had now contracted new variant Creutzfeldt-Jakob Disease (CJD). Whilst all were sceptical of the medical profession because of how they had contracted HIV, each story-teller assumed an active role in their HIV health care and believed they had a 'tolerant' or good working relationship with their current HIV medical practitioners. To these narratives we now turn:

SPIKE

Spike aged 27 was the youngest member of the study and was therefore only a child when he discovered his HIV-positive status somewhere around 1981 to 1983. He contracted HIV and HCV through contaminated Factor VIII blood products and he started HIV combination therapy in 1997. Spike accesses a Haematology unit in his local area and regularly attends health checks for all his illness conditions. His own active involvement with the medical profession from the onset of his diagnosis is somewhat different to other individuals in this story-of-stories; Spike was only about 8 or 10 years old when he was diagnosed with HTLVIII. He did however speak about his Mother's involvement around issues surrounding how he contracted HIV through contaminated blood products and subsequent encounters with the medical profession. He tells us:

"My Mum got other Mothers together and stuff in relation to Haemophiliacs and got a support group together in our local area because she wanted to know why this had happened… there weren't any treatments about at this time… there was nothing on the scene except perhaps a pressure group but the Haemophilia Society didn't do anything at this time… they were pretty apathetic and so they [the pressure group] had to do it themselves… my Mum was never given any answers; she was always just sort of fobbed off and then there were compensation claims… the MacFarlane Trust was set up to distribute funds and they're still going but we Haemophiliacs were initially given like £20,000… I was probably a bit older then when me and Mum… I was probably about 13… this was about 1988… me and my Mum we were going to get the money and we were looked down upon by the people at the hospital because we were basically suing them almost if you know what I mean… you know suing them or blaming them for what happened to us… I was only quite young then but I knew it caused a ruction between my consultant at the Children's hospital and the people who were claiming… I suppose claiming is the right word… well perhaps not all the medical profession, but I know where I was my Mum said that they frowned upon us going with the legal side because Haemophiliacs went in one group to claim against the medical profession and they frowned upon us for joining this group."

When I asked Spike about his relationship with the medical profession he told me:

"You have to pick things up along the way and find out information otherwise you don't learn anything. Doctors tell you minimal amounts; they don't like to empower their patients. My current consultant I have a really good relationship with and I wouldn't change that. I know some Haemophiliacs who don't like their consultants but I am really comfortable with him… he listens to what I have got to say and we discuss any changes to my health care together. He doesn't predominate what happens to my health care… but that's only because I have got to that position because I have gone out of my way to learn about HIV, HIV treatments and Hepatitis C and stuff… you have to go out and learn about these issues. I have a friend in London who is a Haemophiliac and co-infected with Hep C and his T-cells are something like 600. He's never touched a tablet in his life; he's never had any trouble and he's been infected for probably 20 years… he doesn't care; he just works and doesn't care much for learning about treatments because he doesn't need to, you see, so I suppose it's dependent upon the position you are in."

Spike spoke further about his perceptions and experiences of medical professionals relating to his own health care management. He tells us:

"I believe if you are considering treatments you need to learn for yourself about these issues because if you are not empowered then you can't look after your own health care needs and if you can't look after yourself then who can? I know doctors are meant to do this but you can rely on them too much…I am quite an easy-going person but I know the consultant I had at the Children's hospital had somewhat of a reputation... he was, well I don't know, not a philistine but he just did things and worried afterwards and stuff; I don't believe he has the real care of his patient at heart... that might be a bit harsh perhaps but he had the nickname of 'Doctor Death' and I'm sure you'll come across other Haemophiliacs who had him as a consultant when they were young... I didn't have too many problems with him but I consider myself now to be miles ahead of him."

Spike recounted how he had encountered problems with his Health Authority in relation to not getting the appropriate treatment he wanted because of lack of funds. He recalled:

"Well I have just been making an application to my Health Authority for funding for the synthetically produced Factor VIII because there are all the issues about the probable transmission of new variant CJD in blood products. I have made quite a succinct argument I believe and my application was rejected. I have appealed and this has now been rejected and it's all because of lack of money and politics. This makes me mad because stuff is still being passed on to us via contaminated blood products. Why haven't lessons been learned?"

Whilst Spike is unsurprisingly rather sceptical of the medical profession because of the way he contracted HIV and HCV, he currently enjoys a comfortable working relationship with his consultant and chooses to access all his health care needs at his Haematology unit.

GLYNN

Glynn aged 37 years lives with Haemophilia and was diagnosed with HTLVIII back in 1983 at the age of 17 or 18. He contracted HIV and HCV through contaminated Factor VIII blood products and is currently not on HIV combination therapy as he is medically defined as asymptomatic. Glynn regularly attends medical health checks every three months for his Haemophilia and every six months for his HIV condition at his local Haemophilia centre. He received compensation from the MacFarlane Trust for the way in which he contracted HIV and is currently awaiting the outcome for his claim for Hepatitis C. When I asked him about his experiences with the medical profession for his HIV, he told me:

"I have got no tablets to take for my HIV so I guess I would listen to them but I would way up the pros and cons... If they came to me now and said I think we need to start medication, even though I am not ill, I would probably say no I'm alright… I would ask them the reasons behind this as I know things have changed and the treatments have improved but I don't think I would start on medication unless I needed to… You know, if I have got a bad bleed I know I need Factor VIII but it is not so easy with HIV because I have never really known a lot about it… I would be guided by the profession but that doesn't mean that I have to bloody do everything they tell me."

I asked Glynn to describe how he felt about the way he contracted HIV and HCV from contaminated blood products and he recounted:

"I am annoyed about it but I also needed the treatment whether or not it was infected if you like… I mean I needed the treatment and it just so happened that the treatment was infected with the HIV virus. How do I feel about the blood products being contaminated? Pissed off about it because of what we had been told about how it got there… they just told us it was through the American sale of blood mainly from those who were injecting drugs and homosexuals… so that was it… we used to hate gays for ages, you know… I don't particularly think like that now but for a time you just didn't mention the word, but then we found out more and more about it and this wasn't necessarily the case…I was angry with the medical profession and we went through a court battle… I wrote to my MP but I was being guided because I was being told what to do through the solicitors and so I was angry that the Government compensated to a certain degree but it wasn't a lot… but we have now contracted this bloody Hep C haven't we and I don't think anything will ever come of that… I am registered with the MacFarlane trust because they sorted out all the compensation… I get like a pension from them every month."

Glynn went on to tell me about his experiences with medical professionals after he had disclosed his HIV-positive status to doctors and nurses during earlier times in his life. He tells us:

"Oh yes! I disclosed my status to doctors and nurses and I mean stupid bloody things used to get me really angry when I was in hospital… you look back and you think… well, I just laugh about it now because it's not that bad now. I mean there were times when I was in an isolation ward or something with bloody great posters and biohazard stickers stuck on the door saying 'Danger of infection' and all these doctors and nurses walked in as though they were bloody going to go to Mars or something… Gowns and masks and gloves and everything… I ate with plastic knives and forks and paper plates and things like this… peeing in cardboard bottles… this was because I had HIV and I mean it never used to happen to me before… it used to make me angry. I swore a lot at them and told them what I thought of them... You know if anyone should be dressed up in a gown with a mask on, it should be me and not them as they gave me the bloody infection."

Because in the past Glynn has lived with rather severe Haemophilia, medical treatment has always been a large part of his life; the medical profession, therefore, 'does not faze' him. He presently has a good working relationship with his medical team and does not consider himself as a passive recipient of medical treatment. His HIV currently causes limited disruption in his life as he has experienced prolonged good health to date.

PAUL

Paul aged 38 lives with Haemophilia and was diagnosed in 1985 with HTLVIII as part of a mass screening process at the age of 21. He contracted HIV and HCV via contaminated Factor VIII blood products and started HIV combination therapy after a severe bout of ill health in late 1996. Like Spike and Glynn, Paul was born with Haemophilia and is therefore used to medical treatment being a part of everyday life. He regularly attends health checks for all his illness conditions and considers his current HIV medical treatment as effective. As we learned previously, Paul held a deep cynicism and mistrust of the pharmaceutical industry (see chapter four). When I asked him about his experiences of the medical profession in relation to his HIV, he told me:

"... my attitude to the doctors has changed over the years, as well as my attitude to my health care workers...the people in charge of my health now aren't the same people that was in charge of my health care when I was infected with HIV... my doctors have all changed... over the years I have become more involved with knowledge and treatments. Going to conferences and getting involved with the medicine side of HIV, I think it is all very interesting and I have got a lot more time for drug companies now... so yeah medicine has got to be a good thing... I think that it is really important to state this, you see, among my HIV friends, hospitals freak them out. I went to hospital when I was about one onwards and I have spent most of my time in hospital wards... I spent my whole life going at least to hospital appointments for blood tests and trips to pick up my Factor VIII from hospital and trips to see Haematologists and so on. Going to hospitals and sitting in clinics has always been part of my life so my HIV has not been much of a problem because all my life I have had medical problems"

Paul spoke further about how unjust it has been to divide people into 'innocent victims' and those who might be considered 'guilty' of contracting HIV. Whilst he had been infected with HIV through contaminated Factor VIII blood products, Paul objected to the fact that as a person living with Haemophilia he had been labelled and tagged as an 'innocent victim'. He told me:

"All the tagging as 'innocent victims' that we have been labelled with, sets people with Haemophilia up against other people who contracted HIV via other transmission routes through no fault of their own... if we are labelled 'innocent' then this presumes that others are guilty... I think that the other thing is the fact that we, as Haemophiliacs, have been given a pay off in 1991 and the MacFarlane Trust was set up for us for financial support. I have been approached and told 'it is alright for you, you have had cash for this virus'. I used to feel guilty."

Prior to Paul experiencing severe bouts of ill health due to his HIV-positive status, he understandably held a deep-rooted cynicism of the medical profession and the Government due to how he contracted HIV and HCV. Since then, Paul's active participation in the HIV field has armed him with the power of knowledge which, in turn, subsequently changed his views in relation to medical practitioners and HIV combination therapies as a whole.

MARTIN

Martin aged 38 was diagnosed with HTLVIII back in September 1985; he was tested as part of the mass screening process for people living with Haemophilia. He contracted HIV and HCV through contaminated Factor VIII blood products and was currently awaiting test results to discover whether he had since contracted new variant CJD via the same route. Martin is medically defined as asymptomatic, is extremely fit and healthy and was not taking combination therapy at the time of our interview. He attends regular medical health checks for Haemophilia, HIV and HCV at his local Haemophilia Centre and considers himself 'lucky', as he has not suffered unduly with severe problems associated with Haemophilia or HIV. Living with Hepatitis C (HCV) however, was becoming problematic for Martin and he was taking Interferon for his HCV-related complications. When I asked Martin how he considered his relationship with the medical profession, he told me:

"I tolerate them I suppose. I find that they don't want to listen; in a sense, they will listen as if they are trying to listen but I don't know if they take in what you say... I think that they follow the book and they don't look at people and they are not as well informed as I would like them to be. For example, I heard about a genetic defect called Delta 32 and my doctor had never heard of it. I had gone to him and said I would like to know if this is the reason why I am alive and my brother is not and how can I get tested? He said if I could get some stuff on it he would have a look. But now he has left and I have to build up a new relationship with my doctor before I approach this again...As a specialist, I suppose, you do tend to expect certain things and when they don't appear to be listening, you do expect them to advise you rather than be advised. "

Martin told me that because he had experienced prolonged periods of good health in relation to his HIV, he had not explored different avenues for HIV care at his Haemophilia Centre as he did not feel it necessary. When I asked him to describe how he felt about the way in which he contracted HIV and HCV, he told me:

"I don't feel strongly either way to be honest. I am not angry. I know a lot of people who are, I suppose, my Dad was angry... I am not. They put labels on people like 'gays', 'lesbians', 'French', 'German' and these are just labels for great big groups and we all say how we hate the French but I have never met an actual French person I have disliked and the same with gay people. I don't blame them at all. If I were to blame anybody it would have to be the Thatcher government because as I understand it, they were aware of the risks of contaminated blood and they didn't do anything about it... so it would be the Establishment but I don't feel any anger to anybody. It happened. I don't blame the medical profession either. What is the point? It is done and hatred would damage me more than it would damage anybody else... in terms of blame it would have to be the Government because they knew about it and didn't introduce measures and I think that was the basis of the compensation. The fact that the Administration said that the UK would be self-sufficient in blood products by a said date and it wasn't and I think that this was the period when most people contracted HIV."

Martin considered his medical care for his Haemophilia as unproblematic and because of his good health had not experienced HIV specialist care other than regular HIV health checks. The treatment of Interferon for Hepatitis C was causing some problems in terms of disruptions to his emotive state; he had a tendency to get emotional for no particular reason which is a known side effect of this drug. For Martin, the crucial search for an explanation as to why he was still alive whilst others were not, especially his brother who died of AIDS some 10 years previously, was something the medical profession could not answer.

Trust, compliance and medics as experts: taking on a passive role

Many of the story-tellers accounts of personal experiences revealed here speak of levels of trust, passivity and compliance during interactions with the medical profession. All believe that they have a good-to-excellent working relationship with the medical profession. Four story-tellers are medically defined as asymptomatic yet three out of the four were taking combination therapy. Only one long-term survivor was not taking combination therapy due to him waiting for salvage therapy. Interestingly, all but two of our story-tellers had been diagnosed from 1990 onwards when advanced scientific knowledge of HIV and AIDS had become more firmly established. Few considered that they had adopted an active role in finding out information about HIV and medical treatments since learning about their diagnoses. We start with those diagnosed the earliest, setting out a chronological order, to learn how medical practitioners and our story-tellers interacted during medical consultations and how knowledge and medical matters were negotiated and shared.

TYLER

Tyler aged 54 was diagnosed with HTLVIII in 1984 at the age of 38 after voluntarily testing following a short bout of ill health. At the time of our interview his health was poor and he was awaiting salvage therapy due to having resistance issues with current HIV medicines; he was therefore not taking combination therapy for HIV at the time of our interview. In the past, Tyler had stopped his HIV treatment for numerous reasons including experiencing severe side effects. He went for regular HIV health checks. When I asked him how best he would describe his relationship with the medical profession he told me:

"Oh, it is good… they have been excellent with me. I mean I had or should I say still have Herpes. All the drugs failed; they had me in hospital for a week, giving me drugs intravenously for it… they have been excellent with me… they are doing all they can under the circumstances so I can't complain about them… I am not one of these who will come and sit at the computer and learn everything about HIV and go to the doctor and say 'this is what I want!' The point is it is their job, they know more than I do and they'll know more than I'll ever pick up on and I might get things the wrong way round... so I listen to them and if they recommend something I will go for it... but if something is doing me harm and I know it, I will stop irrespective of the doctors. I will listen to my body."

Tyler considered his relationship with his HIV health care practitioners as excellent and did not believe he had a good working knowledge of HIV-related issues. He did not report or recall any experiences of prejudice or discrimination on the grounds of his HIV-positive status and trusted the medical profession as 'experts'.

CHRISTOPHER

Christopher aged 51 was diagnosed in 1988 at the age of 36 whilst in hospital for an arthritic problem. He is medically defined as asymptomatic and has not experienced any HIV-related illness since diagnosis; Christopher is currently taking combination therapy for HIV and is very healthy and fit and works full time. He has the utmost trust in the medical profession and has a good working relationship with all his health professionals. When I asked him about his knowledge and awareness of HIV-related issues and his relationship with the medical profession, he told me:

"I don't read stuff very well, so I have attended some talks and joined groups where you can discuss health issues... I have had nothing but excellent support through the hospitals and with my GPs. I consider myself very lucky because if I wanted to know anything I just sort of ask... I am not that bothered about stuff, if this makes sense... I suppose I am quite ignorant still about my own condition. I know about me and my body but I don't know that much about the illness really... I shut things out. That is the way I am... a little knowledge can be dangerous. I trust the medical profession so therefore I trust the experts. I will go with what they say. I mean I do go to them with questions: for example, if somebody is just taking one drug whereas I have to take six, eight, nine or ten tablets a day I might say to my doctor, 'I have met somebody who only takes this and that, what are my chances of going on this treatment?' and my consultant will say: 'that might be right for them, but you are healthy and doing well without side effects, so why rock the boat? So we just leave things as they are."

Christopher had an extremely positive mental approach to life and has remained healthy in relation to HIV since diagnosis. His HIV treatment is effective with no adverse side effects and he considers himself lucky despite having had two strokes (unrelated to HIV). He told me:

A forgotten generation: Long-term survivors' experiences of HIV and AIDS

"My relationship with the medical profession is very open, honest and very supportive. I am totally me with my consultant and I have an absolutely amazing GP as well; she is absolutely wonderful... when I went to sign up with her she said 'you probably know more about HIV than I will ever know so therefore don't be afraid to tell me if I am speaking to you in the wrong manner'...she's lovely... And my dentist too! I go via the hospital to a dentist and it was in a sterile environment so they were all gowned up but I see this as for my protection as well because I don't want to pick up infections when I am in the dentist's chair. My dentist tells me that she wears gloves with all of her patients... but I feel that my attitude is a big benefit as well... I like to have a chat with my health care team and I don't have any issues at all. If they have gloves on and have to gown up then it is a two-way street, for my protection as well as their own."

Christopher describes himself as 'dying to live rather than living to die' and has maintained an amazing positive attitude to health and emotional issues. His relationship with the medical and health professionals is built on mutual trust and he considers himself as compliant with his HIV medication. Christopher wishes, however, he could be more open about his HIV-positive status in general, as he uses other illness conditions, such as his arthritis and previous strokes as 'a smoke screen' for regular HIV hospital appointments.

PABLO

Pablo aged 32 was diagnosed in 1990 at the age of 20 following a bout of ill health. Like Christopher, Pablo is medically defined as asymptomatic, has only experienced HIV-related ill health for a short period of time and has taken combination therapy since 1997. He is medically retired, goes for regular HIV check ups at the hospital and considers his treatment as unproblematic and effective at the time of our interview. Pablo has a good working relationship with the medical profession and considers he knows 'enough' about HIV-related matters to 'get him by'. When I asked him to describe his relationship with the medical profession he told me:

"I have always had good consultants; they have always been knowledgeable... they spend time with you and explain things quite clearly and if you decide to ask questions or if you don't understand, they will give you answers. But I think General Practitioners need to be more knowledgeable about what's going on. I mean I have got a brilliant GP, she is lovely, but she hasn't got a bloody clue about HIV. I mean she is good at everything else that she does, but if she wants to know anything when I go in and say something, she will be phoning my bloody consultant. Now she shouldn't have to do that. Why doesn't the Government provide training in HIV for doctors? I spoke to a nurse when I was in hospital… I was quite ill and it had lasted a long time so I ended up in hospital. I was on a general ward and this nurse actually admitted to me that she had only had one hour's training in HIV… being a nurse, she got one hour on HIV… I was disgusted."

When I asked Pablo to expand upon his knowledge of HIV-related issues and how this was 'enough to get him by' within his medical encounters, he told me:

"I think I know enough… I mean some people read manuals and articles all the time and things do get out of context and it becomes quite scary… I mean too much knowledge can be scary… I sort of listen to the experts, the people that really know like the medical profession. I mean sometimes they tell you something and you think, 'well hang on a minute! I have heard something different' from a certain source… I can't quite remember the details but something happened with my consultant. She said something to me and I said hang on I read an article somewhere and it clearly said the opposite to what you are saying, so who is right and who is wrong?... She told me that this is what she has learned from a Conference and she believed she was right; I said, OK fair enough. She said that this had come from top experts from this or that hospital and I accepted what she told me. But even so I mean sometimes even the doctors don't always get it right."

In spite of his overall positive experiences of the medical profession, Pablo did encounter problems with dental treatment as a result of his HIV-positive status. This was experienced by others too and will be explored further under a separate heading within this chapter.

PERRY

Perry aged 40 was diagnosed back in 1990 at the age of 28 years whilst being treated for a sexually transmitted disease. He works part-time, goes for regular three-monthly HIV check ups and is taking combination therapy for HIV. Perry considers himself to be reasonably healthy and is sometimes unsure how to separate out his experiences of living with HIV with those relating to his mental health condition. Perry revealed that prior to him learning of his HIV-positive status, he was mild mannered and quiet in character. Following diagnosis his behaviour spiralled out of control which was totally out of character and he was incarcerated in the mental health system for three years. He told me:

"I was treated provisionally for Schizophrenia by a doctor who saw me... and was placed in a psychiatric hospital... I built up a lot of resentment towards others; I mean I was just trying to find reasons for my HIV status. I thought because of lack of treatment, death and dying was around the corner and I felt that I had not really had much of a life... these were serious thoughts about my mortality... I felt all these emotions and they were aggravated because of the diagnosis... everybody was shocked because I was always so mild mannered. I would never hurt anybody in my life. It was a tremendous shock for everybody concerned... Nowadays I am a lot more contented with myself. I am more even-minded and calmer and am not so emotional. But I am on anti-psychotics and anti-depressants so it is difficult to understand what the reason is for the changes in me. The psychiatrist says that it is a product of the treatment that I am taking and I am sure that this is difficult to refute."

Perry spoke openly and candidly about his emotional state and feelings prior to and following diagnosis. He recalled how he often used to outwardly put on a 'happy front' for people around him but inwardly he was unhappy when he was younger. Perry further supposed that whilst the discovery of his HIV-positive status seriously affected his mental health and potentially triggered harmful behaviour, his 'unbalanced emotional state and the resentment towards others' were already in place prior to diagnosis. When I asked Perry to describe his relationship with the medical profession, he recounted:

"I went on medication for HIV and it was the doctor's decision but I was quite happy to go along with it... as with any illness you go along to your doctor and they put you on medication and you don't argue because you assume that they are doing the best thing for you at the time. I had quite a low white blood count... I was on injections for my mental health condition and it makes you very compliant in that sense so I wasn't worried... I just take whatever they tell me to take. But I do make my own judgements of the doctor. I have changed hospitals because I didn't like the set up... the old hospital seemed very sloppy and very casual and they didn't seem professional at all; whereas my new hospital is the other way round... I feel that I get much better treatment. I don't know what stuff they give me; I don't know all about the science and veins, blood cells or anything like that... but I make a judgement of the general situation and make my decisions accordingly in terms of whether I want to access treatment and health care. I mean when you go and see a doctor you expect it to be one-to-one; in the old hospital there were nurses popping in and out of the room all the time, giving messages to the doctor and it is not what you expect really when you are in consultation… it was very distracting; not just for me but for the doctor as well who is treating you, the patient, and there were people popping in and out all the time and it was just a very sloppy atmosphere… I made the decision to move from there… I am quite happy now… I got a bad feeling from the other hospital and I am sure that this hospital knows what they are on about, so I feel happier now."

Perry spoke of relief since the advent of effective HIV treatment became more widely available; he recounted how he now feels more 'even-minded about things' and accepts his current situation without resentment or bitterness.

MARC

Marc aged 38 years was diagnosed in 1990 at the age of 26 following a short bout of ill health. He has never taken combination therapy for HIV, is medically defined as asymptomatic and attends regular HIV health check ups. Marc was looking for work at the time of our interview and was experiencing good health. When I asked Marc to describe his relationship with the medical profession, he recounted:

"I haven't had any medical treatment at all… I trust the medical profession, well I mean I have a meaningful conversation with them and they are people like anybody else and they only know a bit more than me about HIV… I mean they obviously know a lot more about HIV than I do but I feel I know already quite a lot myself… I have got a responsibility in relation to pushing them and pressurizing them to give me information. And that is the idea of a good relationship with me. And if I don't really respect them or they make a mistake then I won't have anything to do with them. I think you can get too hooked up in HIV and well it is not the life that I would want to have."

Marc considers himself as 'lucky' in terms of his good health and the fact that medical treatment plays no part in his life. He now lives healthily by following a good diet, taking regular exercise and gets plenty of sleep. Marc stated previously that he lived each day 'as if he was going to die' but now he approaches life more positively.

TONY

At the age of 32 following a prolonged period of ill health Tony, now aged 40, learned of his HIV-positive diagnosis in 1994, after spending three years in denial. He regularly attends HIV health checks, is currently on combination therapy and is medically retired. Tony was 'fairly healthy' but did complain of feelings of lethargy and a distinct lack of energy which had become a cause for concern. He did not consider his medical treatment as too problematic and was awaiting possible new treatment options at the time of our interview. When I asked him to describe his experiences of the medical profession, he recounted:

"We have a humorous relationship I suppose my doctor and me… I can bounce my ideas off to her…I would say it is very good. It is like a family there with all the staff, but I wish they would be more direct and honest with me about the treatments. I trust them and I trust their judgement. There's a bit of confusion about whether to change my medication at the moment. I have two doctors and I have two different opinions but if their opinion is the same I will consider changing my medication and if it is different I would toss a coin…my state of mind for the last year is a bit confused and so I find it hard to absorb information… I am feeling very tired."

Tony stated that he was unsure if all the medication he was taking were the primary cause of his lethargy and lack of energy. He would like to ask his doctor: *'please can I stop the medication for a bit'* to see if this changes how he feels on a daily basis. Tony believes that his HIV consultant and doctor would not be prepared to do this, as they advise him to 'hang on in there with the current regime'. As he has limited knowledge of HIV-related issues and medical treatments, he feels he must comply with the advice from the medical professionals at this time.

JAY

Jay aged 35 was diagnosed in 1992 at the age of 25 years after experiencing a period of ill health and learning that his male partner was HIV-positive. He is medically defined as asymptomatic and has taken combination therapy since 1998 without experiencing any adverse side effects. He is unemployed, in good health and regularly attends health checks at an HIV clinic. Jay recounted how by choice he has failed to acquire knowledge around HIV and AIDS. When I asked him to describe his relationship with the medical profession, he told me:

"My relationship is excellent… my doctor at the moment is fantastic and he's quite honest and I mean I don't understand CD4 counts and I don't understand viral loads and all that kind of thing. He just tells me a number and I mean if the CD4 rises then I'm happy and if the viral load goes down then I'm even happier… at the moment my viral load is undetectable and my CD4 is starting to climb up pretty well as it was only in the 90s not too long ago… I think it is about 200 or something now… my doctor has kind of worked my medication around my lifestyle as opposed to me working my lifestyle around my medication. This is why it works for me."

Jay told me he believed his consultant to be the expert and would not necessarily challenge the medical profession unless *'there was something that really niggled me about it'*. He stated:

"I always talk to my best mate. I always tell him about what goes on at my appointments and he knows a hell of a lot about HIV and so he may put something into my head and I may ask a question when I go to the doctors but nine times out of ten it is very unlikely."

Jay's positive mental attitude and outlook on life is extraordinary and he feels that his HIV-positive status has had a limited impact on his lifestyle or on his sense of self.

Experiencing prejudice and discrimination within medical encounters

In this section we expose the extent to which some long-term survivors have experienced prejudice and discrimination on the basis of their HIV-positive status within a medical encounter. We learn how these interactions have been internalized and negotiated by the story-tellers. What do we mean when we speak of 'prejudice' and 'discrimination'? When we think about how we define prejudice it is generally regarded as the formation of an attitude, opinion or preconception which is biased either in favour of or against a person, group or thing. Whilst a biased attitude can be positive, it is usually a negative or unfavourable attitude towards a social group or individual member of that group. Prejudice is characterised by stereotypical beliefs that are not necessarily authentic or legitimate and so it is more to do with personal feelings and attitudes. HIV prejudice within a clinical encounter therefore might be perceived as being a somewhat unexpected phenomenon but it is not necessarily rare.

Discrimination, on the other hand, usually refers to our behaviour in terms of different or unfair treatment towards a person or group of people: it is to do with our behaviour rather than our attitude. Often our prejudiced attitudes are accompanied by discriminatory behaviour. Whilst some story-tellers appear elsewhere in this chapter during our exploration of different personal experiences, it is valuable to explore how discriminatory medical practices have been experienced within an HIV context. As before, we will start with those diagnosed the earliest.

MINNIE

Minnie aged 42 was diagnosed with HTLVIII at the age of 21 years in November of 1981. He is reliant on a wheelchair for mobility due to peripheral neuropathy and vasculitis and was relatively healthy at the time of our interview. Minnie attends regular HIV health checks and was on combination therapy at the time of our interview. He describes his relationship with the medical profession as excellent and takes an active role in his involvement with HIV health care. When I asked about any experiences of prejudice and discrimination he may have encountered on the basis of his HIV condition he told me:

"Oh yes! Quite outrageous with bank nurses in hospitals…you know, for example, hospitals have staff who work on all the wards and when some of those staff go sick or they're short staffed each hospital within it has what they call a 'bank back up' and they're general or specialist nurses; they don't work on any specific ward. They're just sent wherever they're needed. Now a lot of the time they are not allowed to do things like IVs… because the Union classes them as 'bank nurses'… I was admitted to hospital in 1996 and this is where I first encountered them… you would get bank nurses on a night duty with a Staff Nurse… I would be in bed and obviously they had read my notes and they would get to the threshold and talk to me from the doorway. They wouldn't come in and there was sheer panic on their faces… I was normally on a ward for infectious diseases so by nature these are individual rooms and not wards... they would not set foot across the door and they were only coming in to do observations such as blood pressure and taking my temperature and pulse... they couldn't bring themselves to do it and would wait until the Staff Nurse had finished doing the IVs... they were completely ignorant and in fear."

Minnie's extensive knowledge and experiences of the medical community were such that he was aware that doctors and nurses had to comply with specific procedures on an infectious ward; the use of gloves, caps and gowns were often standard medical practice. On some occasions doctors should have to remove their white coats to avoid spreading diseases from room to room, but this was often not practiced. We explore more about Minnie's experiences of the medical profession later in this chapter.

JO

Jo aged 53 discovered he was HIV-positive in 1982 at the age of 33 following a short bout of illness. He regularly attends HIV health checks, is in good health and was on his third combination therapy at the time of our interview. Jo considers he has a good working relationship with the medical profession and has significant support from his own brother who is an Oncologist. When asked about his relationship with the HIV medical profession in general he recounted:

"I suppose I have a very good relationship with the practitioners at the sharp end... I am very sceptical of the drug companies. I'm furious with the drug companies in terms of the profits that they are turning out and the fact that there are countries that are not able to access treatments. There are times when I just want to say I don't want to take any more medication. I do not want to be giving them these vast profits when there are millions and millions of people in Africa and the Far East who can't access them. I think that it should be a human right... it sticks in my gall that someone can have a Prime Minister who can uphold the right of the drug companies against the people of South Africa... it's appalling! And I mean these Governments are encouraging the drug companies to bring cases against countries like Brazil and India who are attempting to produce generic treatments for impoverished communities who cannot pay...I am aware that I am really, really fortunate and there are times when I feel guilty and it affects me and I can't help it. It is a major issue for me and affects my health because of the stress and therefore depletes the immune system."

Jo recounted how fortunate he was in terms of not having a problem with dealing with authority. He told me:

"Whether this is because of going through the private schooling system instead of the State system I don't know… It's never been an issue for me to speak out. I'm not passive and have the confidence to speak out when I feel it necessary… I sort of lose it as I get so angry sometimes but I'm prepared to challenge issues that I believe to be unfair… my younger brother has changed direction so I am fortunate in that he always wanted to do something in medicine and so became a doctor and now he's an Oncologist… so I always have someone to talk to about HIV issues… I think I've been really fortunate because I'm up front."

Jo continues to describe how in the early days he encountered prejudice and discrimination based on his HIV-positive status back in 1985 when he needed dental treatment. He revealed:

"I went to a dentist for treatment and told her that I was HIV-positive and that I had had Hepatitis B previously but that I was not sort of a carrier because I had antibodies… she refused to treat me and told me that it was because of the Hep B and she hadn't got appropriate equipment which sort of shocked me… she was adamant it was not because of the HIV but I don't believe this to be true. I was having dental problems and needed treatment and could not get a dentist to treat me. Ultimately I had to go to a dental clinic within my local hospital and I remember they were gowned and gloved… they were wearing visors and almost everything was wrapped in cling-film. I mean it was a horrible experience! Then one of the people just took off the mask and it was like they were trying to break down the barrier or something, you know… in point of fact I just thought this is ridiculous because if the mask is there for a reason, which made sense if they were doing drilling and if there was blood hitting them, why take it off? It was totally wrong."

Jo identified how inconsistent medical practices were around HIV as he recalled an incident whilst he was on holiday in Crete with a group of friends. He was involved in an accident which required stitches in his arm; as a matter of course all the nurses and doctors dealing with the injury wore gloves and protective clothing. When he returned to the UK he went to his own GP and the nurse in the clinic did not put on gloves to examine the wound, despite him telling them he was HIV-positive. Other than these incidents, Jo considers his relationship with the medical profession as good.

A forgotten generation: Long-term survivors' experiences of HIV and AIDS

TOM

Tom aged 55 was diagnosed in 1986 after voluntarily testing and is experiencing relatively good health. He is on combination therapy, goes for regular HIV health checks and is medically retired. Tom has, in the past, been a human face for HIV; his picture was in all the city's newspapers during one of the World AIDS Day week. He is unsurprisingly extremely proud of his political involvement in earlier AIDS awareness campaigns. He has an excellent knowledge of HIV and AIDS matters, has been an HIV trainer and takes an active role in learning about HIV medication. He has a good working relationship with his HIV medical practitioners, as we will see later in this chapter. When I asked him about any experiences of prejudice or discrimination on the basis of his HIV status, he recalled:

"I told you about the incident with the X-Ray with the rubber gloves? No? Well, they took me for an X-Ray and then they realised I was the wrong person [they had someone else with the same surname]… In the middle of the afternoon, living with this bleeding colon thing, the nurse said I was due for an X-Ray and I thought that was strange because my consultant had never mentioned it in the morning… anyway they got me down to X-Ray and I was sitting there for ages and ages… I realised that they had made a mistake when they told me… and they had seen my medical notes by now. Oh! They just went on and on because they couldn't get anyone to take me back upstairs. Eventually a porter put on rubber gloves and gingerly took me back upstairs… this was about 1987 or 1988… nobody wanted to take me back upstairs because they had seen the biohazard sticker, you know the yellow thing on my file… I was working for the City Council by then and later I got in touch with the Health Authorities and asked them if they had done any HIV training and I offered them HIV training… of course they hadn't done any training and that was discrimination in a way… It was maybe the second morning I was in there and the two things that seemed to be really obvious was the fact that 1) doctors wouldn't look you in the eyes when they were talking and 2) tea ladies wouldn't bring tea anywhere near you."

An interesting point was made later, when Tom spoke about training experiences within his Local Authority. At one particular Health Unit, the HIV team were rapidly expanding and had become patient advocates for people living with HIV. Tom was aware that his team needed training on ethnicity and racism in order to broaden their understanding and awareness of these issues in relation to HIV. When two of his members, a gay man and a lesbian, attended a training session on Race and Ethnicity they reported back to Tom how the session had separated Black and White people in terms of oppression. The trainers had promoted a hierarchy of oppression in terms of health placing Black people at the top. One of Tom's team objected to this type of structure of oppression and mentioned how women and the gay community might be equally oppressed in terms of health and this was dismissed. Tom went on to tell me:

"One member of my team stated that it was offensive to be referred to as a 'batty man' and this was just shrugged off… the trainers were two Black women and a Black guy… then I was told by another Black guy in the Health Unit that someone had raised the issue of HIV and this training at a party… they must have been City Council employees, and he overhead the same male trainer saying, 'Oh don't bloody bother with them it's two batty men and a dyke'… I brought this up with the Head of the Unit… all this experience did was stop two parts of the same unit from talking to each other… I repeated this to others and I tried to make several appointments with the woman who managed the team of patient advocates and she just kept fobbing me off… it was not good, it wasn't justifiable… it really split the HIV unit… it was prejudice and discrimination on the basis that any validity we might have had about HIV was automatically taken away by the fact that we were all gay… I really resented it because as I stated to them, we have more in common than we have got differences… I don't think that per se just because you are a gay man it doesn't mean that you can't have a degree of empathy with those people living with HIV in different communities… in the context of health as soon as we start to compartmentalise people, placing them into groups then things start to become rather competitive and it is politically divisive."

Tom believes he is an Idealist and would like to see an HIV community right across the board in the UK. With the experiences of living with HIV and a deeper understanding of each other, he would like to dispel all the myths and stereotypes we have all been brought up with and make decisions together between each member of his idealistic HIV community.

LISETTE

Lisette aged 51 was diagnosed with HIV after voluntarily testing in the USA whilst travelling in 1990; she was 39 years old. Lisette was medically defined as asymptomatic at the time of our interview and was consciously avoiding taking combination therapy for a number of reasons (see chapter six). When I asked her how she would describe her relationship with the medical profession, she told me:

"Turbulent perhaps... I've never been a very passive patient. I told him it was a partnership. Take it or leave it. We're in partnership to deal with my HIV and that's final and they know that we are in a partnership. I always get the last word."

When I asked Lisette if she had ever encountered negative experiences with the medical profession in relation to her HIV she recounted:

"I had a traumatic time when I went to the local hospital. I had a fire in my house and it was a couple of years after I had been diagnosed and the GP came out to me at the house which was completely filled with smoke and she said that she needed to send me to the local hospital because she was worried about PCP and my lungs...I got put into a ward with four women who were in their nineties and not a soul came near me for the whole day. And this was in 1992 and on the Saturday night I got moved from this little ward to the Maternity ward because they were short of beds... I didn't realise I was having a bit of a trauma about not having more kids, not that I wanted any more... but it was just another thing I kind of felt that had been taken away from me, you know, the choice of whether or not to have any more was removed because of the HIV... so to find myself on a Maternity ward I became quite upset and so I remember being in tears and this nurse coming up to me and saying 'Oh! What's the matter?' I tried to say to her, 'is there somewhere where I could go?' because there was a woman in the next bed... so she took me to the nurses station, which is right in the middle of the ward and I felt... I assumed that because I was a patient on the ward that she must know what's wrong with me and why I was there. I turned round and I said that I just couldn't believe that they had brought me on to this ward because I am having this problem because I've got HIV... And she completely flipped and she turned round and asked me if I was a threat to her patients...I just ran away and phoned a friend. It was about midnight and I asked my friend to come and get me. I wanted to leave the hospital immediately... I ended up staying the night and going home the following day. It was absolutely diabolical."

Lisette went on to tell me about the prejudice and discrimination she had experienced the year before she was diagnosed with HIV when she had to have a back operation at a different local hospital. She told me:

"The year before I was diagnosed I had a back operation and because I'd done drugs there was definitely a question as to whether or not I'd got HIV and at one point they were suggesting that if I didn't get tested that they wouldn't do my operation. I remember this chap coming in who happened to be the GU nurse and had set up an AIDS support group in the area... he came to my bedside and started chatting and telling me that the staff were out of order and that I didn't need to get tested if I didn't want to. They had to do my operation but he told me that they might treat me differently if I refused... I asked him what he meant and he told me they'd probably put me either first or last on the list. It was because of this that made me wonder about universal precautions because they were treating me differently but they were not asking anybody else to get tested who were waiting for an operation. You know, they didn't know other people's history of sexual practices or drug use... So I didn't get tested out of spite in a way because I thought I am not going to give them the satisfaction of knowing one way or another. I have to say, though, that I honestly didn't believe that I had anything to worry about... I came back from the operation and I was just lying there and the nurse came in to give me a cup of tea and the Sister screamed at her because she didn't have any gloves on... she was horrible."

Lisette went on to tell me other discriminatory practices she had experienced because of her HIV-positive status:

"Oh yes! My GP she won't allow the nurses to do my smear testing. I have to go to her and I had to fight her to get her to do the testing every year which is what is medically recommended. My consultant in London is screaming and shouting because it should be done at least once a year and my GP wants me to come back in three years because the results show there is nothing wrong... anyway I went and had the test in the GP's room as opposed to the clinic where everybody else goes... she did the test and I kid you not, when she had finished she got all the bits in a bottle, right? And she had them in a bucket and she took the bucket with the gloves on gingerly out of the room and said 'I'm sorry to leave you now but I have to run because I don't want the nurses to touch this.' And she ran to wherever they take it to go and get it all sterilised. So... if that doesn't make you feel different I don't know what does... And my attitude is that is OK because they know about me being HIV but what is all this about? Why aren't they treating everybody else the same? You know I have been going to that GP practice for at least ten years and they never did that before... it makes me so angry and I can't help it. Those and dentists drive me mad."

Lisette then went on to recall the problems she had experienced with dentists in the past. HIV prejudice and discriminatory practices associated with the dental profession have been identified many times during many of our conversations with long-term survivors and we touch on other personal experiences, such as Lisette's, throughout this chapter. Here Lisette went on to reveal:

"They're like a breed apart... I almost feel with dentists that they know something that they're not telling the rest of us... that HIV is spread through the air or something. Do you know what I mean? There is something really serious because dentists have a real problem, even more of a problem than the GP has, and I don't really understand it because in reality, you know, again they're only worried about people they know about, the people who are already diagnosed and that's a crazy way to be... because the danger of that is a lot of people won't tell them. I've had a dentist that looks at your teeth but they won't do any of the work, they send you to the hospital to get a filling... I had a tooth taken out in a surgical theatre in hospital and all the guys were in gowns. And I didn't even bleed. And yet where my daughter lives in New Mexico the dentist there, his practice is next door to the drug and alcohol unit, so he can't know but the chances are that somebody that comes through there is going to be HIV, so he treats everybody all the same and he treats them all as if they're HIV positive. And that is what you have to do. I just don't understand why in this country it seems to be so hard for either GPs or dentists to do that. It's like a different world."

Lisette goes on to reveal how local medical practices are different to those she accesses in London. Whenever she is required to access health care with her local GP, she describes the medical practitioners as always 'on edge' because of her HIV-positive status. In comparison, the hospital in London where she accesses most of her HIV treatment is 'so laid back'. Lisette continues on the subject of dentists and GPs and recounts the following:

"I know there's a problem with national health dentists anyway regardless of HIV... it just makes it twice as hard. It is hard enough because you're a national health patient but you don't need the added HIV bit. What also makes me laugh is that the dentist I had once I was positive, my GP decided to phone them up and tell them... and they would not treat me after that and yet they again were treating me for the last ten years with HIV. That's what caused all my dental problems in the first place because I would have just carried on going to the one I'd been going to before, after I moved here. There wasn't any reason why I shouldn't keep going to my old dentist and my GP decided that she better tell her and the funny thing was that she [the dentist] turned round at that point and said that had I only had HIV then she could have probably treated me, but it was the Hepatitis... but in reality they'd never tested me for Hepatitis so although I did have it, nobody knew that. I tried to tell the dentist that and of course she had to then back-peddle because it was nothing to do with Hepatitis because I didn't know I had it at the time. The GP had said I'd had it but I didn't. You know I'd never been tested for it. The GP must have absolutely assumed I had it because she phoned the dentist and said I had Hepatitis and HIV. Now what gave her the right to phone the bloody dentist? I definitely wasn't tested in them days a) because there wasn't a test of Hepatitis C and b) I'd been vaccinated at the hospital for Hepatitis B so according to them I'd never had it and was never gonna get it."

Whilst Lisette does not reveal the year this incident took place, it was most probably around 1990. It is totally outrageous for her GP to inform other health practitioners about the HIV status of a patient. Such HIV discrimination as this is utterly inappropriate and unacceptable behaviour. Lisette has had more than fifteen dentists over the past five years as a result of her HIV-positive status. Unsurprisingly, Lisette had a deep-rooted scepticism for the medical profession on the basis of her personal experiences and, in particular, the pharmaceutical industry on the basis that she is a woman. She had avoided taking any medical treatments for HIV to date and maintained she would always take an extremely 'active and leading role 'in her own health care.

PABLO

We have learned about Pablo's experiences earlier in this chapter. Pablo is 32 years old and was diagnosed in 1990. He is medically retired, asymptomatic and in extremely good health*. Pablo has been on combination therapy since 1997 and has a good relationship with his HIV medical practitioners. He believes, however, that GPs and nurses in hospitals should have more training around HIV issues and it angers him that sufficient funds are not available for more extensive HIV training. When I asked him to recount any problems he might have encountered because of his HIV-positive status within a medical or health encounter, he told me:

"I have heard some horrific stories about people that have stayed in hospital and the way they have been treated, but dentists are terrible... Do you know how hard it is to get a dentist if you are positive in my local area? It is so hard because most of the dentists here will not take you if you are HIV... I had one dentist which I got referred to through the hospital but I had to change because he scared me to death. He really really scared me, I mean I am not very good with dentists anyway but he made me worse... I went in and if you wanted an appointment he would only see you at half past four in the afternoon, you were the last person in the surgery. I sort of questioned him about this and asked: 'why am I always the last person in the surgery?' and he said it was because I was HIV-positive and obviously you were going to bleed more in the gums and stuff and we need to clear up. And I said: 'excuse me but shouldn't you be taking the same procedure for everyone? I told him he could have somebody coming through his door that didn't know their status, they could be everywhere, so I said you shouldn't just be taking the procedure on me, I said you should be doing the same for everybody that comes through the door… He just looked at me sort of gob smacked that I'd made this comment… what really got me, what really pissed me off a bit because I don't know if he'd done this with everyone but the whole of the worktop was cling-filmed. Even the chair that I sat in had this cling-film sheet all over it. It was everywhere… He'd got these bloody visor things on and he was like, God, it was so scary… I just thought to myself I am being treated like a leper, you know it is a dentist surgery, fair enough, you have got to be careful but I thought to myself, after every patient that's in here don't you have to sterilise everything anyway? You have to clean up after each person anyway and destroy whatever… so I mean, yes obviously because I am HIV-positive there's a slight chance of infection so you have to be careful but you should be careful with everyone… how many people does he get through his door in a day that he doesn't possibly know if they could be infected… I have changed now but I have been to eight dentist surgeries and not one of them would take me on… I had to go through the hospital for them to find one and I was disgusted, I felt disgusting really… It is discrimination but there is a lack of knowledge because they don't know enough about HIV people… I think they need more training."

Other than negative experiences of discrimination with dentists, Pablo was happy with his overall medical health care for his HIV. He had a good relationship with his HIV consultant and his local GP but believed there should be more training on HIV knowledge generally amid health care practitioners.

RICK

Rick aged 32 was diagnosed in 1990 after voluntarily testing for a second time using his proper name. We learn more about Rick's experiences with the medical profession later in this chapter. He regularly attended HIV health checks, and was not taking combination therapy at the time of our interview; he was awaiting salvage therapy. Rick had taken up to 10 different HIV combination therapies over the years and has experienced resistance and allergies to certain drug treatments along with severe side effects. He has taken an active role in learning about HIV treatments and is knowledgeable about HIV and AIDS matters. When I asked Rick if he had encountered any HIV-related prejudice or discrimination within a medical encounter, he recounted:

"If you look at my case conference notes, the heart specialist was extremely rude… obviously he hadn't had an HIV patient before, and he was very nasty towards me. He asked me to ask questions whenever I wanted and he also asked me what side effects I was getting, so I told him. He said really nastily, 'Excuse me! I don't want to know about your HIV side effects.' And I didn't know which side effects he wanted to know about, so he asked me which medication I was on and I gave him a list and he said, 'I don't want to know anything about your HIV'. It was so confusing I mean he asked me which medication I was on and I gave him a list…He was the heart specialist and my heart condition is hereditary but it is made worse by the HIV… Like he said, 'stop me at any time when I tell you about the read outs that we've done' because I had loads of tests and monitors done so when I started to ask him a question, he said, 'Excuse me! Can you just let me finish?' He was really snotty and everybody tells me he is normally such a lovely specialist and I was really lucky to get him in the first place. We have come to the conclusion that he hasn't treated an HIV patient before… as was said in the case conference, I don't deserve to be spoken to like that whether I am HIV-positive or not but I believe that he was prejudiced against me and my being HIV… because he really didn't want to examine me and he washed his hands so many times, it was unbelievable… he washed his hands after he had just checked my heart… he washed his hands about three times… the friend who was with me couldn't believe it was the same specialist because she thinks he is wonderful. She came with me because she was with the same specialist and she can't believe that he was like that with me… all he did was snap, snap, snap at me… he would ask me a question, then snap at me again and then said I was answering the wrong questions."

Rick was rather upset with this medical encounter and will explore other problems he had been experiencing with his current HIV health care later in this chapter. He had always maintained an active role in learning as much as possible about HIV and AIDS and had been told by doctors and nurses, in the past, that perhaps he knew too much. Unsurprisingly, he did not feel he could know too much about HIV and stated on a number of occasions: 'I am not a hypochondriac – that is one thing I am not'.

RACHEL

Rachel aged 39 years was diagnosed with HIV in 1993. She is married and has two children and is a sero-concordant relationship. Rachel attends regular HIV health checks, takes combination therapy and has a good relationship with medical professionals. She is *'in total control of all decision-making in relation to treatments'* she will and will not take for HIV. Rachel praises HAART as it enabled her to plan her family and she now believes that she will probably live to see her children grow up; HAART is a very positive thing which brings with it positive life chances. Rachel believes the medical profession is slow to change especially in relation to women and pregnancy. She has a medical background, is extremely assertive and *'will not be brow beaten into making decisions I am not willing to hastily make without being appropriately persuaded'*. When I asked her if she had encountered any prejudice or discrimination in relation to her HIV-positive status, she told me:

"When one of my children was born in hospital, I erm… a midwife who wasn't on my team came into the room that I was in, and she didn't obviously know anything about me and hadn't bothered to check. She saw me bottle feeding… She said, 'How dare you bottle feed, don't you know breast is best? You ought to be ashamed of yourself especially somebody with your education and so on…' I actually hit the roof and said 'how dare you make assumptions like that! You know, you do not come in here a) you are not one of my midwives and so you are not looking after me and you do not have the right to judge what I am doing and b) you should have more understanding and awareness, especially in this hospital, as there might be a medical reason why I am not breastfeeding and in my case there actually is - I am HIV-positive.' Well, she was horrified and she ran out of the room and never came back. I mean that was probably the worse bit of prejudice. What made it so horrifying, quite honestly, why I was so cross was because it was a specialist hospital… OK at that stage there weren't an awful lot of women who were having babies, who were positive and having babies, but there were some and she should have been more aware of the possibilities. I think my colour being a White woman, and educated probably made her think that it was unlikely and she just didn't expect it."

Rachel then went on to tell me about her work in HIV training with health care workers in her local area, she recounted:

"I actually spend a lot of time doing talks to a lot of health care workers around what we call 'eyeball screening'… you know you look at somebody and you say: 'Oh, well, she is White, she is professional, she is well educated, she couldn't possibly be HIV-positive.' This is 'eyeball screening' and is a talk I do to midwives; I point out that if they do that, they will miss the ones *like me* and if they miss the ones like me and the baby is born positive then they are going to be blamed because they should have told the patient and they should have given the patient choices. They seem to take on board what I am saying remarkably well simply because it is coming from somebody who they might not expect to be positive. So they feel very open to ask questions and so on. I have been very lucky and had very little prejudice really."

Rachel's relationship with her HIV medical team is very good and she decides on all her own combination treatments by researching them first and involves her doctor and consultant during the decision making process.

SANDRA

Sandra, aged 37 years, was voluntarily tested and diagnosed as late as 1994 after her five month old child became ill and later died in hospital with an AIDS-related illness. She is medically retired, symptomatic, attends regular HIV health checks and is on combination therapy. Sandra describes her current health as reasonable and assumes an active role in her HIV health care. When I asked if she had encountered any problems in relation to her being HIV-positive she told me:

"It is when you go outside of the HIV clinic for other treatments when I have problems, for example, eye tests. HIV causes havoc with the rest of your body and I have come across discriminatory practices amongst so-called health care professionals… I have problems with dentists too. That was the first shocking thing, for my own protection I warned the dentist that I am on combination therapy, not because I want them to know, it is to protect myself: it is purely selfish. I want to be safe in case they give me an anaesthetic that will clash with my medication, so I will tell them. The first time I went to this clinic, one that was supposed to be HIV-friendly…you access these clinics through the specialist nurses so obviously they know when you go there… it is like a community dental clinic which caters for all the odd type of people I suppose. That is a terrible thing to say, isn't it? But anyway, I went in there and filled in this form, told him all the medication I was on and apart from getting looks from people at the reception and people poking their heads through the door to see… they obviously had access to the form I had filled in. I had an appointment made for the last appointment in the day which clearly makes sense, but they should clean the equipment anyway! I thought it was fair enough but then I went into the dentist's office and found an armchair completely covered with cling-film and I had to sit on the cling-film. That was a nightmare and was my first experience. This was in 1998... cling-film all over the dentist's chair and the dental assistant was clothed in an apron and everything and had a visor... she came into the waiting room and there were a lot of other people sitting there, kitted out like that... can you imagine how that feels? It was awful, it was awful. I was thinking I wish I hadn't told you, you bastards, pardon the expression. You know I am positive and they shouldn't think like that. They don't know who they are dealing with when others are sat in the chair... but I did make a complaint. So you are discriminated against for being honest about your status. I had my treatment and thought: 'well just sit there' and he got his drill and whatever out and I got my treatment and at the end of it, when it was all done, I said: 'you can get the bleach out now, can't you?' and walked out... I went back for more treatment after I had made a complaint, and this time there wasn't any cling-film in sight. I have moved now and so that is the only reason I don't go to that particular clinic. The thought of going to an independent dentist and having to go through all that again is too much hassle... It is better the devil you know, even though he is a real devil. I now live in a small village and I do not have a dentist. I daren't go here so I will wait until I am desperate and then possibly try the nearest city or somewhere."

Sandra keeps her HIV-positive status to herself as much as is practicably possible due to extremely unpleasant past personal experiences of prejudice within social relationships. Her relationship with the medical profession is based on mutual participation. She takes on an active role in her HIV medical health care and is an equal participant in any decision making on combination treatments. This makes Sandra feel particularly good because *'for the first time in a long time, I felt like I had some kind of control over this alien.'*

Sandra recounts how other discriminatory experiences based on her HIV-positive status have affected her. She told me:

"At the eye clinic, this was another one where I informed them that I was HIV-positive because there is a virus called CMV, which, erm, is linked to HIV and it can affect your eye sight, I mean you can go blind from it and I am concerned about my health and so I have to have my eyes tested every year, so I informed the optometrist that I had HIV and he was terrible. As soon as I told him he would not even touch me. Can you imagine somebody trying to examine your eyes without actually touching you? It was awful, it was awful. You feel abused almost. You think 'how much do I have to put up with?' Sometimes you feel so low you can't fight and you just give up."

Sandra had previously made an attempt on her life and she recounts how she felt when she encountered a psychiatrist afterwards. She recalls:

"A psychiatrist who treats you as though you are a criminal, you know, who interrogates you about your sex life; I had gone there to get, you know after my suicide attempt, I had gone to ask for a prescription for a suitable anti-depressant and he was interrogating me about my sex life. I was so angry at the time and I stood up and I said: 'I am not fucking coming to see you again'. I went back to my doctor, told him what happened and a letter was written to him. The next time I went he was falling over himself, which was even worse, because I knew that the reason he was acting like that was because I told on him... you do face things like that... I think sometimes it doesn't help well it doesn't help when people see your colour and certain things kick in and the way that they treat you depends on whatever ideas they have got about you and colour, being Black... It is disheartening sometimes; you go somewhere with a shield already there, which is terrible because you end up getting angry with the wrong people because you are kind of *always* expecting people to be negative towards you... There are a lot of us who get very defensive because of what we have been through with HIV. It is exhausting!"

Sandra's experiences certainly encapsulate other long-term survivors' experiences of prejudice and discrimination in relation to HIV. But, as she points out, this is perhaps further exacerbated by her ethnic identity, by being Black, which subsequently impacts on negative and harmful attitudes and discriminatory behaviour. In spite of Sandra's personal experiences, I was so pleased to hear her say she was 'at peace' with herself psychologically in terms of the new home in the country.

Healthy scepticism of HIV medicines: relationships can still work

This section explores how story-tellers have maintained a degree of healthy scepticism of HIV medicines and the pharmaceutical industry and have, at times, refused or stopped taking prescribed medication. Whilst Elisabeth and Richard have embarked upon HIV combination therapies due to ill health and being medically defined as symptomatic, David has always resisted HIV medicine and taken alternative or complementary therapies for his HIV. Interestingly, both story-tellers who have taken combination therapy have experienced rather severe side effects from HIV drugs and have stopped taking medication due to quality of life issues. For David, taking combination therapy would have to be the last resort as he considers HIV drugs as 'poison'. Cynicism and scepticism of HIV drugs is therefore not surprising. All three story-tellers assume an extremely active role in managing their HIV-health care and are knowledgeable about HIV and AIDS matters. Challenging the medical profession during medical consultations is considered essential for maintaining a good working relationship.

ELISABETH

Elisabeth aged 48 years was diagnosed in 1985 after voluntarily testing. During this time, and for eight years after diagnosis, she was a practising IV-drug user taking heroin. At the time of our interview, Elisabeth was taking HIV monotherapy and had previously taken combination therapies which were problematic due to severe side effects. She had been admitted to hospital on three occasions in the past year with a serious liver condition and haemorrhaging due to HCV and problems associated with her taking Interferon. She was awaiting a liver transplant. Elisabeth regularly attends HIV health checks, is self-employed and takes complementary therapies which include: acupressure, massage, reflexology and aqua detox. She has a deep mistrust for the pharmaceutical industry, especially in relation to the viral load test which she believes was invented by the drug companies; and has a healthy scepticism of the medical profession yet enjoys a good working relationship with her HIV medical team. When I asked her how she considered her relationship with the HIV medical profession, she recounted:

"A healthy cynicism and a healthy scepticism I think... I mean we can't help it ...I certainly don't listen to a word they say anymore... I've changed my doctor after about 10 years because I got fed up with her telling me I was going to die if I didn't go on the combination therapy. I really didn't appreciate being told that, so I changed my doctor and I explained to this new one what my problem was, and he's been great. He gives me my options and then just leaves me. I really appreciate that and I'm more likely to do what he wants that way...I am on medication now but I've had terrible trouble with prescribed medication with lots of side effects, rashes, feeling sick and I mean even with... the Interferon nearly killed me. I believe that nearly killed me rather than my liver... I probably believe in the combination medication, but in a lot of ways it's not helping us... a lot of people when the medication came out sort of gave up looking after themselves. And that's hard to find a balance, to still do alternative therapies and give them a chance, to still eat well and to still listen to your own body when it doesn't feel like it is your own body any more... the medication I am on gives you diarrhoea and then it makes you constipated and then I'm busy trying to figure out what I'm eating and what I can do to better this, but my doctor says well there's nothing you can do because it's the Kaletra... thanks for telling me!"

Elisabeth went on to talk about how she is not compliant with her drug taking and how she likes to organise her medication around her own life. Her life comes first, she said:

"I often wonder if I could come off them but probably they won't let me, you know I often come off pills. I only really stay on them for six months and then bring myself off them for a couple of years. That is my choice and the doctors hate me... but there is always that niggling doubt: 'Well, if only I had listened to my doctor'. But hey, you just don't know... I took a new drug once, it was unregistered, I can't remember what it was but it made me quite sick. I couldn't eat. I would want to eat but two spoons of food and I would be full up and I was losing loads of weight... I took myself off that medication and doctor said he would find me a new one. I said don't bother I will stay on two... I will not go on a new pill because I know that a new pill will cause a problem. The doctor said that this was OK and research thought it was strong enough on its own, and he was quite happy because indications are that my viral load is negative and my T-cells have gone up. So, he's actually listening to me... I can understand how easy it is to get pushed into things... the side effects I've suffered have always been so horrendous... I'm allergic to quite a lot of them... so with the Hepatitis C it was me who pushed to go on Interferon; they said it would kill me... I really pushed and I got on it and it did nearly kill me but you know at least I tried."

Elisabeth had a deep-rooted cynicism and scepticism about the viral load as a health indicator. She told me:

"I just have this thing about the viral load test and it's peculiar that we didn't have one before. I think the Pharmaceutical companies thought it out and it's just a ploy to ware their drugs... I mean it's just ridiculous because when I first got told my viral load was about 43,000 and my doctor said: 'Oh! That's fine, it's not bad' and you see we didn't know any better. But now if you're told you have a viral load of 43,000 they'd have buried you... and it's crazy, like you know a friend of mine goes absolutely mad if she gets a 500 viral load and I mean 'Whoa! It's fucking nothing, you know, people have got millions... the knowledge can kill you instead of the HIV... It's hard to remain in control and make the doctors listen to you, you know, because they're not always right... I suppose your experiences have a lot to do with the way you do things... my doctor says it's not the HIV that will kill me it's my liver."

Elisabeth's active role in HIV medication is based, she believes, upon her past experiences of life too. She was a heroin addict long before she was HIV-positive and that has been the most overriding thing in her life that she has had to fight. She describes herself as a 'determined long-term survivor'.

DAVID

David was diagnosed in 1990 at the age of 52 and is the oldest member in this study at 65 years old. He has never taken combination therapy, goes for regular HIV health checks and uses complementary therapy in conjunction with a well-balanced vegetarian diet to maintain his healthy status. David is medically defined as asymptomatic and whilst participating in a plasma scheme he discovered he had contracted Hepatitis C (HCV). He then decided to embark upon Interferon treatment for his liver, which has now ceased. His liver is functioning well and he refuses to take any HIV medication until it is the last resort. He describes his relationship with the medical profession as a very good working relationship. When I asked him about medical treatment and how he interacts with the medical profession, he told me:

"I made a positive decision not to have anything until I have tried all the alternative options and the only treatment I have had has been Interferon for Hepatitis, because I felt I had to have a healthy liver in case I had to go on combination therapy; that date can't be far away because I have been offered it for at least eight years, but I have always declined. My relationship with the HIV medical profession is extremely good... I still go back to the London hospital even though I don't live nearby because the relationship is so good and although they have never actually condoned the fact that I am having complementary therapies, they do in fact give massage and a few other therapies there. I don't use them because it means travelling 40 minutes each way on a nasty motorway, so any good that came out of it would be lost by the time I get home... I am still not convinced about combination therapies. If I do take it, it would be really the last resort and I will be expecting that I am taking a poison. That is the way I see it, so I am very, very reluctant to start."

David emphasises the importance of a good healthy vegetarian diet in conjunction with numerous vitamin supplements, which includes Spirulina. He has introduced a number of his friends to Spirulina, including myself and believes it is a contributory factor to his good health. He also takes acupuncture and herbal remedies to promote good health and improve his immune system. Evidence suggests that David's alternative therapies are working effectively, as when he is unable to access his alternative therapies, his CD4 count goes down and his viral load increases. David firmly believes as Primary Care Trusts (PCTs) are paying for HIV medical treatments from their budgets, then individuals seeking alternative therapies rather than opting for medical treatments, should be offered these without having to pay out of their own pockets.

RICHARD

Richard aged 32 was diagnosed in 1990 whilst living in London. He had lived with an AIDS diagnosis for many years, had experienced severe side effects and was therefore not always fully compliant with previous HIV drug treatments. He went for regular HIV health checks, worked part-time in the HIV field and was extremely knowledgeable about HIV and AIDS matters. Richard believed the advent of HAART was life-saving but, at the same time, he was initially frightened by its effectiveness because it constantly changed 'the goal posts' and created even more medical uncertainty. He struggled to maintain a good, healthy diet and found it difficult to 'survive alone'. There are times when Richard had refused or resisted medical treatment, but at the time of interview he was taking combination therapy. When I asked him to expand upon why he actively chose to resist medical treatment in the past, he told me:

"Because I am an arrogant fuck and I don't listen to doctors. Well, the start of my resistance began when they were giving out monotherapy... I stated that I would not continue to take Zidovudine (AZT)... So I told my doctor, 'No', and he said how did I expect him to treat me if I was not prepared to take any medication? I said that there were plenty of other things to treat me with if I did get ill... the doctors were downright rude if you did not conform to the treatments they wanted you to take. Things have now changed an awful lot and people generally are much more aware about treatment and not because of doctors giving it out. Organisations and the internet are a brilliant source of information on treatment. It has become much easier if you want to be more assertive and constructive with medical professionals about how you are actually treated because of the availability of information... I would always assume my right to make choices about my treatment. I know I have a right to choose and express my views but those views are only any good if they are informed views. I certainly don't feel confident about taking something I don't understand. If I don't know about it, or understand it to a reasonable level about what it is going to do to my body, or I am unaware of the risk factor, then I am not sure that I would want to be launching in and taking whatever anyone offers me willy-nilly. The other thing is that choices around whether you choose to take treatment or not is clearly linked to the quality of life you might have... your quality of life has to outweigh the issues that arise from those medications. So, if you end up on a drug regime that requires you to have an empty stomach an awful lot, and you are unable to eat, and as a result of that you lose a considerable amount of weight, and look dreadful and all your friends fall out with you, then that is going to affect your quality of life. The tablets might be working but if it is going to affect your quality of life, emotionally you are not going to be in a good place."

Richard believed, like many others, that quality of life issues were extremely important and therefore taking an active role in making decisions on treatment options was paramount. There were many times when Richard was in conflict with medical practitioners and he resisted treatments if he was uncomfortable with what was on offer. Other factors he touched upon when taking control in medical encounters were based on accurate information. He recounted:

"Other factors that might influence my decision to take or not to take medication are based around correct, up-to-date and accurate information. Without this I would probably refuse medication... I need accurate information from doctors, the scientists, clinical trials and probably organisations dealing with issues of HIV...they all provide good information... The medical profession have gone through a very steep learning curve, very steep, but I still feel there is an over reliance on the use of HAART medication and I think we will see evidence of this in time. The levels of resistance and multiple resistant viruses are now coming to light. I don't think that HAART will always be the answer. I think we will reach a stage, in the not too distant future, when people who become infected, well even now this is showing, are already resistant to the majority of treatments, if not them all."

Richard experienced a great deal of animosity amid some HIV medical practitioners and I was unfortunate enough to be present during many of these medical encounters, particularly when he was very ill, weak and tired. His reluctance to be a passive recipient of medical treatment and his assertive character made the medical encounter uncomfortable and at times the doctor was quite hostile.

Experiences of positive relationships: maintaining a challenging role

This segment of the chapter uncovers how four long-term survivors have renegotiated successful working relationships with HIV medical practitioners over time. Our story-tellers speak of: empowerment; taking control; the necessity of knowing about relevant HIV-related knowledge; and, the benefits of learning from each other, in order to establish mutual respect and trust within medical consultations. It is also a firm belief by those who share their experiences that adopting an active role in all aspects of HIV health care and being prepared to challenge medics is vital to build favourable relationships within medical encounters. All our story-tellers acquired an enormous amount of knowledge about HIV and AIDS over a prolonged period of time and believe that they know as much, if not more, about issues pertaining to HIV as their HIV consultants. Many had also worked in the field of HIV for many years and all believe it crucial to take total control of HIV health matters. Whilst it is sometimes necessary to confront the medical profession, 'telling them off' and being assertive strengthens relationships and initiates mutual participation in any decision making processes on HIV-related health matters.

MINNIE

As we recall earlier in this chapter Minnie aged 42 was diagnosed with HTLVIII at the age of 21 years in November of 1981. He was reliant on a wheelchair for mobility due to peripheral neuropathy and vasculitis and was relatively healthy at the time of our interview. Minnie was on combination therapy and has had AIDS-defining illnesses since 1996 onwards. He described himself as a 'control freak' and regarded his on-going relationship with the medical profession as excellent. He revealed:

"Well clearly I think we have completely set a precedent within the medical profession with this whole arena of HIV and AIDS because a lot of the long-term survivors have learned at the same pace as the doctors about this illness, particularly myself... in a lot of cases I might know more about specific areas than certain doctors that are not specifically specialist in this area... you know, they understand the chest or something else but they don't understand the virus and we know more than they do and it's taken a while but it is now working between us as patients and our consultants... you know, when you're an in-patient and have a chest infection, for example, you're going to be under a chest team, albeit that you are primarily under your own HIV consultant as well. But she's got to rely on the chest team to get you sorted out and it is there where you come up against the problems with the medical profession because they don't like being told their jobs... unfortunately we have had to do that... it's just empowerment I think... Patients for years and years have been just patients; they don't take control over what is wrong with them. They leave it to their doctors and, for me, the biggest thing about any terminal condition that anybody might face is, for crying out loud, the taking of control. It is your illness not theirs... as soon as you take control they give you information that you need and you glean information that you need and then you can make informed choices with your own consultant... I now think 'Yeah I have a very good relationship with my team here'; I have two community nurses who tend to be over protective and I know they listen to me and so I do have a good relationship with both my consultants and my nurses."

Minnie recounted that between him and his consultant they would discuss the causes of any illnesses he experienced; his current combination therapy was he believed effective. He can identify what might make him unwell and listens to his body and has actively gained information on HIV and medicine throughout the years. Minnie is in total control of managing his own health and is empowered by the knowledge he has acquired over time. He tells us:

"I feel strongly about 'we' as patients actually taking control of our terminal condition. You have to! If you let somebody else do it and take it out of your own hands then you know there isn't much hope for you... I certainly know that my own consultant has learned from me as she's told me because you know who better to teach her than her own patient... but a lot of patients are patients and need guidance and are not able to take all the information on board and be empowered enough to make informed choices and decisions about their own treatment. I know this, of course, because they don't fundamentally understand it and that isn't their fault... but my consultant, in particular, is very good at directing to a different level if she has to do that... You know she can put things into good layman's terms for those who are not equipped to understand the medical terms... people get bombarded with medications and they don't always know what they are taking... I am amazed at this because I need to know what I am taking because I like to know how it works on my body and on the virus... but more to the point I want to know what I am putting into my body... I only read what's necessary for me; I don't read about everybody else's medication."

To be fair, Minnie does have a background in bioscience yet he fully comprehends and appreciates how some people might struggle when faced with biomedical terms and combination therapy within an HIV context. He will therefore challenge the medical profession and is active and empowered in every aspect of his HIV and other health-related illness conditions.

COLIN

At the time of our interview, Colin aged 46 years, was relatively healthy, was on combination therapy and attended regular HIV health checks. Diagnosed in 1985, he cared for his partner who had AIDS until he died. Colin has at times barely escaped death but describes his current treatment as effective and sees HAART as a positive thing. He has a vast amount of knowledge around HIV and AIDS matters and has *'made it my business to know all new information and developments in the field'*. He has a very good relationship with his current HIV medial practitioner and has always taken an extremely active role in medical decisions and health care. When I asked him to describe his relationship with his HIV medical practitioners, he recounted:

"I like my doctor a lot. We are kind of... almost friends. Now one of the things I credit to my survival is that I wasn't in awe of doctors and was perfectly prepared to change clinics if I decided that I was not getting on with my doctor and was getting bad advice. And as I have gone on, I've kind of moved up to the top. I am not prepared to put up with some junior doctor who doesn't know his stuff... I have changed clinics seven times throughout my HIV career. The first time because they wouldn't give me an HIV test, the second one was because they kept nagging me to take AZT and I was refusing to. He was a lovely doctor, a really sweet man, he couldn't care enough for his patients but I just wouldn't take it and in the end I just got tired of him nagging me. It is funny I met him at an AIDS conference a couple of years later and he said, 'You were right, you were right to have refused to take AZT monotherapy.' Then I went somewhere else and demanded to see a certain professor and they actually saw me through the very worst period with my AIDS symptoms. And this doctor was a brilliant doctor when you were in a genuine medical crisis... I remember I nearly got my guts whipped out at one point, because I was having desperate abdominal pain. I turned up actually crying in pain and was poked and prodded and they said we think you have got CMV of the gut which was a really, really serious AIDS-related illness. It is the one that makes people go blind but it can also get into your guts, and if it gets into your guts it can literally punch holes in your intestines within hours. They said we are going to have to whip out your intestines and they phoned up the professor and he said that he was not convinced that it is CMV by the sound of it. He thought that Crypto has got into my bile duct and I had essentially got gall stones, blockage of the bile duct and he was right and they were wrong. I didn't have my guts ripped out... I know somebody that this did happen to... so that was good. But he was very conservative when it came to prescribing combination therapy so I went elsewhere and this doctor is very much the other way. He is prepared to prescribe quite experimental regimes... I will take what works; if it works I will take it. It was difficult because literally in those days you had to, well doctors were going by guess work, not exactly guess work but they were going on their hunches and this doctor is prepared to go on his scientific hunches and he doesn't wait until all the info comes in. They are scientific hunches, it is not guess work but 9 times out of 10 his hunches turn out to become standard treatment... I am very confident in his judgement. I had known this doctor beforehand anyway so it is a supportive relationship really. He tells me if he is depressed and I tell him if I am feeling ill.'

Colin has worked in the HIV field for many years and so takes an active role in learning about HIV and AIDS matters, particularly in relation to HIV medicines. He had worked with the National AIDS helpline during 1987/1988 and had been trained in up-to-date information about HIV transmission at a time when the Iceberg and Tombstone awareness campaigns were prevalent, as discussed in chapter one. Colin enjoys a good working relationship with his current HIV medical practitioners.

TOM

We have heard from Tom earlier in this chapter on matters of HIV prejudice and discrimination. Diagnosed in 1986, he takes combination therapy, attends regular HIV health checks and is reasonably healthy. He has an excellent knowledge and understanding of HIV and AIDS matters. Whilst he sees HAART as a positive thing, he did initially lack confidence in HIV medicines; he will also challenge medical professionals if he disagrees with medical advice or guidance. When I asked him to describe his relationship with the HIV medical profession, he told me:

"It is very good, very good. But I acknowledge that it is because I'm quite an empowered person who asks questions and I would say that it does give you more successful treatment options. My doctor is not very popular here, he says it how it is, but I like it... I told him when we first began a relationship that I don't want him to know anything significant about my health that I myself don't know... if there's a problem tell me and I'll deal with it. He gives me advice and maps out options and I'm always the one that makes the ultimate decision but it's his job to inform me and that includes giving me bad news as well as good news... I mean in 1991 when I got an AIDS diagnosis, I got a bottle of Dom Perignon that I'd been saving for years for when I got an AIDS diagnosis... I could tell when he called me through for consultation, it was only when I got home that it kind of hit me... AIDS is such a powerfully evocative word and I thought 'I'm no different!' so I am going to give that label back. I much prefer to think of myself as somebody living with HIV and I'm glad to say that this seems to be a general trend. You don't hear very many people talking about AIDS now... I'm a remarkably optimistic person really, and no doctor can say categorically this or that because we are all a product of something that has never been experienced before, so you know, it makes us all very individual patients because we have all experienced different things "

To the best of his knowledge, Tom has not experienced too many severe side effects from HIV treatment in the past. He believes that medical uncertainties of living with HIV is a big feature in his life and he struggles with planning for the future but deals with the present using a positive approach to everyday life.

LARRY

Larry was 56 at the time of our interview and was diagnosed in 1992 after voluntarily testing following the onset of illness. His route of transmission remains a mystery although he believes it might have been as a result of infected blood products. Larry is feeling very healthy at present since he recently embarked upon combination therapy and he attends regular HIV health checks. He has a good working relationship with the HIV medical profession and has taken an active role in learning about HIV matters. After two weeks of starting his combination therapy, Larry noticed a subtle difference in his health. When I asked him how he considered his relationship with the HIV medical profession, he recounted:

"I tell them off... I do. I went up there one day and I was sick to death of sort of feeling he wasn't listening or doing anything when my body was saying, 'Larry, someone needs to do something now.' So I sat there and I said to him, 'Excuse me, I've been living with this longer than you've been learning about it... and he started shaking poor lad. No, he actually started to respect me more. I feel there's a sense of respect there because he actually said to me since then, 'If you went [he didn't mean die], but if you went we'd miss you.' And I thought, bless him. No, I don't beat around the bush not when it's my body and health. I think I've probably got a more in-depth relationship than a lot of people could expect to have, yes. I am not always happy with the relationship though, only sometimes. I've never had a problem with other health professionals and dentists are marvellous. It was the dentist who discovered I had systemic thrush. I get on wonderfully with them."

Larry believes that to the best of his knowledge he has never experienced prejudice or discrimination on the basis of his HIV-positive status. Interestingly, Larry used to work as a volunteer in the HIV field before he learned of his own status and he loves to help people; people are the most important aspect of life. He firmly believes he knows as much if not more about HIV matters than health professionals and is always willing to adopt a challenging role in negotiating his own health care and medical needs.

Experiencing changes in HIV health care: stress and anxiety

We explore here how long-term survivors' have personally experienced radical changes in HIV health care which, as a consequence, is producing levels of stress, uncertainty and anxiety for future HIV-related treatment. Changes in HIV health care practice along with restricted funding and changes in budgets are now impacting on how HIV health care is being experienced within medical consultations. Our story-tellers speak of how medical practitioners are discussing their budgets with patients and how limited funding is affecting treatment options. Changes in medical practices now means HIV consultants working in hospitals who, in the past, have treated HIV-positive patients for certain reoccurring illness conditions, are now referring them back to the General Practitioner; this means it takes longer to access medical treatments and GPs are not HIV specialists. When HIV consultants move on from their permanent posts and temporary staff are drafted in, this creates instability and patients have to renegotiate relationships during multiple consultations. One of our story-tellers reveals how no-one is willing to take the responsibility for his HIV medication because there is no continuity with his HIV medical team. It is to these narratives we now turn.

NEIL

Neil is 42 years old and was diagnosed with HTLV III back in 1985 after involuntarily testing. He is medically retired, attends regular HIV health checks, is on combination therapy and has experienced few side effects from treatment. He describes living with HIV as 'a battle' and was currently experiencing visible signs of body fat redistribution, known as lipodystrophy, which was causing distress and considerable concern. When I asked him about how he considers his relationship with the HIV medical profession, he told me:

"Yes, it is good, it is good, I mean in a sense that I trust that they will do their best. I believe that they will do what they can for you... I have had very different treatments and I always got to see people fairly quickly if I had a problem but there has certainly been a change in the last few years, possibly the last three years. They certainly have started talking to me as a patient about their budgets and budget needs and this affects my treatment... for example, being able to go in and see if the doctor is available to talk about anything. Now they are saying that I should go and speak to my GP about certain things. Each winter I tend to get a really bad cough which goes into the tracheitus: it's not a big problem, it just needs antibiotics to clear up, but in the past I have always gone to the hospital and now they are saying: 'well you can come to us' but they are sort of saying well look to your GP as well. The problem is that you certainly have to wait longer for the GP, you know, to see the doctor, and in the past, I have always been able to go and see the consultant the same day or the next day to clear things up. You know there is always the possibility that it is not the same problem but is something else...finances and budgets were never discussed with me before as a patient but that sort of thing is now discussed and I read about this in the paper too, about changes to HIV funding and the NHS. I have asked the doctor about this and they just said: 'well yes, that's what's happening in theory but in practice it's not, it shouldn't really affect the service we provide'. I don't know that I believe this though... funding is not being allocated to HIV - they are to compete with everybody else. I mean the nurses I've actually chatted to when I have been down for blood tests, as a patient, they're saying to me that the number of patients they have on their books, most of them are on HAART and the cost of that per patient is coming from the budget... the fact that they're talking about it makes me wonder if this is obviously becoming a big problem."

Having conversations about funding and budgets with his HIV medical health care team is clearly worrying Neil as a patient. He continues:

"I am worried about my future in a sense... it remains to be a question as to whether funds will be available, for example, to pay for drugs. From what I understand the drugs I am on cost several thousand pounds a year and so I do wonder how long that can continue for; especially if I have to be on them for the rest of my life, I mean I am 42 years old now and that could be for another 40 years."

Neil explained that he is on his fourth combination therapy now and considers this regimen as more effective with fewer side effects. He takes an active role in his learning about HIV issues and has a good working relationship with his HIV medical team. His concerns, however, over budgets and financial matters do cause him distress and anxiety. Neil has not experienced prejudice or discriminatory practices on the basis of HIV status within any medical encounters.

PETER

Peter is 48 years old and was diagnosed in 1987 after volunteering to take part in a clinical trial. He is experiencing relatively good health and is medically defined as symptomatic and is taking combination therapy. Peter regularly attends HIV checks and is medically retired. His HIV medicine is relatively unproblematic but he has experienced horrendous side effects previously. Peter has had a good working relationship with the medical profession in the past but will challenge them when necessary. He told me how he is reluctant to see his GP; instead he prefers to attend his HIV clinic for medical matters:

"I am not particularly friendly with the new doctor. I mean the trouble with so many of these professionals is unfortunately they have become so specialised that if something is not specific to what they are precisely trained in, then that's that… it is not a very holistic approach; it is not an all-encompassing approach that I would value. I suppose the National Health would like me to spend more time seeing my GP now, with all the changes in budgets and funding… my GP making appropriate decisions and suggestions as to where we might go with this and that?…let's face it GPs are over-worked and I don't think the average GP knows very much more about HIV than I do after 17 years of living with it… I know my particular GP is quite happy for me to go to my HIV clinic for all my treatment that I feel I need, it is a Centre of Excellence, … or for investigations that I may need because it is sort of like cutting out the middle man to go to the HIV clinic to access some of the best treatment in the world than to go to my local GP who is well over-worked… what with a whole surgery full of germs that I can well do without sitting amongst with a compromised immune system…my relationship with my GP is sort of distant and a rare connection… but it is there by our mutual agreement for the purpose of my getting repeat prescriptions of things… I mean even if I had a bad cough I wouldn't go to my GP with it, I would go to the HIV clinic because I firmly believe that the HIV clinic would probably suggest a particular antibiotic to deal with it rather than another one which they may choose to hold in reserve for something more sinister...you know a GP might give you a fire engine to put out a candle and it is not necessary. The HIV clinic will give you a cup of water to pour over the candle... that's how I see it...I don't have a key person involved in my overall medical well-being in a way that the National Health Service wishes to provide... perhaps I am an awkward old sod because I think that what I do is best and is in my best interest."

Peter believes the medical profession do not really want to help him overcome some of his medical conditions, like sexual dysfunction, as they put it down to an inevitable aspect of the HIV treatment. Peter prefers to access the HIV clinic for health matters; the HIV clinic prefers that he goes to his GP. In terms of his sexual dysfunction, he no longer engages in sexual activities but this does not bother him at all. He has a good working knowledge of HIV issues and will challenge medics whenever necessary.

JOHN

John is 48 years old and was diagnosed with HIV in 1989 after voluntarily testing. He is experiencing good health, is medically defined as asymptomatic and is not on combination therapy. John regularly attends HIV health checks and works full time. John had recently moved from the South of England to the Manchester area and told me how surprised he was at the differences between medical provision in Manchester and his old city. He told me:

"Where I came from it had changed over the last 12 years from being a bit stiff and starchy, you know, you shouldn't have unprotected sex; you shouldn't be having sex at all. But this changed and my old clinic acknowledged that gay men, positive gay men will have unprotected sex sometimes, all the time or whatever... now you feel that you can go and talk about it without being looked down on or disapproved of... the provision in Manchester is not the same. I was shocked to discover that considering it has the third or fourth largest population in the country, there is no drop-in clinic in Manchester... If you want to go to a GUM clinic you have to wait for a week for an appointment... Yes, unless you go along and present yourself to a triage nurse you won't be seen for a week. When I spoke to one of the nurses she was shocked as well. She had come from London... there is even one in Rochdale, I think [laughing]...but there is not one in Manchester... I think if you are an existing patient you can go along and ring up the ward at North Manchester Infirmary and they will see you but there is no drop-in clinic. I mean the whole attitude is like it was 12 years ago in my old locality... for a start, in North Manchester the HIV clinic is in the infectious diseases unit. It is not in the GUM clinic... I mean what really pisses me off is that I work and I don't start until 10 so I have to go at 9 o'clock and at 9.40am you hear the nurse on the phone saying, 'who is taking the morning clinic? Doctor so-and-so... you can hear all this... where is he? I don't know he is on the train somewhere... no-one comes along and you have been waiting for 40 minutes but the doctor won't actually be coming... it also applies to medicine in all sorts of other ways too and if you don't feel able to take control over your own life they just assume you can hang around all day... this of course does not encourage certain people to have an independent life... I don't feel I need medication, certainly for me I feel that quality of life is more important than longevity. I don't want to live as long as possible just for the sake of living as long as possible."

John does not want to take HIV medication until he feels it is absolutely necessary and certainly not until medical markers indicate that his health has been compromised. He finds the differences and changes to medical health care for HIV in the North somewhat surprising and unaccommodating for people in full time employment.

RICK

Rick aged 32 was diagnosed in 1990 after voluntarily testing for the second time using his proper name; he was aware of his HIV-positive status in 1987 following his first test result. He regularly attended HIV health checks, was medically retired and was not taking combination therapy at the time of our interview, as he was awaiting salvage therapy. Rick recalled how he had taken up to 10 different combination therapies over the years and was unsure of all of the different names. He had experienced severe side effects from his HIV treatment in the past and he was currently experiencing bouts of ill health and was dealing with anxiety and stress due to current changes with his HIV health care. When I asked him to describe his relationship with his HIV medical practitioners, he told me:

"Where I was before it was brilliant, but because of recent changes I have to go elsewhere and where I am we have got Locum after Locum after Locum... the one at the moment has been there quite a while. We don't really see eye-to-eye and that is why I take someone with me. He doesn't seem to write any notes down and if you say I have got diarrhoea, you know where I was before, they would say I would need to see a gastro-entrologist but in the meantime we will try you on this or that to see if it calms down. He doesn't do this where I am now, he just says wait till you see palliative care. If you say you are coughing up blood, something used to be done about it where I was before and they would send you somewhere and in the meantime give you antibiotics or something, but he doesn't, he just says he will refer me and that's it. I told him in October I was coughing up blood and I got an appointment in May and when I asked him about it he said that he didn't put me down as urgent. That is because he didn't believe me... I ended up getting really upset after I came back from America cos I said about coughing up blood again and he hadn't even referred me by then and he asked me 'Are you sure?' I said well I am colour-blind and he is aware I am colour-blind but I know what blood is and I do get my partner to check everything, my stools, my wee and my sputum. And I was definitely coughing up blood in America... so I got really upset and I said that my partner is next door and I asked the Locum if he wanted to speak with him. He asked me if I was sure that it was as bad as I said it was... I was getting so upset with it all, he didn't believe me. You see, it is not very often that my partner shows his emotions but the other night he was crying in bed and I thought it was because of something else, but it wasn't it was over me, he is so worried about me... so I asked the Locum yet again if he wanted to speak to my partner because I was coughing up blood and I was having night sweats. And he said to me, 'Are you sure they were night sweats?' I don't believe it! The whole bed and my partner's side of the bed and the pillows were waterlogged and my partner was kept awake all night because he was wet through... I asked him again if he wanted to speak with my partner... Now, instead of the Locum giving me *Sometadine*, I had to wait two weeks until palliative care gave me *Sometadine* and it has cut the sweats down to nearly nothing. Now he knows that *Sometadine* helps the sweats... it is the not the same care now with all the doctors changing and the funding problems... I mean until they get a proper doctor working there... I mean there is a proper doctor there but he has to rush here, there and everywhere... we keep getting Locums and they have no knowledge of my background history and so it has got to be all gone through again... one doctor has been there quite a while now and he has got to know me quite well but he doesn't write anything down... but like I said I was coughing up blood three appointments before I went to America but it is not in his notes and he has no knowledge of me saying this... And the sweats, I mean I was in America in queen-sized beds which were absolutely soaked and I was sleeping on towels. It is not fair when he could have prescribed me *Sometadine* which works well for sweats... I am always passed from pillar to post, which is why I am having this case conference... why isn't the HIV doctor doing something? Why does he always say, 'wait until you see somebody else'... since I last saw you, Judy, we have two more doctors there and one of them has just taken a permanent post elsewhere, so we are now getting yet another stand-in Locum... so I guess I will have to give him a couple of chances to try and sort something out and if not I am definitely going to move from here as it seems to be getting worse and worse."

As Rick was waiting for salvage therapy due to his past HIV combination therapies no longer working effectively, he was reluctant to change his HIV clinic. He was refusing to take Protease Inhibitors unless he had a lipid management specialist due to the severe side effects he had experienced in the past. Rick had been informed that if he took Protease Inhibitors again it would be effective in managing his viral load and would increase his CD4 cell count but he was at risk of a heart attack or Pancreatis. He was informed that this could be medically managed. He told me:

"I need proper lipid management within seven to ten days of taking Protease Inhibitors because I have problems with lipids, triglycerides and cholesterol… but if they can't sort it out within seven days of my taking new treatment I will refuse to go on them because I am not putting my life at risk. I am not going to take life-threatening or fatal risks… I ought to go back on them because they gave me good blood results but it is no good if it is going to give me a heart attack or pancreatis…I took the trouble to discuss this in detail with one doctor, but as he was leaving a couple of weeks after our appointment, he wasn't really interested… nobody is prepared to take any responsibility because they are not there long enough. I am just sat here waiting whilst my viral load goes flying up to what we call a wild virus and my CD4 count keeps going down… I am just sat there waiting for a doctor to make a decision."

Rick recalled how his HIV health care had gone from good to bad and from 'worse to crap'. He did not see eye-to-eye with many of the doctors passing through the clinic and because there was a tendency for doctors not writing things down, he always took someone with him who took notes. During consultations he takes a folder with his notes and is desperately awaiting a decision on new HIV medication. As you will recall, Rick died a few years later.

WOODY

Woody aged 45 was diagnosed at the age of 32 back in 1992 after voluntarily taking the test because of embarking on a new relationship at the time. Woody underwent pre-counselling prior to taking his HIV test. He goes for regular health checks, is very healthy and is in full time employment. He is taking combination therapy and has experienced mild side effects in the past. At the time of our interview, Woody was experiencing rapid weight loss which was becoming more noticeable to others around him; he considered this visible change as problematic. When I asked him to describe his relationship with the medical profession over time he told me:

"Well, that's changed over the years. It used to be very good now it's OK because in the last ten years all the doctors and people at the local clinic have changed. The main consultant retired and they got somebody else in who's an HIV specialist. The whole staff has basically changed and it's a part-time clinic where the staff share their time between so many days here and so many days in another city…it's not a specialist HIV unit it's the GUM clinic and it has got increasingly busy with other sexually transmitted diseases… so there are several consultants and a couple of them specialise in HIV and everybody is a lot busier and all the systems have changed… No it is not as good as it used to be because I think they had more time. I don't feel as I get as much time as I probably should do but then that's not altogether their fault because I don't insist on it… I don't push it and I suppose they don't either. I don't have thorough sessions with doctors. I have a doctors appointment may be once or twice a year whereas I should have one every three months. Other people have appointments with their consultant when they go for their blood tests… I'm not too sure because different people do different things but I try and fit mine in. I don't have them as a matter of course, I have a couple a year… there have been no immediate problems since I went on Protease Inhibitors as my CD4 count and viral load tests have been much better… I mean if I was poorly and I had to see someone then I guess it would be alright. It's not that thorough but that might be my fault as well, because as I said I don't go as often as I should but then again they don't push it and say you must come every three months."

Woody revealed that he didn't feel as though he had a good relationship in general with the medical profession as he had experienced five or ten years previously. Over the past couple of years he stated:

"Different staff, different ways of doing things and the whole clinic is busy with HIV and other medical issues… there are dozens and dozens of people sitting all down the corridors in the waiting rooms and the place is packed with people. It is like half the population of my local area."

Woody is extremely cautious and secretive about his HIV-positive status, he therefore chooses not to disclose his status to others around him. As a consequence, he finds the changes in his health care provision difficult to successfully negotiate and therefore only attends HIV check ups once or twice a year unless he feels particularly unwell. He is currently enjoying good health apart from recent weight loss and takes regular exercise and maintains a good diet.

Medical errors: on still being alive

This last story stands alone as it is somewhat different to others above. Whist it is unrelated to HIV, John does speak about quality of life issues, challenging the medics, doctors not having enough time and medical mistakes that can be made and so on. We reveal how John experienced the medical profession in relation to his diagnosis and treatment for cancer, which was unrelated to his HIV condition. I believe that in spite of his experience not necessarily 'fitting in' with other long-term survivors' experiences, it should not be overlooked and therefore is included in this chapter.

JOHN

As we have seen earlier, John is 48 years old and was diagnosed with HIV in 1989 after voluntarily testing. He is experiencing good health, is medically defined as asymptomatic and is not on combination therapy. John regularly attends HIV health checks. A few years previously, he was medically diagnosed and treated for cancer, which was unrelated to his HIV condition. Due to chemotherapy treatment and its known effect of depressing the immune system, he was advised to go on combination therapy for two or three years. He did not experience side effects and *'is not totally absorbed in learning about HIV issues'*. John's personal experiences of the medical profession that he recounts here are not directly related to his HIV but instead convey his experiences of living with and overcoming cancer. When I asked him to describe his relationship with the medical profession, he told me:

"Well some people are better than others, as in everything. They are human beings, they make mistakes and they don't have enough time. The cancer experience was very, very strange because I went to the doctor and said I think I have got a hernia, and the doctor said, 'Yes'. I went to the specialist and he said 'Yes'. So I decided I would pay privately to have a hernia operation and woke up and was told by the same doctor who would have done it on the NHS, some two years later, that he had removed 14 ounces of malignant tumour from my groin... so if I hadn't paid I would be dead. This is very unsatisfactory and then I was told I had Lymphoma which is very nasty... it is one of those things that spreads throughout the body and they were going to give me chemotherapy and I wasn't going to be treated for it until I had got more information. They were a bit sniffy about this. I asked what were the chances of this treatment succeeding? And they said it was 30% on people who are otherwise healthy, which by their terms I wasn't healthy. So I said: 'can we find out how far it has spread? So treatment was delayed and I spent about 3 weeks thinking I was going to die. I went in to work on a Monday morning and there was a message on the answering machine asking me to call the surgeon at home. And most surgeons don't give you their home number. So I rang him and he said it was really good news! He says: 'I was playing golf on Sunday with the Pathologist' and I said 'yeeeeeeeeessssss', and he's changed his diagnosis. You have seminoma and that is really good news. So, what is that then? I ask and he said I have got testicular cancer and that is really good news... it had a 97% cure rate and so yes it was good news and I am now approaching the 5 years following the end of treatment, after which they stop monitoring you."

John was not presumed to be healthy on account of him being HIV-positive and he resisted going ahead with further cancer treatment and went against the advice of the medical practitioners. He went on to tell me:

"I can imagine there are people, probably quite a lot of people, who believe doctors are one step ahead or whatever, and they will do exactly what their doctors say... I don't... I personally don't feel that being treated for whatever illness is necessarily a good thing. It depends on quality of life and, you know, chemotherapy. At that point, I felt perfectly well but I wasn't going to have chemotherapy and feel grim for whatever time I had got left. I don't want that. I would rather just enjoy another few weeks, few months and then that's the end of it."

John is not particularly interested in matters pertaining to HIV. He is aware of different combination therapies and if he can '*carry on in life without thinking about it then that is absolutely fine. It is not a subject that interests me for its own sake at all*'. He takes a confident and active role in his health care, has not experienced HIV-related ill health and would take total control in any medical decisions he might have to take in the future.

In closing this chapter, I reflect on some of the issues brought to light by the personal experiences of our story-tellers. We have learned how long-term survivors approach the medical profession in various ways and how relationships have been maintained during multiple consultations due to

A forgotten generation: Long-term survivors' experiences of HIV and AIDS

HIV being medically defined as a chronic illness. All our story-tellers attend regular HIV health checks and many are taking combination therapies whether they are symptomatic or asymptomatic. We have witnessed how prejudice and discriminatory practices have been experienced within a medical setting and how this has impacted on those who have experienced such encounters. Changes in HIV-related health care over the years are causing undue stress, uncertainty and anxiety for future treatment options. Many of our story-tellers speak of empowerment and actively involving themselves in decision-making strategies for HIV medication and health care. Challenging medical practitioners is perhaps considered essential by almost all long-term survivors, as knowledge and awareness of HIV-related matters becomes more prolific. A healthy scepticism and deep-rooted mistrust of the medics and pharmaceutical industry seems widespread amid our story-tellers which is not surprising in the context of HIV.

Many of our long-term survivors have successfully negotiated a good working relationship with HIV medical practitioners; yet have had to be prepared to change HIV clinics, change HIV consultants, take control over their medical destinies and challenge medical advice wherever necessary. It is evident that medical practitioners must continue to learn from long-term survivors about HIV matters, as mutual participation is essential for good working relationships built on mutual respect and trust. Some of the experiences uncovered in this chapter are shamefully inappropriate, unjust and quite alarming and I hope that lessons can be learned from exposing these experiences publicly.

Again, I ask you the reader to reflect on how these stories have impacted on your personal attitudes and beliefs. Who do you consider is the HIV expert? Do you take an active or passive role during medical consultations? How might you have coped with the challenges of living with HIV during medical consultations? What is your opinion of medical practitioners? How might you feel if you had experienced prejudice and discrimination on the basis of your chronic illness condition? Can you empathise with our story-tellers and their personal experiences? Critically reflect on what you have learned after reading this chapter and, as I ask in every chapter, consider your own feelings, opinions and positions in relation to these experiences and reflect on whether these remain constant or have changed and if so why?

A forgotten generation: Long-term survivors' experiences of HIV and AIDS

CHAPTER EIGHT

Me, myself and HIV: exploring networks of support

∞

"Friendship is born at that moment when one person says to another: What! You too? I thought I was the only one."

C. S. Lewis

"You have not lived today until you have done something for someone who can never repay you."

John Bunyan

Introduction

How we socially integrate within our cultural and sub-cultural 'communities' is crucial for sustaining our health and psychological well-being as we explored in chapter one. If we accept that dominant social factors influence and shape our perceptions of health and illness, then it is crucial that we develop a meaningful understanding of how living long-term with HIV impacts on the social lives of human beings living with this chronic illness. Experiences of illness transcend beyond medical matters and taking medicine; illness is a social state. We have acknowledged throughout these chapters how our story-tellers have experienced degrees of loss at various levels of their personal and social lives since diagnosis. Losses occur throughout our daily lives and these can include: loss of jobs; loss of a loved one; loss of established friendships; loss of health; loss of self-worth and self-esteem, and loss of social status in our social world, to name a few. In the face of loss we may become isolated and vulnerable; and when we are vulnerable we often find that resources to help us overcome our losses become limited.

The presence of social support via an assortment of 'networks' is recognised by almost all as playing a vital role in enabling us to draw upon particular resources that we might feel are unobtainable during personal experiences of loss, uncertainty and periods of ill health. When we have sources of support available we can seek assistance from others and have the knowledge that we are being cared for. Networks of support provide us with essential resources which can comprise: companionship, giving us a sense of belonging; emotional and practical support in terms of care-giving and nurture; financial support in the face of economic hardship, and the provision of vital information and expert advice. When there is no presence of social support in our lives, we may become isolated, alienated and vulnerable which can lead us towards a poor sense of well-being and ill health. What kind of support do you offer to friends, family and other members in your social environment?

Social networks of support provide essential encouragement and assistance that may facilitate motivational inspiration to adopt positive attitudes and behaviours that are beneficial to those seeking support. When we think of the term 'network of support' this conjures up the idea of a social structure that consists of individuals or organisations who are linked or connected by social relationships with significant others; these links form social networks. Types of relationship links might include: family or kinship relationships; communication relationships; friendship relationships; intimate relationships; workplace relationships and more recently, social networking sites and forums located on the Internet.

During times of need and crises, we require the co-operation and support of others to give us a more balanced and focussed outlook on life and help maintain a positive self-image. When we socially interact with others whether it is a trusted social group or a valued individual, we enhance our quality of life and psychological well-being in the face of loss and adverse life events. Along our journey so far, we have learned about how some long-term survivors have faced varying degrees of: loss of self-esteem; emotional insecurity; financial insecurity and poverty; significant loss of quality of life; loss of physical intimacy; loss of privacy; depression; anxiety and a distinct lack of motivation in the face of living with HIV and AIDS. Arguably, facing such adverse life events brings with it a degree of vulnerability in terms of how we experience everyday life. In our private lives, we as human beings may believe we are facing our problems alone and that there is no-one 'out there' facing the same social predicaments or dilemmas.

In this chapter we find out how living long-term with HIV has impacted on our story-tellers' sense of 'self' and uncover the dynamics that influence whether HIV is a big or small part of who-you-are. We also expose how our long-term survivors have maintained and negotiated family and friendship relationships and whether these have been affected by HIV. Are family and friends a good source of support around HIV issues? Our story-tellers speak of their personal experiences and active involvement with other sources of support in relation to HIV and reveal to what extent these have provided appropriate resources and valuable assistance. We learn about how our long-term survivors view the notion of a 'HIV community' and other kinds of communities where there might be a perceived sense of belonging. Whilst examining family, friendships and other networks of support, we also aim to explore any other social concerns that were raised by our story-tellers as part of living long-term with HIV and how this impacts on social life. Towards the end of the chapter, we pay particular attention to the *National Long-term Survivors' Group* (NLTSG) in the UK with a collection of quotes. A number of story-tellers identified with and were members of this social group and had attended at least one residential weekend.

On being asymptomatic: HIV, networks of support and other pressing matters

All ten of our story-tellers in this collection of personal experiences were diagnosed between 1983 and 1993 and were medically defined as asymptomatic: showing no clinical symptoms of HIV. Seven story-tellers were not taking any HIV medication at the time of our interview, and five had never been recipients of HIV combination therapy since diagnosis. Many long-term survivors in this section have not experienced frequent bouts of HIV-related illness since the onset of diagnosis. We start with our story-tellers who were diagnosed the earliest.

GLYNN

Glynn, aged 37, describes himself as a White, middle class heterosexual man and his religious affiliation is Church of England (non-practising). He was diagnosed with HTLV III in 1983 and the route of transmission was via contaminated Factor VIII blood products. At the time of our interview Glynn was working as a volunteer co-ordinator in a charitable organisation. He had previously qualified in a different occupation. Glynn lives with Haemophilia, HIV and HCV; he is divorced, has one child and is currently single and lives alone. When I asked him how HIV impacted on his sense of self, he told me:

"I would say it is a small part of me... it's like saying, 'do I think Haemophilia is a large or small part of my identity?' I would say it is small, I suppose... because you learn to live with it, don't you? You know with Haemophilia I don't know any different. With HIV I suppose I did know a difference but because of the age when I was diagnosed, well it is different because of sexual matters and women... It does impact in certain ways, you know if I hear a friend dies well that affects us, doesn't it? Although I think that you get hardened to it. My best mate died of it and I mean that was bloody awful... I thought Christ it could just as easily have been me... I don't know the answer to it, really."

As mentioned previously, Glynn was one of 65 people living with Haemophilia who were diagnosed at the same time; he was one of only three survivors at his local Haemophilia centre. I asked Glynn about whether HIV had affected friendship relationships and he recounted:

"There are friends of mine that I knew before I got HIV and HCV and then there are others who are no longer friends... it was their choice. I mean it was probably ignorance and it was a long time ago. Probably if I were in touch with them now they may think differently, I don't know... I used to know them, I used to go to the pub with them... I don't know whether they thought it was the gay plague or whatever... they just decided that they didn't want to be, well [long sigh]... we just weren't friendly any more basically. We didn't hate each other or anything like that, they just said they didn't want to..."

Glynn did not complete the sentence and believed this loss of friendship was predominantly based on ignorance and fear. He went on to say:

"I was pretty pissed off really but then I am not going to force them to be my friend. If that is what they wanna do then that's up to them... there was nothing I could do about it... it was only two people so there were plenty of other friends that didn't give a toss. I was still Glynn so that was that and I've still got a lot of friends now... but then a lot of my friends were Haemophiliacs or those with Christmas disease so a lot of them have HIV anyway. I have more friends that were involved with HIV than not, if you know what I mean."

Glynn did not access any support groups for HIV but did have involvement with the MacFarlane trust in relation to compensation matters. He is registered with the Trust, is in receipt of a monthly pension and he reads the newsletter. There is the Haemophilia society and a local Haemophilia group at his Haemophilia centre but he actively chooses not to participate in these support networks.

MARTIN

Martin, aged 38, describes himself as *'an individual like everybody else, rather than a sufferer of Haemophilia, HIV, HCV and possibly new variant*

CJD; but it doesn't start with 'H' so I can't have got that'. He also describes himself as a White, heterosexual Yorkshire man who is an Agnostic. Martin was diagnosed with HTLV III in 1985 and the route of transmission was via contaminated blood products for Factor VIII. He is married, lives with his wife and child and was working at the time of our interview. When I asked Martin about networks of support in relation to HIV, he told me that everybody he had told had been brilliant and totally supportive. He believed he was very lucky. When I asked him about family support, he told me:

" That's another subject for discussion… How are you? Fine… that's as far as it goes… I often wonder how much they understand. No, it was never: how is your HIV going? How are you feeling about it? It was never raised… I always thought that AIDS kills individuals but it also kills families. I believe it certainly killed mine, not my family here, no! AIDS killed my brother and I believe it killed my father indirectly and it caused the break up of everything… it devastated my Mum, it took her a long time to get over my brother."

As we recall, Martin's younger brother died from an AIDS-related illness and he understandably continues to search for a medical explanation as to why this happened whilst he is so healthy. I asked Martin about whether he accessed support groups and if he perceived there to be an HIV community, he told me:

"I believe there is. I don't believe I belong to it. I tried to. Well, I tried to be interested in it, to see what it is all about and I went to the Lighthouse once to one of the support groups, but I found that I came away from support groups feeling worse than I did before I went to them. I think some people define themselves as HIV-positive above every other aspect of themselves. But I also think it is easy for me to sit here and say that when I am totally fine at the moment. People are ill and they are living with it everyday and they need that support. They need to belong to that because society has said, 'You're ill, you are HIV-positive, go and support yourselves.' So I can see their point of view but I don't consider I belong to any of that at the moment… When I first moved to London and was on my own I went to a support group and I must admit it was great to start with. My first meeting, listening to people voicing what I had been thinking; I had never come across that before, it was amazing! I got a lot out of those meetings and I hope other people did. Then it became a case of, well, people started dropping off, meetings were fewer and then when you met you left wondering, 'Oh, my God! Is so-and-so going to be there? How are they looking? Oh, he looks ill. So I backed off… this was for positive Haemophiliacs."

Martin went on to tell me about his perceptions of the HIV community as a whole. He recounted:

"I think there is a difference between positive Haemophiliacs and positive gays, definitely… I mean there was a lot of talk about a lot of support being given for positive gay men but very little for positive Haemophiliacs who are heterosexuals, so I see a difference… I do think there is an HIV community out there… I think people do get together for common purposes. I know that relationships are built around more than one thing, but I think there is a chance to get together, because HIV is such a big thing and people feel shunned by general society. You know, stigmatised but when they get together with other people with the same problem you can be more open about it. I think the gay community has done a lot of work around health and HIV."

Martin's wife also participated in our interview and she reminded him of previous conversations that had taken place between them about being involved in the HIV community. She told me:

"I am not actually putting words in your mouth but you have felt out of it, we have talked about this before. You couldn't become part of that because of not being accepted. Haemophiliacs had nothing in common… you know there is only about 3,000 in the UK and so you are never going to meet because of a genetic disorder because you have nothing in common. If you are gay, you are part of something where you have already had to fight prejudice. And you meet because you have social interests and a commonality, whereas what Martin was part of there was no commonality just because you had a genetic problem… I think one positive feature that has come out of it is support groups for Haemophiliac children… they do lots of things… but even with the Haemophiliac community, newsletters… there is a lot of criticism and attitudes that have now changed… newsletters did not mention about HIV and Haemophiliacs because they had parents who are non HIV Haemophiliacs who didn't want to know. There was almost a sense of embarrassment and the sooner you die off the better."

Martin agreed with this and further considered that HIV did, in part, bring the Haemophilia community together during the 1980s and early 1990s but he believed that it is not as 'tight-knit' as before. The Haemophilia Society has given space for a page on HIV matters in their newsletter, says Martin, so they are 'getting their act together'.

A forgotten generation: Long-term survivors' experiences of HIV and AIDS

CLAIR

Clair, aged 40, describes herself as a White, heterosexual, Irish, practising catholic who is from an 'ordinary' social class background. She was diagnosed in 1987 and the route of transmission was sexual from her husband who contracted HIV from contaminated blood products. She was working at the time of our interview, was not in a relationship and lived alone. She had been involved in one intimate relationship after her husband's death and found it difficult to 'find the right man'. Clair believes HIV is only a small part of who she is and she classes HIV as a label she does not really like. When I asked her about social networks of support, she recounted:

"I have worked in the HIV field before... the politics I have been involved in... there were other issues around as well as it being very much a gay thing... many good things have come out of what has happened, so you need to stand back a bit and there's a huge bond, certainly psychologically...one of the things I have come to understand myself is that I have a notion of uncertainty and I know a lot of people don't want that... they actually want certainty... some people like to be told this is the drug they want... it's about responsibility, as well. Somebody else then takes care of the problem and I am not from that culture, it is really your own responsibility, and uncertainty means we don't know how long... there's been nothing wrong with me. They might call me 'not dead yet'."

Clair continued to reflect on how she felt living with HIV by stating that it had changed and broadened her mind through her questioning it all and challenging dominant viewpoints. She has 'had the most wonderful experiences' yet wonders what kind of life she might have had without HIV. I asked Clair about her family as a network of support, and she told me:

"I don't even talk about it. I talk to my brothers: I have four brothers and two sisters. Well, I talk to two of my brothers openly, particularly about the work I have done and some of the nonsense and it has been really good as a sounding board. I think I come from a cynical family and I come from a nursing background too. Generally, I don't sort of bother them."

Clair told me that she did not personally access support centres and did not read any HIV press, such as: Positive Nation. However, in the past, she had worked in the field and attended global conferences; she shared some of her personal experiences:

"I was working for a health support centre and there was certainly a community there... I suppose there are different circles of communities, like support for women, gay men, Black African groups, where people come together for social support... I don't feel part of it, no! I know hundreds of people across the world, but one of the great things is that you do get to talk to people at a more personal level... you know about your hopes and fears... but I also realise the dangers too... I went to a conference as part of the Global Network of Positive People and I went to a workshop on grief... I didn't know the women sitting around and we had to throw roses into the centre and say the names of people who had died... I just thought, 'Oh no! It's just not me!' I mean I could have lied and they were all balling their eyes out... then there was one woman she was reeling off about twenty names, but I mean she was working in the field, she'd organised the workshop... then they came out with names of people who hadn't died from HIV but had died from lupus or cancer or died from a blood clot... all the ones that had died and there was wailing and people lighting candles... OK maybe sometimes we need to go through processes like that but I think some of it is self-contained."

Clair has no desire to be part of any community but believes there are different communities and support groups for those who might need them. She believes she is too questioning, critical and challenging to belong anywhere and refuses to label herself or be labelled by others.

CHRISTOPHER

Christopher, aged 51, describes himself as a working class, *'dying to live rather than living to die'*, gay man. He was diagnosed in 1988 and the route of transmission was sexual. Christopher was not in a relationship, lived alone and was working at the time of our interview. He is a practising Christian and describes his ethnicity as White and English. Christopher has remained healthy since diagnosis and to the best of his knowledge has not experienced HIV-related illness. He believes that HIV is a fairly large part of who he is but he deals with this covertly, he told me:

"I don't hide it from myself in a denial way, I just shove it in its box and it doesn't need to come out unless I talk about it... I think it is big as far as the sex side of things are concerned...I had a lot of fear, a lot of guilt, a lot of moral dilemmas, well, religious dilemmas at the start... I have grown as a human being in the last sort of three years and first of all I learned to like myself and then learned to love myself because I think it is just part of me now, it's just there."

I asked Christopher about HIV networks of support and he told me:

"There are certain pockets of support here where I live… I have been an active member of my local positive support group and I go whenever I can to meetings and drop-ins and things like that and it allows me to make friendships with people… I believe I belong to the gay community here where I live… I have got a social worker who has become a friend as well… I don't feel I need support from many other agencies that might be available to me, like Buddies and things… purely and simply because I do feel that other people are in more need of this than me so they should have that… so I try not to be selfish… whilst I am healthy let other people who need them have this support and should the time come when I need them then I will access them."

Christopher has told members of his family about his HIV-positive status and some of his close friends. He does not want to tell his Mother because he does not want to burden her with this knowledge; his family have a practice of shielding his Mum because she is over 80 years old. He does, however, wish he could be more open and less secretive in wider friendship relationships.

JOHN

John, aged 48, describes himself as a middle class, gay man and a member of the Bear club. He was diagnosed in 1989 and the route of transmission was sexual. He is currently single, lives with a lodger and works full time. His religious affiliation is Church of England (non-practising) and he describes his ethnicity as White, UK. He is healthy and lives well with HIV, but is fearful of the prospect of future HIV-related illness. When I asked him whether HIV was a big or small part of his life on a scale of one to ten, he told me that it varied but most of the time it was on a scale of 3; this changed when he was embarking on an intimate relationship with a new man when it hovered around the 8 or 9 mark. When I asked him about networks of support and the HIV community, he told me:

"The HIV community certainly exists and there are people who, either when they are diagnosed or some time after they are diagnosed, revolve their whole life around being HIV-positive. Most of the support is used by them and certainly most of the support is available during normal working hours so it isn't very readily accessible to people who work full time… early on I went to the local Body Positive group because I was encouraged to go along... there were probably about seven or eight of us sitting in a kitchen round a circular white melamine table which had a lamp directly above it. Those seven people all knew one another and the facilitator... they went around the table and they talked about their benefits being insufficient and the medication they were on. Then it got to me and I thought: not on medication, I earn quite a lot of money, I shouldn't be here. I don't belong to this group. The only thing I have got in common with them is that I am positive. I never went again... there were a lot of people in my old city who were diagnosed at a similar time to me and they stopped working because it was easier then to stop working and get DS1500 and all the benefits... when you see them out looking perfectly well and driving around in their 4x4s which are on Mobility, you know... the person I used to live with stopped working because he was not particularly well but was on much more money with benefits than he ever had when he was working. This would not be the case for me if I stopped working... these people having nothing else to do with their lives [short pause] than complain about their lifestyles. In fact they feel hard done by and they are not really... a lot of them spend a huge amount of time and money in the pub. I am not saying that I don't drink because I do drink quite a lot... but I am glad that I haven't given up work and my whole life isn't based around being positive and waiting to die... every so often I wished I did not work so I didn't have to worry about things, but I am glad I didn't give up working."

John has a positive mental outlook on living life with HIV and is open and honest about his status when it is necessary. If he can carry on in everyday life without thinking too much about living with HIV then this is absolutely fine for John.

MARC

Marc, aged 38, describes himself as a middle class, gay/bisexual man who is currently pursing sexual relationships with women, as he has had enough of men. He believes *'men are dogs'*. Marc was diagnosed in 1990 and the route of transmission was sexual. He is currently single, works part-time and lives alone. He describes his religion as Jewish and his ethnicity as White. Marc considers himself to be lucky because he is healthy and has never taken combination therapy. HIV is a small part of his life but it could be a large part if he allowed it to be, he told me with a sense of irony:

"It could be a big part of my life if I let it... the way I would like it to be a big part is I would like to be on the board of directors of an HIV organisation and have an OBE and be friendly with the *'great and the good'* and have nice parties and earn a little cash all on the strength of some kind of HIV expert or Guru... I don't care, I just want the money. So, in that sense I would quite like HIV to be a big part of my life, but apart from that I would rather keep it, well not in the closet, but you know firmly keeping a hand on it. You know the jack-in-the-box neurosis could spring up from it... so I try to be quite strict and keep that box firmly closed; because you are worrying about nothing really."

Marc has been involved in HIV support networks in the past and has also participated in group therapy around drug use. He told me:

"I found it easier to be a volunteer than a service user, so from very early on after my diagnosis I started volunteering with lots of organisations and I still volunteer today and that is how I get support... I am more comfortable being a volunteer than a service user...I have been in a support group around not taking drugs with people who were HIV-positive... you just went along to this meeting and shared experiences to help us stay clean... HIV community, erm, there is an HIV gravy train. Definitely I have seen that with my own eyes and I am mighty pissed off that I am not on it...there are lots of HIV organisations and I used to, well I am involved with a couple at the moment. I am quite happy although there are lots of others, and you know after a while you see the same faces... I guess I don't really have lots of HIV-positive friends. I know quite a few who are but I don't see them often. I know more people who are HIV-negative... I was born in London and have always lived in London... there was a time when I was going to HIV meetings with NA [narcotics anonymous] and I was volunteering in the sector regularly and I did have a full time job and I had a car. So in those days I was very involved; I knew lots of people and have relationships with people that go way back, because I have always lived here."

Established long-term friendships have not been problematic for Marc; he did not refer to any members of his family as a network of support. He had a preference to be a volunteer rather than a service user in key HIV organisations and claimed this is how he accessed support. Marc was very healthy and he maintained his health by following a good diet, exercising regularly and getting plenty of sleep.

PABLO

Pablo, aged 32, describes himself as a working class, gay man who has experienced a bisexual phase in earlier life. He was diagnosed is 1990 and the route of transmission was sexual. Pablo was medically retired, in a long-term intimate relationship and lived alone. He is currently very healthy; he takes combination therapy as a preventative measure and describes himself as lucky. Pablo spoke about family matters and was adopted after his mother left him at six months old; members of family are aware of his HIV-positive status, he told me:

"I think that it's quite important to know you have support from your family. I mean some people have got that and some people haven't. My sister is quite supportive... My adoptive parents know but they don't want to talk about it basically. It is sort of not mentioned and being gay is not mentioned either... my sister is really good about it. I think she is brilliant. She's turned round and said if I ever get to where I am ill and can't cope then I can come and live with her and she will look after me. I wouldn't want that, I wouldn't put that on her anyway...all I bother about is my partner and someone taking care of him at the end of the day. I'm not sort of bothered about dying when the time comes it'll come. I suppose at the back of my mind, if I was to be honest, is the fear of suffering... I think that is probably the case for a lot of people."

Pablo does not see himself 'any differently to anybody else, apart from having a terminal illness'. This is his illness; it does not belong to anybody else and he controls it in his own way. He has a positive attitude and outlook on living life with HIV and only tells people he needs to tell. He spoke about losing friendships in the past:

"I didn't really have a big network of friends when I was younger; it was just a few close friends. I told about four or five of them about my HIV status and their initial reaction was: 'Oh! Don't worry about it, it'll all come out in the wash' type of thing. I suppose they didn't realise how serious it was. A couple of them were really supportive and still are to this day, although I don't see them that often but they always phone up to see how you are. It's amazing what a simple phone call once in a blue moon can do for somebody... then there's the others who sort of turned round and said, 'you're dirty, it's your own fault, you shouldn't have been messing around here, there and everywhere'... they just didn't want to know so I thought obviously they are not true friends, sod them... I suppose at the time it did affect me because I was living in such a small tight-knit community but now I think it is their problem and I have still got my other friends who are supportive."

Pablo does not consider HIV is a big part of his life. He recounted:

"I don't class it as a major part of my life. It is sometimes there and I don't dwell on it. I do what I have to do to keep myself healthy and that's it. I would just describe myself as gay and living life to the full. I don't turn round and say that I am an HIV gay man living life to the full because HIV doesn't come into it... yes, every morning and every night I am reminded that I have got it because I am taking my tablets. I take every day as it comes and there is more and more information available and support so you become less panicky. You don't panic about it"

I asked Pablo about networks of support and whether he believed in the existence of an HIV community. He told me:

"No I don't think there is an HIV community, I mean obviously there is a gay community wherever you go. Where I lived before, the gay community and the HIV community worked all in one area and it was quite bizarre. They had a big HIV problem there and not just within the gay community either, but in the heterosexual community. Heterosexual HIV is on the increase anyway amongst young people so it's getting quite scary. I worked as a volunteer in the HIV field but I don't think it's a community. I don't feel I belong to any community I am just a person... it makes me angry sometimes because I suppose we belong to many communities. If you belong to the gay community does it mean you don't belong to any other community? I think everybody is one community regardless of whether they are straight, gay, bloody bisexual or whatever... it's like when they say about 'poofs' – that's a gay poof and that's a straight poof. Why can't we just say he's a bloody poof?"

Pablo no longer volunteers in the HIV field and feels he does not require to access networks of support for his HIV. He is healthy and knowledgeable about HIV matters and has his partner who is a big support. Pablo maintains a healthy state with a positive mental attitude.

LISETTE

Lisette, aged 51, described herself as a working class, heterosexual woman. She was diagnosed in 1990 and the route of transmission has three possibilities: IV drug use, sexual or from an operation. She gave up using drugs in 1979. Lisette was medically retired and used to work in the porn industry as well as other jobs; she was not in a relationship and lived alone. She had no religious beliefs but leaned towards spirituality and described her ethnicity as White, European. Lisette was reasonably healthy but had a back-related problem which was not HIV-related. She had never taken HIV medicine since diagnosis. When I asked Lisette about networks of support for HIV she told me of her experiences with social workers:

"I have a problem with social workers or social workers definitely have a problem with me... I get this ILF money which is independent living fund; I've had this since 1993... just recently they've come to review it and it's the first time they've done it in all these years. And when I got ILF there definitely was a feeling around if you had an AIDS diagnosis you didn't have to do very much. I got a visit from a visiting social worker who came out and said he would give me the help with this and this and then he left... I was quite worried about it and I wanted someone to represent me. It said I was entitled to representation on the form, to have someone to explain about my care to the ILF body. So I phoned the social work department and they had someone who worked with a special remit for HIV. This person was new and was on holiday. So the day she's back from her holiday I phone up. Then she was on sick leave. So I left all these messages, having to tell the whole bloody story to the secretary... I ended up telling my story seven times and I said this is so not confidential. You know I am talking to duty social workers and I never did get a social worker to come out. I got a message from my social worker that I'd met in the past and she said: 'what on earth was I doing with ILF and who did I think I was trying to get a social worker in two days?' ... this was not true. I had not phoned for two weeks beforehand because I was told the woman was on holiday and then on sick leave. She wasn't very nice to me and personally I think it's because I can speak for myself... she was really angry on the message she left. She was saying, 'there was no way they could get anybody out there and anyway I didn't qualify for ILF.' But actually I did... I used to get home care at one time but they couldn't get anybody to come in to somebody with HIV, so I didn't get it anymore."

I asked Lisette about friendship and family relationships as networks of support. She recounted:

"I had a couple of friends at the beginning, I told them about my positive status and after meeting up a few times after I told one of them, she came on this final occasion and said she couldn't be my friend anymore; the reason was because she felt she had put herself at risk as a divorced woman in her 40s and she'd been out with many partners... and she couldn't see me because every time she saw me she thought it might be her and she couldn't cope with that and she didn't want to get tested...I just got shut of the cow. She couldn't look at me because all she could see was this HIV diagnosis and what she actually saw was her; she was terrified it was her and she was too scared to go and get tested to find out. We went our separate ways... My family, I had a bit of trouble with my sister. I mean I get on with all my sisters but I'm friends with one and she's six years younger than me and when I found out I went to visit her and I told her. She was very sad but she was really freaked out because she'd never known I took drugs... I found out later that she had me on some kind of pedestal and so this was a double whammy that I took drugs and I'd got HIV. It did her head in... to let you understand, she had phoned the GP to see if there's anything she should do different to protect me. She said to him, 'my sister's coming up, she's got HIV is there anything I should do? And he turned round and told her about cups and knives and forks and spoons and towels should all be separate. We were having this party, right? This was in 1990... and she later decided that she'd eaten a bit of cake at this party off the same fork and we got back from the party at 4am in the morning and she started screaming at me that I'd infected her. I couldn't believe that she was saying this. I couldn't figure out how she thought I had infected her and the whole story came out about what the GP had told her. I actually made her phone National AIDS helpline at 5am in the morning. Bloody sin getting some poor woman out of her bed for my sister; she turned round to my sister and said, 'Well, have you ever told your sister that it's OK?' My sister was in shock and once again the GP had done no good whatsoever... and now she is absolutely fine and she's been a really good support, she has been really helpful."

Lisette stated that where her sister lives there appears to be the same attitude towards HIV now as there was ten years ago. The fear and prejudice still remains. Lisette continues talking about family matters:

"My grandson goes to school just round the corner and they were desperate for people to come in and help with certain kids for reading and it was something that I would have done at the drop of a hat. I did think about it and then I thought it was far too dangerous. In the sense that if I go in there and anybody finds out about the HIV then is that OK? If I am going to listen to the kids read do I have to tell the school? If I tell them will there be a backlash that involves my grandson? So it's just a can of worms that I wasn't prepared to deal with so I end up not doing it, being a helper at school... I am the person who stayed at the school gate one day waiting to pick up my grandson and one of the local childminders had been on a course and was proudly acknowledging that she'd been on a course about HIV and taking care of kids. She announced it to every mother waiting and said that she didn't really have to go on the course because nobody in this locality had it and she was never going to meet anybody with HIV... To be honest I was desperate to talk to her and say, 'Well, I've got it'. It's like that, you know, it makes me think that her attitude and the attitude of my sister that things aren't really any different."

Lisette recalled her experiences of other networks of support in terms of HIV in earlier times. She told me:

"The community thing I have a problem with because I kind of feel that all the people, when I was first diagnosed, who should have been on my side, if that's the right expression, were Positively Women. In reality I had such a negative experience with them in the early 90s that it's affected me after all these years. And basically that was because I rang them up to try and see if I could go to a meeting or something… and they more or less told me that unless I went in there and slagged men off and hated men, there wasn't any point in coming… it's about that initial contact and how easy it is to just get put off… and once you get put off how difficult it is to go and do it again because I've never ever gone to Positively Women. I get the Mag and I know what's going on and I know a few of the girls that have worked there and still work there and I meet them at different things. At conferences and whatever and I get on fine with them but I've always had that problem and I've always perceived it as being like that, because that's what was said to me the very first time I phoned up… I belong to a support group called Thames Valley Positive Support TVPS and in the beginning when I was diagnosed I was really involved with them. But there's definitely a feeling that if nothing happens to you in terms of illness you are just left to get on with it. And I think that's a thing they do to women. I remember years ago there was a guy living not far from me and we both accessed the same support group and he really was no different to me. We had been diagnosed around the same time and our health was the same. The support group in my area wasn't made up of many women although there were many women volunteers and I discovered that this chap used to get a phone call every other day asking how he was. I never got a phone call. And still to this day I haven't. The contact I have with them is when I ring them up… they have a drop-in and do lunch but I haven't got transport and I have never been able to get there because they can't provide transport…They asked me if I wanted a buddy about five years ago and I said, 'yes' but they still haven't materialised."

Lisette believed that support was different for men than for women. She was disheartened with her negative experiences of networks of support for HIV. She considers herself as a woman who knows what she wants.

DAVID

David, aged 65, describes himself as a very lucky, middle class, gay man. He was diagnosed in 1990 and the route of transmission was sexual. He is retired from his work in the finance sector and lives with his partner in a long-term intimate relationship. He describes his religion as Church of England (non-practising) and is of White European ethnicity. He has never taken medical treatment for HIV; instead he uses alternative therapies and follows a healthy vegetarian diet. He is extremely healthy and has a wonderful positive mental attitude about his positive status and his role in life. When I asked him about networks of support he told me:

"We looked around at the kind of HIV official support that there was and we found a group called Positively Healthy which was run by Cass Mann. Well, Cass Mann has lots of faults and you may know them or you may have heard rumours about him but he was the right person in my life [I had heard of him and had only heard positive comments about him]... Absolutely brilliant and he led us into the Asian or the oriental or the Eastern way of thinking about things, respecting and loving yourself, which is so alien to male culture in this country... we had about six or seven years with Positively Healthy; having weekends away or weeks away in Scotland... and going to regular group sessions like 15 weeks at a time; every week for about three or four hours. It was a marvellous experience and of course he was vegetarian so that was one of the influences on us with organic food and just healthy lifestyle, apart from my cigarettes."

David was told he had about two years to live when he was diagnosed in 1990 and he chose to believe that he would not die as he had too much to do. He started to volunteer in the HIV field. He recounted:

"I became involved in the HIV community in London and there were a lot of very healthy young lads who were getting diagnosed and just giving up... they were getting benefits and they were giving up work and they were just sitting at home in their flats, watching TV and waiting to die. I was determined I wasn't going to do that... at that time it was a big thing, the 'gay disease' and I knew people who wouldn't admit that they had got it and who were eventually dying and having pretty horrendous deaths as well but none of them would sort of come out... they were told you were HIV-positive and you would move onto ARC, AIDS-related conditions and then you would get sort of full blown AIDS. This ARC thing seems to have disappeared now... HIV was a big part of my life at the beginning especially when I was involved in a lot of voluntary work and my partner would say, 'could we not just have one day where there are no phone calls with people wanting help?' So we moved out of London and it was a positive decision to do less for other people and more for myself and my immediate friends. I am still involved with voluntary work of course."

David continued to reflect on family and friendship relationships as networks of support, and recounted:

"I have loving support, financial security and a nice home. And because of being gay all my life I have made family of my friends; and in talking to you about my past relationships, you realise that these are more than just friends, they are family; and those six people that were initially told of my diagnosis are people, in a broader context, you would say is family... My partner and I are very lucky people as everything always seems to work in our favour... With my immediate family I had wonderful parents, who both recently died, so they are gone. My lover's so very supportive; the four close friends through previous relationships and the other couple are absolutely amazingly supportive. But they don't quite understand what it is like being diagnosed; they try to understand but I think from time to time you need contact with other HIV-positive people... I do go to a local support group here but it is not that well attended; and I am also involved with another group that is based in Slough... so we went last weekend to a BBQ that was organised by the local group. But Thames Valley covers beyond Slough, so it covers quite a large area."

David still volunteers in the HIV field and gets all he needs in terms of networks of support from his family of friends, his partner and his local support group. He does not need anything, he says, other than what he has already. However he is aware that his needs might change over time.

JAY

Jay, aged 35, describes himself as a gay, working class, 'one hundred per cent poof'. He was diagnosed in 1992 and the route of transmission was sexual. He describes his religion as Church of England (non-practising) and his ethnicity as White and British. He was medically retired and had previously worked in the service industry in bars and public houses. He is extremely healthy and has a wonderful positive mental attitude and outlook on life. He is happily living with HIV and feels that this has not impacted on his life in any great way. When I asked Jay about family relationships and networks of support, he recounted:

"Well not one member of my family knows about my status… My father is dead so I'd need Doris Stokes to tell him and my Mum is a whinging old, no… she is really old and she's not in the best of health anyway; and the chances are really that I will outlive my Mum even though I have been diagnosed so long; so I don't see the point in ruining her health any more that it has to. What's the point of telling her and then it goes to my sister and everyone just rings and I just can't put my family through that kind of thing. I think it's best if they don't know. They haven't got a clue and I don't go round that often and when I do I make sure that I'm going there when I am well, so I don't see the point in bothering them."

Jay stated that he would do the same if he had cancer or some other illness; it was nothing to do with the fact that he was living with HIV and bound up in prejudice and stigma. Jay lost a few friends to AIDS who were diagnosed around the same time as he was, yet they died within six months. He recounted:

"A few friends who were diagnosed same time as me, they died within six months…I mean they were really, really nice and good friends as well. I miss them so much but you just can't let that kind of thing get to you too much. You've got to sort of pick yourself up and move along… if you wallow in it you just make yourself more ill… It doesn't matter how they ended up dead whether it is terminal illness or accident, it is still a loss and it makes no difference what you die of… I tried not to get that low down and sometimes you have to be stiff upper lip."

Jay had moved from London and most of his friends were based there; he did talk about possibly moving back to his old area. When I asked him about HIV networks of support, he told me:

"No, I never use them. I did go to Landmark once but it's just not my kind of thing… there's so many people with HIV I mean it's outrageous [laughing]…I knew quite a lot of people that were there… it's just like, 'Oh, I didn't know you were' and I just thought I don't need this every time so I didn't bother going back. It just didn't work for me and I don't want to know that much about HIV. I think actually the majority of my friends are probably negative not positive… I don't think you can build a friendship on status though and I don't stick to certain groups."

Jay believes he is just a normal, everyday kind of person and does not access HIV networks of support in his local area because they are 'not really for me'.

On being symptomatic: HIV, networks of support and other pressing matters

The remaining eighteen long-term survivors in this collection of personal experiences were diagnosed between 1981 and 1994 and, at the time of our interview, were medically defined as symptomatic: showing clinical symptoms associated with HIV. Sixteen story-tellers were taking HIV combination therapy and two were awaiting salvage therapy due to complications with past HIV medicine. Many long-term survivors in this section have experienced periods of HIV-related illness since the onset of diagnosis. We start with our story-tellers who were diagnosed the earliest.

MINNIE

Minnie, aged 42, described himself as an upper middle class, gay man who is celibate. He mentioned his upbringing as typically working class and was medically retired; his previous occupations were: a professional opera singer and Chef. He was diagnosed in 1981 and the route of transmission was sexual. He described himself as an Anglican but was not a regular churchgoer and perceived himself facing a dilemma because of his sexuality. He described his ethnicity as British, White Caucasian. Minnie was medically retired, not in an established relationship and lived alone. He was reliant upon a wheelchair for mobility purposes due to vasculitis and peripheral neuropathy and his health had been further compromised by dietary problems. He was physically well enough to negotiate everyday life, he told me:

"I still function because I am able to get around with a car… AIDS sort of doubles the fight in lots of ways… I have to wheel myself around in this thing and I can't afford to be weak otherwise I have to rely on being pushed by someone…I like my own company; I like living alone with the dog and just pleasing myself and doing what I want to do, when I want to do it. I've said on many occasion, I've never felt or been as happy in my life as I am now. HIV is a very small part of who I am…I won't be drawn into the 'virus scene', it's very dangerous and people get too engrossed around issues and things… it can be all-consuming and we have all met people who have been consumed by it… but for me, no, it's never been a big part of my life since 1981. I have never allowed it to be, apart from the political issues that one has to fight for in this climate… I'm talking about local Social Services and health services and the implications this has for HIV, especially Primary Care Trusts."

I asked him about his family and friendships and whether these relationships had been affected by HIV, he recounted:

"You know with close, close friends of which we only ever have a handful in life because there isn't room for more than that, I believe you cultivate a certain number of dearest friends and we can only have space in our lives for a few. I have a best friend who is my chosen next of kin, and that relationship has gone through hard times because of the diagnosis... she didn't want to believe that HIV would one day have an effect on my life... I am talking mid 80s now and she was right, nothing did happen to me for many years...and I have seen her children grow. My close friendships have not been affected and my best friend has my Power of Attorney in the event of any medical decisions that need to be made if I am not mentally capable... she agreed to do it because she knows what I want and we have discussed it for years...I have a mother that can override my chosen next of kin. I can only trust my best friend because I've lived a very solitary life for many years away from my family, my mother in particular, and she's learned to know whatever I say goes and she wouldn't interfere... I specifically say in the Living Will you know where it says do you want to be kept alive whilst a particular person arrives... do they keep me alive just for my mother to get there? No thank you! She might be mortified but people are gonna be there when it happens... those people that matter so I don't want to be kept going for the sake of my mother or anybody else; even if my best friend is not there, then what will be will be. People sometimes need permission to die. I've given them permission... I've been in the situation where I have seen friends die and they almost ask for permission to go and when you give it to them, they go... and other positions where people will fight it and they can't face it... I've seen many angles of death."

Minnie spoke of how he and his partner encountered a breach of confidentiality which led to HIV-related harassment in relation to housing in earlier times, he told me:

"When I was with my partner, we were together but not living together, albeit I was either at the flat or we might be at the house... anyway he was waiting for a property from the Housing Association because his illness was progressing... he needed a two-bedroom property and they only had one-bedroom on offer for the interim... he was given a flat by the Housing Association and back then they weren't particularly confidential... we moved into it and above us lived a Black guy and his White Australian girlfriend... there really isn't a need for me to particularly say he was a 'Black guy' but I'm just giving you the scenario... he was dealing and I knew that and didn't have a problem with it at all. But more to the point, his girlfriend had already been after the flat that my partner had been given downstairs. So, she went mouthing round to the Housing Association asking what had happened. And they told her why he had been given the flat so quickly… from then on, every couple of nights the car window would be smashed or we were accused of leaving the doors open in the communal hallway and bicycles had been stolen and you name it… it was horrendous. I used to hate going back there and I knew it wasn't him it was her… this was between 1988-89; the Housing Association had told this woman that Paul was living with AIDS… she just went ape shit and I know it was her that smashed the car window… He was dealing and there were people in and out all the time and anybody could have stolen the bicycle. We were accused of it and we got people banging on our door… saying we have so many days to pay up. We experienced a lot of harassment."

Minnie did not get involved with HIV organisations and the 'viral scene' but recounted one of his personal experiences of accessing HIV support shortly after his diagnosis:

"The Lighthouse I found were very discriminatory if you were a positive person and claiming but you weren't ill, you were made to feel very uncomfortable in the early days there… if you weren't presenting symptoms or didn't have opportunistic infections but you'd been diagnosed as positive…they were very hostile. Don't ask me why they were hostile, it was almost as if they didn't believe you… you'd go there and yes I know I have had experiences… because people are 'wannabe's' out there, people who go out of their way to get in, they wannabe positive because they think we get all these benefits that give us this lovely luxurious lifestyle… and unfortunately it's not the case any more. It might have been in the early days but not any more; there aren't those benefits available now. But more to the point, you'd think who on earth would want to fiddle their way into anything like that, but they do… and whether this was the Lighthouse's opinion in those days, I don't know… I don't think so; I don't think they'd had enough time to think long enough about it. It hadn't been around for long enough for them to have developed that kind of attitude… it was just as if, you know, they needed proof and the only proof they could have was visible proof and that meant the classic portrayal of a 'victim', you know, who was skeletal and 'dead next week' type thing… then they were all open arms, but if you were healthy and fit looking, asymptomatic and springing in and out of the Lighthouse with your partner, they had no time for you whatsoever… I found that only at the Lighthouse."

A forgotten generation: Long-term survivors' experiences of HIV and AIDS

Minnie was happy living in a rural community and never felt lonely or isolated. He only felt cut off when he was unable to drive during periods of severe illness. Whilst Minnie did not access HIV organisations for social support, he did have help with personal care in his home from Social Services. He recalled:

" I get good care in my local community, on-going care and in saying that there is a price to pay and that is you have to be discrete about your diagnosis and that's all there is to it. As much as it pains me not to educate people in my own village that live here, I have to give them another five to ten years – nobody knows! Well I hope they don't know… all my carers know. In the very early days of me being assessed for personal care and housekeeping… I insisted that whoever was going to be my carer had to know my status because I wasn't going to hide my life every time they came in the door… it defeats the object. You know they wouldn't look at stuff in my office but I had stuff in there and things with logo's on it that might reveal what I was reading about… so they had to know. The woman went round my place, checked all the rooms, made a care plan with safety hazards… the woman who is my present carer she is great and we get on like a house on fire."

Minnie was content with his 'chosen family' of very close friends and was not particularly close with his biological family. He enjoyed his 'quite reclusive lifestyle' and felt part of the community where he lived.

SPIKE

Spike, aged 27, describes himself as a working class, heterosexual man and is a MA student in social research. He was diagnosed as a young child between 1981-1983 and the route of transmission was contaminated Factor VIII blood products. Spike does not prescribe to any religion and describes his ethnicity as White English. He is in a long-term relationship and lives alone. He is extremely healthy and has lived with Haemophilia all his life. HIV is a big part of his life but it does not prevent him from doing things he wants to do, anymore or less than his other conditions. Spike believes that HCV is likely to become more of a problem than HIV. When I asked him about relationships with his family and friends, he told me:

"My sister and my parents know but I have never spoken to my grandparents. My Mum has spoken to some of her friends about it, which doesn't really bother me…It has been so long now that I don't really care who knows but I still don't tell people. It's funny… I have got relationships with people for reasons I have got relationships with them, not because of my HIV and stuff... I like those relationships and all my friends would probably be most accepting of my status, I know they would. But I still don't tell them, it's my choice... It's a large part of me but it isn't dominating all the things that I do... but it's moulded me and gives me the perception of the way I think. So to that extent, it's part of me but it's not me in the way I've stopped doing something. It's never stopped me having a relationship when I was a teenager. It never stopped me going out and having a good bunch of friends who I have still got; and going out and getting pissed for the first time. Physically it's never stopped me but it's probably moulded me psychologically perhaps... I have probably only told a few of my friends locally and I have told a couple who live elsewhere...I even had girlfriends but nothing has been affected... It's probably improved my relationships because I am still in touch with my two previous girlfriends; we are good friends... everyone I have told have never discussed it with anyone. I might not see people for months but it's not an issue."

Spike spoke about the media attention around the link between HIV and Haemophilia and recalled:

"When it came out in the News I would have been in Middle school around 1984 or 1985... I was probably about 9 or 10 and as far as I know no-one was informed about it; they didn't have to be as far as I am aware...it was never mentioned. But my Mum was saying recently, in the last few years, that she'd heard somebody had mentioned to her that another parent had written to the local newspaper saying that there was a child at my school who was a Haemophiliac and had AIDS and stuff... apparently they were going to run it on their front page; and luckily Mum heard about it first and managed to phone the Editor and got him to stop it... It would have been directed at me as there were no other Haemophiliacs... obviously it was speculation because no other parent would have known this anyway, so I guess they thought most Haemophiliacs had HIV anyway, even though it was 1 in 4 when it first happened...I can't remember what the quotient is, but 1,240 Haemophiliacs were infected with HIV and at the moment there is only 416 still alive... well that was the last time I heard so it might be even less now."

Spike was fortunate to have a mortgage for his own home which had been organised by the Mortgage Advisor at the MacFarlane Trust; he was however unable to obtain life insurance. The MacFarlane Trust is an organisation of support for people living with Haemophilia. I asked Spike about other sources of support he might access or belong to, he told me:

A forgotten generation: Long-term survivors' experiences of HIV and AIDS

"I am a volunteer with an AIDS foundation nearby; I am a trustee. I wanted to do something voluntarily... I thought I could help and offer my experience and I wanted to learn more for myself and that's been a big part of me. Empowering myself and with the HIV it is important... I don't know how long I will stay but I think I want to do more with an organisation called Birchgrove, for Haemophiliacs with HIV. I find it hard to get into these organisations and offer my services... it's not a closed network but I don't know what really happens apart from the Newsletter...I have never really accessed other support networks... I am happy with my position and my networks are my family and friends...When I did voluntary work nearby, there's one person actually diagnosed each week which might not be much compared to other areas, but it's quite a lot for this area and it's a lot for the Health Authority to cope with... there should be more networks in place but the voluntary base is quite good actually. There's the empowerment group going on and that's really good... for myself I am happy being there but it's not me. My community is my friends and my family here and that will always be the same."

Spike spoke of the 1990s when many people living with Haemophilia were dying of AIDS and he remained alive. He talked of survival and being a survivor and yet HIV has not particularly affected his lifestyle; his voluntary work helps to empower him whilst simultaneously helping others.

JO

Jo, aged 52, describes himself as a middle class gay man who is medically retired: he was previously in the acting and the tailoring profession. He was diagnosed in 1982 and the route of transmission is sexual. Jo was born into a Jewish family but describes himself as spiritual rather than orthodox. He is in a long-term relationship and lives in the same complex but in a separate flat to his partner. Jo describes himself as White European because he is Jewish not English. He is currently healthy but has experienced severe ill health in the past. When I asked how HIV impacted on his sense of self, he told me:

"It's a huge part and in a way it can't be anything other than a huge part. Maybe it shouldn't be. Maybe it's unhealthy I don't know but there are still issues... it is still a form of stigmatisation, what can you do about it? That exists; it's a fact of life just in the same way one is stigmatised because one's gay and wants to be 'out'... I suppose it's become part of my identity but maybe it's because of longevity and being around it for so long... twice a day you've got to do pills and you've gotta make sure that if you're going out you've got your pills with you."

Jo recounted his experiences of networks of support for HIV and how these had changed over the years. He told me:

"...the whole thing of finances around the epidemic has changed. So whereas before there had been amazing self-help groups offering support like the Lighthouse, Landmark, Body Positive and Terrence Higgins Trust, all these institutions gradually lost funding because the funding needed to go towards medication, which also meant that again empowerment started going... before you had felt empowered now you are feeling less empowered... twenty years on suddenly there are no drop-in places; there are one or two places that offer peer support... I used to go to the Landmark, which was local and there was a drop-in essentially seven days a week. That has all gone. It doesn't exist anymore... if you want help you have to access it via a phone line to THT direct...that's not face-to-face interaction; there was always peer support where you just met people; there was food and you would meet people and discuss issues and if someone was going through something you could say 'well I went through that too' and this would help. Suddenly it became so that unless it was somehow quantifiable and they had facilitators it wasn't seen as being important. That wasn't peer support, peer support was something that was concrete... it just seems like madness now... as gay men we were already stigmatised and used to dealing with that and were very forceful in setting things up. THT and Body Positive were set up by gay men and the global perspective has come in and the nature of the disease changed... everything's changed."

Jo has a younger brother in the medical profession and feels he always has someone he can talk to. His parents did not know of his HIV status and they have both since died; for Jo in one sense this has been 'an extraordinary sort of relief' because of the issue of secrecy. Whilst he was working he did disclose his status to others around him, he recounted:

"I just didn't want to distress my parents and there was so much mis-information and part of me felt terrible but I just thought why should I add to their grief? After their death, because that lie no longer had to be perpetuated I remember the first day I saw my eldest brother who I hadn't told because he would have told them, I just told him; poor love he had to deal with that when he was already dealing with grief for my father, so it was difficult. In a way it was selfish but I just wanted to do it... everybody that I knew, certainly my friends, they knew... after three of four years I told people where I worked because when we were doing new shows we sometimes worked fourteen or fifteen hours a day, seven days a week; it was non-stop... I got Shingles and I got over that – it was horrendous. So I told the manager about my status and she was brilliant...then I became ill again and my CD4 count went below 200 and I felt I just couldn't go on... I'd lost a huge amount of weight... it was great at work; it wasn't an issue it was extraordinary...I try to protect myself in terms of who I tell but I have been really fortunate. I've been fortunate in terms of living in a housing co-operative... everybody I live around everybody knows I'm HIV so it's not an issue."

Jo moved on to talk about benefits and having to deal with social workers at a time when he could no longer carry on with work, due to bouts of severe illness. He recounted:

"I was really fortunate in getting all my benefits very early on... Nowadays it's really difficult for people to get hold of benefits, having to deal with social workers, all that has changed. I can understand why that has changed but they are real issues... I have DLA but it's like being stuck in a benefit trap because there's part of me that feels maybe I could go back to work, but at the age of 53 to put myself back in the job market is hard... what kind of job could I do? I would lose my benefits and if I lose them then this makes it difficult later on so it's horrible... it sort of affects one's whole sense of well-being and self-worth... I do voluntary work for people; I am involved in maintenance so that keeps me busy. I used to volunteer at Landmark until that was all done away with. I used to feel at least I was actively involved in something and was giving something back... I have being doing computer courses as a handy skill."

Jo felt that there was always confusion living with HIV in terms of whether a cold was simply a cold or something else. He was not as fit as he once was and therefore was unsure if this was part of the natural ageing process. He has a good sense of belonging where he lives and has a good network of support around him. He reads Positive Nation and is aware of how the changes in networks of support have impacted on HIV as a whole.

TYLER

Tyler, aged 54, described himself as a middle class, gay man who was medically retired. He previously ran his own businesses before he was diagnosed back in 1984; the route of transmission was sexual. Tyler described himself as a Christian who practised inside his head and was a firm believer in 'life after death'. He described his ethnicity as English and White. Tyler was experiencing ill health at the time of our interview and was awaiting salvage therapy due to complications with previous HIV medicines. He was not in a relationship and lived alone; he took one day at a time and was told he did not have long to live. When I asked him about friendship relationships as a network of support, he recounted:

"All my friends have gone. The friends I have now are through Positive groups... the friends I had were people I chose to be with and people who chose to be with me; those I am surrounded by now aren't friends at that level... I have lost life-style friendships and now I've replaced them with 'illness-friendships which is totally different."

As we recall in chapter three, Tyler had feelings of 'survivor guilt' [although he did not use this term] as a result of experiencing great losses in relation to close friends dying of AIDS. HIV was his 'entire identity' as he had to live his daily life around it because of problems of illness, low energy levels and memory impairment. I asked him about other networks of support he belonged to, and he told me:

"If we didn't have Body Positive I probably wouldn't have any friends now because they're all dead. So there is a community but I am not sure... remember it's not a situation where you are mixing with someone because you are just so in love with their sense of humour or their intellect. You are mixing with them because they have an illness that you have...everything else we have to fight for. If you want to obtain a friendship out of someone you have to fight for it... it is a support network I feel part of... I am the Treasurer of this group... I have turned a couple of friendships into something deeper but it's not natural...with one friend at the end of five years we've actually ended up with a bit of a friendship that's gone a bit deeper... his relationship finished and he was in a state and stayed here for a week. So he was very grateful for that and I ended up ill and he looked after me, moved in for a week and looked after me. We got to know each other on a different level and found we could tolerate each other much better than what we originally thought... we are not in each other's pockets but we are much better at supporting each other than we were... he's still an HIV friend, not like my other friends... I mean most of my friends were absolutely mental because I had a mental lifestyle... we went all around Europe and even down to North Africa and we used to go camping in all these wild places... we were all irresponsible, wild but still held down good jobs and had a responsible life in our irresponsibility, do you know what I mean?... they were a special breed of people and I was lucky to be one of them... you can't join an HIV group and meet people like that."

Tyler clearly differentiated between his old friendship relationships which he considered as 'natural' to those that were connected by illness. He had made several attempts at taking his own life and was passionate about wanting to choose his time to die; when his quality of life was no longer bearable and taken over by pain and discomfort it was time to go.

PAUL

Paul, aged 38, describes himself as a middle class, heterosexual man who is voluntarily unemployed; he used to be a school teacher. He was diagnosed in 1985 and the route of transmission was via Factor VIII contaminated blood products. Paul describes his ethnicity as British and White and is a non-believer in religion and God. He is in an established intimate relationship and lives with his partner. Paul is relatively healthy and has lived with Haemophilia all his life. HIV is a large part of his life, as he would have liked to have children and continued to work; he believes living with HIV prohibits this, he told me:

"I think you have just got to live with it, as it is part of you and I don't think there is ever a day goes by when you don't think of it; so yes, it does have an effect on my life. Whatever you do you have to think, 'how will that affect my HIV?'…it is a large part of who I am, I think it is…because if I hadn't got HIV I wouldn't be doing what I am doing now. If I hadn't got HIV I would probably be having kids and I would probably be at work, so yes it does affect me and I'd give it an 8 out of 10… but psychologically it doesn't have the same impact that it had in the 1980s when I was diagnosed… people were dying of AIDS."

Paul told me of how it took over 12 years to tell his close friends about his HIV status; the longer you leave it the harder it becomes. He has, however, not experienced adverse reactions from any of his close friends following disclosure. I asked him about other social networks of support for HIV, he told me:

"If there was anything I could say as the most positive aspect of HIV it is getting the proper support from other people. I felt so isolated in the first few years. Being heterosexual as well, I feel isolated further because anything I ever got from any HIV organisation was related to gay men and gay sex. I couldn't even get condoms from a hospital; the only condoms I had access to were extra strong from a clinic. I didn't feel I was being catered for as a heterosexual man… well it probably still isn't balanced… I don't want to sort of sound like I am picking fault with any organisations, but THT only last year brought out a leaflet on safer sex for heterosexual men and women. I have been diagnosed now for 17 years and I think it is a bit late in the day to provide the only booklet ever on safer sex for heterosexual men and women… In 1989 I first saw my psychologist… and this had the biggest impact on my life… she actually set up a support group for haemophiliacs in this area. She was quite instrumental in getting us together and that was the first time I had ever met other haemophiliacs with HIV… I was the youngest out of the lot but only by a few years; we used to meet up once a month for a couple of years. Until about 1991 or 1992… over that time every single person who went to the group except me died and most had been really quite ill… there was only AZT around at the time and their symptoms got worse. They died from things like PCP, brain tumours… all the things that people die of with HIV… initially I got so much support from others, feeling that I wasn't on my own; there were other guys out there that did feel the same things as I did and did feel like their life had been robbed and all the rest. It was absolutely a brilliant experience… I was off-loading to the group but I spoke to the psychologist at the time as well… it was quite instrumental in my life but because everybody in the group died… this did reinforce the fact that I had not got long to live… HIV kills people there's no doubt about it… I didn't have contact with anybody with HIV for a number of years after that because of my experiences that everybody I get to know and eventually, I get to like, we are going to share a lot of very personal things and one of us is going to die. I thought I didn't want to go through that again. It completed devastated me and my partner at the time. We got to know their partners and you know every time one of them died, she supported their partners through hospital visits and so it also reinforced things for my partner… it was quite a traumatic time towards the end. I stuck my head in the sand; I got on with my life. I did as many nice things as I could for a number of years until I became ill… this is when I needed support… it was like the shit had hit the fan again and I needed help and I needed someone to talk to. I had Haemophilia and I have got Hep C… so I basically started to get in touch with other guys with Haemophilia again and I got in touch with a self-help group supporting Haemophilia and HIV. I have met some absolutely brilliant mates through this support group over the last 4 or 5 years."

Paul continued to talk about his involvement with other HIV-related support groups, he recounted:

"I am also involved with my local HIV support group which caters for people in my area. I go there and get advice and there are IV drug users, gay guys and other different members which is a completely different dynamic. I am

A forgotten generation: Long-term survivors' experiences of HIV and AIDS

the only Haemophiliac there. I fit in and I don't feel I am ostracised otherwise I wouldn't stay, it is very open…there is one closer to where I live but it doesn't cater for me and my HIV; it's for Men who have Sex with Men (MSM). I am not homophobic and I don't have sex with men. I feel it is going back to the old days when HIV support groups were basically a knocking shop for gay guys and I know a lot of gay guys who have said this to me themselves… they just turn up and see who they can cop off with… I do get loads of support but it is not the same as other people who have Haemophilia, Hep C and HIV… it is interesting because a lot of IV drug users that I know talk to me about Hep C… they don't know anybody else who has got Hep C apart from other drug users… I am quite good mates with a lot of gay guys that I know from the drop-in. We do socialise occasionally… you can't go around making sweeping statements… there are some gay guys out there that just don't understand I am heterosexual, and you know, at Christmas parties they still want to cop off with me, they still want to touch me up and I know that is down to personality and not being gay… there are other gay guys that completely and utterly respect my personal space and respect the fact that I am heterosexual… yeah, I have got some good support there… it's not just about sexuality it's about personality; who you get on with, who you click with and who you don't… overall, there is no body who understands your situation, how you feel and what you experience unless they have similar issues. How can I have a conversation with a gay guy about issues in your sex life relating to women? And how do you talk about your feelings on being infected with a disease that is so unjust? I've got deep feelings of injustice hanging over me still… all this tagging as 'innocent victims'… I think that this sets people with Haemophilia up against gay guys with HIV at the end of the day."

Paul commented on how networks of support for HIV are largely concentrated in London and elsewhere in the UK has limited resources, he told me:

"I get the HIV press and if you look inside everything is London based. If I had lived in London for many years I would have been able to get free complementary therapy, I would have been able to have meals delivered free to my door… you know the food chain only works in London [laughing]. Support groups are better in London, home help and everything. I know people in London will say it depends on which Borough of London you live in and I know the situation changed drastically after the funding pulled out of the HIV sector… I am well aware of that as I have contacts in London as well as other areas… Yes, I feel where you live is quite an important part of a social support network. But an important part of my life is my friends and my family and I don't want to move away from them. I have given up enough with this virus. I don't want to give up my friends and family just to live near a decent clinic... I used to go to Body Positive in London when they were running... if I wanted a second opinion from somebody who was a bit more experienced."

Overall, Paul believed he had access to appropriate social networks of support for his HIV and Haemophilia and HCV; his family and friendship relationships were extremely important sources of support. He did have feelings of being ostracised, at times, on the basis of his heterosexuality when accessing HIV organisations. Paul continues to be actively involved in HIV, Haemophilia and HCV social support networks.

ELISABETH

Elisabeth, aged 46, describes herself as a working class, heterosexual woman who works part-time. She was diagnosed in 1985 and the route of transmission was likely to be either from sharing needles or sexual or both. Elisabeth describes her ethnicity as White and Scottish. She was not in a relationship and lived alone. Her health was compromised with a serious liver complaint and she had been admitted to hospital on three occasions in recent times at the time of our interview. When I asked her how HIV had impacted on daily life, she told me:

"I was an addict long before I was HIV-positive. That had been the overriding thing in my life that I've had to fight... HIV was a secondary illness as far as I was concerned. I couldn't see any difference because I wasn't sick and the heroin took up so much of my life that most of my decisions were based around that rather than HIV...I actually used more heroin because I thought I was gonna die anyway, so in that way it did affect me. On quite an unconscious level I think, it's weird... it's a real paradox cos I remember at one point I got so fed up with using and so annoyed with myself and I wished I could stop but I didn't know how to and every time I had a hit, I would look at the syringe and the heroin and I'd think 'this is gonna kill me'... I made this pact with myself that I wasn't gonna die until my daughter was 16... it doesn't make any sense when you say it out loud, but to me it made a lot of sense... I was to all intent and purposes killing myself... I was a determined long-term survivor really."

Elisabeth went on to tell me about family issues and networks of support for HIV, she told me:

A forgotten generation: Long-term survivors' experiences of HIV and AIDS

"Along the years I've been with Positively Women and ICW and I've met other women and discussed things and made up my own mind about a lot of things... there were no medications although this was never an issue... my health was absolutely fine; it was a lot easier to deal with than for other people because there were no health issues... there was the secrecy and the privacy of keeping it quiet and that was always a big thing because of my kids... there was a place called the Landmark which was for positive people and I used to go to the support group there... it was close to my kid's school and I was really scared that someone might see me going into that place... it was OK to go at night but through the day you used to go and have therapies and have lunch and meet people... I went on three occasions but I was too scared to go and you know it dominated my life and how much care I took of myself in a lot of ways... I was working at Positively Women and it became very easy for me to talk about it and to acknowledge myself as being HIV-positive and to be confident in that... but then I had to come home and play a different role and I couldn't mention it... I was still scared I'd get sick in case the kids put two-and-two together...I was just too tired to keep secrets and told my daughter when she was 16... she's wonderful, she's been great ever since... she runs me to hospital and does not appear to have any fear around it... I told my other sons when they needed to know; my eldest wasn't at home anyway."

I asked Elisabeth if she had any other matters of concern in relation to living long-term with HIV, she recounted:

"It's stopped me from travelling any length of time and that's just the reality. I'm not saying I would have done but now I can't... I've got this big plan of going away for a year and I've had that for a few years now, but I can't do that... I want to go out to see family in Australia but I'd have to go for three months and come back...I've been to World AIDS conferences before... before it used to be absolutely horrendous if Customs Officers found my pills and said, 'what are these?' I'd get really embarrassed and ashamed but now I just say and leave it up to them as to how they react... I went to America and you are meant to tell them if you've got any infectious diseases and I just said, 'no'. That was crazy because I was going out there for an AIDS conference. I mean they had the Worlds AIDS conference in Japan one year didn't they and they wouldn't let anybody in that was positive... it's crazy isn't it?"

Elisabeth believed that her attitude had helped her to live positively with HIV. She said she was 'too bloody minded' and stubborn. She reflects on these issues:

"I think attitude has quite a lot to do with prolonging life with HIV...I have really had a good run for my money...I look at this guy who knew Terrence Higgins and he's a gay man and he goes to the gym nearly every day, he's got muscles bulging everywhere. He's never worked a day in his life. He was a drug user, he was on the game when he got diagnosed and he's persistent with everything. I mean he gets loads of money and they've just taken away quite a big chunk of it because they realise he's not gonna die. He's had all this money for about 10 or 12 years...he gets DLA and has got something called ILF and that was an atrocious amount of money... I really used to resent him. He is twenty years diagnosed, not on medication and is fit and healthy... he could be out working and I look at him and I think 'how come I'm on medication and my liver's collapsed?' and his attitude is like, 'well the world owes me a living' so I guess therefore that sometimes attitude has nothing to do with it. I can't see it. I feel that my attitude has helped but then when I look at other people I don't know, is it luck?"

Elisabeth does take a positive approach to life and has a sense of belonging in support networks for HIV in her locality. She is a member of Narcotics Anonymous and regularly attends meeting and this is her primary 'community'.

COLIN

Colin, aged 46, describes himself as a middle class, gay man who works in journalism; he previously trained as a social worker. He was diagnosed in 1985 and the route of transmission was sexual. He is an agnostic and describes his ethnicity as UK and White. He was in an established intimate relationship and was cohabiting with his partner at the time of our interview. He is relatively healthy but has, at times, barely escaped death as a consequence of living with AIDS. When I asked him whether HIV was a large or small part of his sense of identity, he told me:

"It is annoyingly a large part of my identity; I would like it to be a smaller part of my identity. It is partially because I actually work in the field and I don't want to work in the field forever... I would love to just escape it and not think about it. Now I have to think about it because I have to take pills twice a day, so that is a twice daily reminder... I am as healthy as your average 46 year old man...It is very difficult... I mean I feel a bit like a blind person feels, I suspect... it is not written on my face, although if I had taken drugs with bad side effects it might be... but it is an identity you can't escape. In other words, at every moment both as a gay man, firstly, which I have always dealt with ever since I was aware that I was gay, and as a positive person... you are faced with the question of whether you are going to tell people or not, which annoys me that it has to be a dilemma. I would much rather operate as a regular human being... No, the fundamental answer is no I am not defined by being HIV-positive or by being a gay man. Those are incidental, they should be incidental in the way that I am half Scottish or I have got freckles or whatever... that's ideally how unimportant HIV should be but of course it is not."

Colin went on to speak about his concerns about going back to work following a prolonged bout of AIDS-related illness, he recalled:

"Despite my positive mental attitude I put myself into the category of being somebody who is going to die and I resigned myself to that fact unconsciously. And I have always said to people it was difficult coming to terms with dying but it wasn't one tenth as difficult as coming back to life again... some people get stuck in that 'AIDS victim' place because it is actually so difficult to rebuild yourself... I am halfway through my life... I was 41 when I actually started recovering. I had been off work for six years with AIDS... who on earth was going to employ me? What on earth was I going to do? I was still afraid that I would not be able to you know... the strain of work would ruin my health but it was that I desperately wanted to have a place in society again, not wanting to be this sort of long-term medical casualty... I didn't want to live on benefits for the rest of my life. I wanted to give something back... I suppose to people with HIV, to society in general... I have always had a fairly strong left-wing political attitude...I ended up volunteering to work within the HIV press and quickly got a job... I had always been able to write and talk... I had always written the odd little pieces for magazines and columns whenever I felt inspired. I am an English graduate... And I work extremely hard. Too bloody hard, sometimes, which is one of the reasons I have been so dozy this weekend...I don't want to work in HIV forever...I am carrying on with other training but it is very difficult to combine that with a demanding full time job, or at least four days a week... I have an enormously supportive team... I have learned a lot; I have got a certain amount of confidence but I don't quite know where I want to take it next. I had dreams about writing for a living but I know how difficult it is."

Colin went on to talk about networks of support for HIV and how he credits these to his continued survival, he recounted:

"There are four people I credit for my continued survival. One is my doctor, one is Cass Mann, one is not a person but the AIDS Mastery and one is my partner who just looked after me very practically when I was ill, he is good...in terms of practical ability to help you in a crisis he really pulled me through... I am in a work environment where I don't have to decide whether to disclose or not; it is very bizarre. I am working in a work environment where you assume people are positive until they say otherwise; I presume people are gay until they say otherwise... it makes me afraid to move out of that environment, it makes it difficult to move out. How do you explain it in a job interview? Do you make a big thing out of it, or do you minimise it? Do you lie about it? Where I work is very rewarding but it does exact a psychological toll as well...I am not necessarily obsessing about my condition anymore but I am for other people, because I am still thinking about HIV far more in the day than I would like to. I would rather like to be thinking about other things some of the time."

Colin recalled how being in the public eye in relation to HIV matters impacted on his social environment. He also spoke about the gay community and changing identities, he told me:

"I have been on TV in the News... I have been asked to appear on popular programmes about HIV and I have declined...in the back of mind I thought, 'I hope none of my neighbours are watching this.' I think most of them would deal with it because I think... if you are a regular person and conduct yourself with confidence and treat people fairly then they will treat you fairly. Some prejudice is created by the victim; this is absolutely true. For every bully you need a victim but there is some just out there... during the really dark years of AIDS gay men found a sort of solidarity and I think we miss that these days...there is a community which is based on shared adversity... shared tragedy really...I think the gay community got a lot of moral legitimacy out of it, we proved that we were capable of looking after each other... a lot of myths were demolished during those years... we showed that we had relationships and it was real and we were as committed as anybody... we are struggling to find a post AIDS-identity...in this country there is a whole bunch of people who are heterosexuals, the newly infected; the Africans in particular, and I think they're struggling to find a new sense of identity because a lot of them are newcomers, immigrants and they have their own issues to deal with. They are often people from desperately poor parts of the world; I meet some of them and some are wonderful people, but they have a huge problem with anti-HIV stigma, much worse than in the gay community... so I don't think there is an HIV community as such."

Colin has acquired a vast amount of knowledge around HIV issues over time and has made it his business to become acquainted with new developments in HIV medicine as they emerge. He works hard and has resumed his social role in society in terms of returning back to the workplace following a prolonged period of ill health. There is a back-to-work programme called Positive Futures which supports positive people who wish to return to the workplace.

NEIL

Neil, aged 42, describes himself as a middle class, gay man who is now medically retired: he used to work in the public sector. He was diagnosed with HTLV III in 1985 and the route of transmission was sexual. Neil is an Agnostic and describes his ethnicity as White and British. He is in a long-term intimate relationship and lives with his partner. Neil is relatively healthy and feels he needs a new challenge in his life. He adopts a positive mental attitude and gets on with life, in spite of experiencing severe bouts of ill health. I asked him about family relationships and if he had support from his friends around HIV, he told me:

"I haven't told my family… when I came out I was 18 and my parents found it very hard to take… there was still a strain in our relationship by 1985 so I didn't want to, I still haven't told them… my sister did actually ask me if I was ill and I just said 'no'… I think my Mum would get terribly upset and start crying and I don't know if I can handle it, I don't want to handle it…she would get really, really upset if I was ill, yeah, and I think the stigma would come into it but I think it would be mainly because I was ill… I would have to try and convince her that I wasn't dying… I find it very hard to even start to think about how I would ever deal with that with her… the other thing too and I feel that it is a bit of a cop out but they are both in their mid 70s; they are both pretty active but they are slowing down and our relationship is changing… and I sort of end up caring for them…I didn't tell friends, my main support was my partner. I told him and we talked about it… actually to do with family, although I never told them, certainly we started getting on a lot better in the 80s and now we get on very, very well."

Neil spoke about accessing networks of support for HIV when he started experiencing severe illness; this was 11 years after his diagnosis, he recalled:

"From about 1996 when I started to get ill I got information from THT and I got in touch with an AIDS network in London…I visited a hospice too where they had lots of peer groups and for the first time I actually met other people with AIDS and HIV… I hadn't really mixed with people with HIV before… it did help but looking back I think there were down sides to it too in that I took on everything that other people were saying about how ill they were and many were very ill, not all of them, but some were very ill and I took on that kind of perception of being ill...it was helpful yes... there was a lot of practical, or should I say financial advice I had obtained, you know, like pensions and private pensions...we had started looking at housing needs and what might change and what we wanted and, to be honest, we bought this house because I thought if I am going to die I want somewhere with a garden... I used to refuse to deal with mortgages because all those years when I was ill I just believed that I would not get a mortgage... we had pensions and we had to start to take out private pensions too because we thought we would be working until 65 at least...I don't think that I'm part of any HIV community because how I see the HIV community is things like support groups and institutions really... like London Lighthouse and Body Positive, and that's closed now but I have never been part of those sorts of support groups... I have never really been one for attending meetings or getting involved with groups... Through the Net certainly I feel more part of something and having talked to other HIV people on the Net... what's interesting on the Net is that a lot of them have got very different experiences... some are working and have never been ill; some have been very ill and have been retired for years... so I feel more involved with that side of things and it is certainly what I prefer... that's how I interact with others."

Neil told me the pressing issues around why he had to consider medical retirement, he recounted:

"I had been on HAART for over a year and the side effects just weren't letting up... I had diarrhoea, and pain in my legs... I just thought that this was going to be for the rest of my life... the prospect of working full time was difficult and my doctor suggested to consider part-time work... the problem with that was if I ever did retire that would affect the pension I got and to be quite honest the system was such that it was easier to retire, completely retire medically than reduce my hours... financially I would miss out if I went part-time, so that is why."

Neil saw living with HIV as a *battle;* sometimes he won and sometimes he lost. He had become anxious about bodily changes as a result of living with HIV and the side effects of HIV medication. He is trying to welcome HIV as being part of his body; instead of thinking 'why do I look so thin in my face?' he was attempting to change his attitude towards 'well, you know, this is how I am.' He used the Internet as a network of support for his HIV; his long-term partner is his main source of strength and support.

A forgotten generation: Long-term survivors' experiences of HIV and AIDS

TOM

Tom, aged 55, describes himself as gay and middle class, but believes *'because he is gay and positive it makes him outside of the class system.'* He was diagnosed in 1986 and the route of transmission was sexual. Tom has no religion but has a leaning towards Buddhism yet does not believe in reincarnation. He describes his ethnicity as White and *'has no nationalistic tendencies'*, he is a human being. Tom was medically retired and previously worked in the public sector and the health service; he has also worked voluntarily in the HIV field. He is not in an established intimate relationship and lives alone. I asked Tom about whether HIV was a big or small part of who he was, he told me:

"It is a total part of my overall identity which is why I have the tattoo, the positive tattoo because it is something that I'm proud of. In sort of physiological terms I think it's a virus, it's in every bit of me; every bit of me is positive. In the way that I live my life as an 'out' gay man living with HIV; it's a comparatively small part but at the same time it's a total part in a sense that it colours everything and how I do everything... but I feel that I've dealt with all the issues... I've devoted so much time and energy to HIV over the years... I've been involved in gay agencies like working the Gay Switchboard and I have been involved in HIV work and tried to resolve HIV issues, as far as they can be resolved... I have now reached that time in life when I feel that there has to be more to all of this... you know occasional dinner parties, Mediterranean holidays twice a year...I have worked through HIV and now I want to get a bit more involved as a gay man. I feel an on-going resentment about HIV and the number of things it's robbed me of in my life... it affects relationships and what you can do with other gay men and day-to-day uncertainty of never knowing what's happening."

Tom told me about relationships with his family:

"When I did finally tell my parents, they were the last people I told really because I had such a hard time with them over the gay thing... with my step-mother in particular... my Dad was an incredible prude... I decided that I needed to tell them because I was doing radio broadcasts so I thought he was going to find out...they'd come from a generation where everything is kept in the family and you don't go outside to social workers and all those kinds of things; it was an expression of inadequacy or failing...I just used to have meaningless telephone conversations with them and I didn't want it to be like they were just called to the hospital if I became ill... I might die before them so I needed them to be prepared for it... I told them and with my Dad it worked wonders, because he was never a very physical, demonstrative guy but after that, after coming out that I was positive, every time I saw him after that we had a hug…eventually something good came out of it… in those 16 years I have had the happiest and saddest moments in my life but I wouldn't take any of them away."

As we recall, Tom had worked in the field of HIV in the early years and he told me his views on HIV networks of support and the idea of community. He stated:

"There aren't that many people who now work in HIV who remember times before there was any money, before 1989, for a lot of understandable reasons. But you know people did things borne out of a sense of commitment to other people not because there was any kudos or payment for these things…because there was just nobody else who was willing, there weren't that many support groups or agencies; it started with people who were prepared to do something, or was roughly in the same sort of psychological state…everything becomes so politicised and things changed.. I mean things have changed dramatically by the influx of large amounts of money and agencies suddenly became more concerned about the well-being of the agency rather than the well-being of the people they were supposed to provide services to… money is going to get more and more scarce and figures are doubling every five years, funding will not match that…I think we will have to go back to more things being voluntary as they were before…My ideal would be if we could have an HIV community right across the board in the UK; we have got the experience and the understanding of each other and realise all the myths and the stereotypes; they don't really exist…and they aren't important to us. Perhaps then, as a body, we could make decisions between ourselves about when money is available, who is going to bid for it, who has got the greatest need and we could regulate this between ourselves. This is my ideal… there are no longer places to go and while that goes on, both the agencies and the departments are quite happy to keep us in separate bunches because we are easier to manage…But it all takes time you see…A few years ago I went to a NAT conference [National Aids Trust] and there was a good workshop looking at services for Black people and gay people… it was great it was roughly 50/50 Black and White. The two facilitators were great from THT…what the workshop sort of led you to believe was that THT realised that only new monies would become available for Black communities and THT were bidding for it all the time because they already had those connections. But my view is that each community should be empowered in itself and what THT should have done, given its resources and connections, is to see that the money sets up a

Black organisation and share with them their experiences and skills... but it's the power thing; the power of this organisation that wants to keep its power and control all the time."

Tom has been extremely active in the HIV field for a great number of years. He does not believe there is an HIV community in the UK and has been a public figure for HIV since the early years. HIV is a large part of his identity in a very positive way and he has an extremely positive mental attitude towards living long-term with HIV.

PETER

Peter, aged 48, describes himself as a middle class gay man who is now medically retired; he previously worked in the transport industry. He was diagnosed in 1987 and the route of transmission was sexual. Peter describes his religion as Christian (non-practising) but states religion heavily influences his life. His ethnicity is English and White. Peter was in an established relationship but did not engage in sexual activities and lived alone. He is reasonably healthy and has worked closely with HIV organisations to help others as a volunteer. I asked him about support networks for HIV and he told me about a close friendship:

"I have one very good friend who I don't know how I would manage without... I am very lucky in that respect; but sometimes I fear that because of my whinging and whining and moaning and groaning...and because of some of the hell I have been through and some of the worries and anxieties I still have, he could possibly decide that enough is enough... that is my greatest fear because he's like a life-line to me... I think this is a deep-rooted fear and I would find life very difficult... I mean I would like to walk away from me if I could."

Peter was very emotional during our conversation about his close friend. He told me how HIV had impacted on his life and his voluntary work in HIV:

"I live it and breathe it all the time basically... you know some people would probably think, 'My God, what planet is he on? How come he seems reasonably intelligent and yet says something like that? He needs to get it in proportion.' But right from the word go I decided that HIV should be seen as a challenge and not as a threat and while I have got breath in my body, I will attempt, at every opportunity, to try my best as far as I am able to continue to see it as a challenge rather than a threat; so I have got the biggest fight of my life...HIV has got to be huge, it's not just for me, it's hopefully for other people too...I have a great love for other people...as a gay man living in London I wanted to do my bit for the Terrence Higgins Trust and I had connections with London Lighthouse and Body Positive as well... I became more and more aware of friends of friends who were dying and those numbers were increasing and they were quite frightening...sometimes they were quite young people and this was something that was devastatingly horrendous...I did try to enforce in myself a positive attitude towards HIV... fighting a fight to educate people about the risks and I mean my life took on a different kind of quality as well...coming to make decisions that enriched the quality of my life and HIV gave it a different dimension and I had a feeling of purpose that I hadn't had previously."

Peter did access support groups and had worked within HIV networks of support for a number of years; he had a genuine desire to help others about HIV matters. He told me:

"Living in London I was able to connect with other positive people and other groups that were starting up and I decided that I wanted to see HIV as a challenge...and get involved in the fight against AIDS so I actually joined the Terrence Higgins Trust and became very actively involved in their work and remained with them for 17 years. In fact I was with them before I knew I was positive... I only stopped working with them last year because of ill health when I was unable to continue to do the work I was doing."

Peter has a good knowledge of HIV matters and accesses networks of support when he feels he needs them. He did not talk about family relationships and we did not raise the issues of prejudice or discrimination during our conversation.

RICHARD

Richard, aged 32, described himself as a working class, gay man and was working part-time in the HIV field; he was previously working as a jeweller. He was diagnosed in 1990 and the route of transmission was sexual. He described himself as a Christian and his ethnicity as British and White. Richard was relatively healthy yet found it difficult to maintain a good diet and look after himself. He was in a long-term intimate relationship and lived alone. He was very knowledgeable on HIV and gay men's issues and had been involved in HIV awareness training from the early years. I asked Richard how HIV had impacted on his sense of who he was, he told me:

"My confidence has, at times, been in tatters... when there is no stigma attached to an illness that you might have, it must be easier to cope with...I think I lost everything really...I guess it would have been easier if I had plenty of money and a good support network: present company accepted [smiling]... To me, H-I-V means Here Implacable Vulnerable...I am stubborn, difficult to sway and if I believe strongly in something then I will not be moved on an issue. I think also 'here' is a big word, as in I am still here in the here-and-now. It has always been told to me that I would not be here. I am not ungrateful that I am here but I never thought I would be here today. I am very vulnerable but in a powerful way. I won't be walked over but I am aware of my status and health...I think I am brave, quite brave for me. I think I have had an impact on a lot of people's lives."

Richard continued to talk about how he believed he had impacted on lives of others in terms of his earlier training experiences, he told me:

"In my training role...I allowed myself to be vulnerable by sitting at the front of workshops and allowing people to ask me questions about HIV and living with HIV. Taking part in HIV awareness training allows people to understand more and I hope that people will read this. I hope to have impacted on people's lives and I am pretty sure that I have. I hope that I have offered people an opportunity to look for themselves at what HIV is and isn't and from that, make choices for themselves."

For a long period of time Richard did not work, as at the onset of diagnosis he lost two jobs in quick succession on the basis of his HIV-positive status. He recounted how HIV had taken away life chances, he told me:

"Because I am quite a long way on with my HIV, it does affect me. I do feel tired. I find it difficult to cope sometimes with the effects of my illness. The drugs and side effects are a problem, especially loose stools. It is very difficult for me to work full time; as a result of that I have to work part-time. Working part-time means that really I am always on the breadline even if I have a good job and work part-time. Whatever I do I will always be on a lower income as a single man, or a man who lives alone. So the real issue for me is that I will always be an ill person and therefore in a poverty trap, which is a hard place to be...I lost my future, my career, my life. It had gone, but it didn't have to be gone; that is what is sad about all of this. It was the doctors who told me that my life would soon be gone. Now 12 years on, I made the decision to go back into work and I am in work, and part of me is furious that if I hadn't have had HIV, where could I have been now? Maybe I wouldn't be working part-time, or if I had have been working part-time I would have been building up a full time pension...those things are not there now. So, 12 years have gone and society told me that I had to stop work, go onto welfare benefits, withdraw from most of life; and during all those years when I was asymptomatic and very little was happening, I could have been doing something. So in a sense, those are the areas where I have deep regrets, but again we all say, 'if I only knew then what I know now'... I think the voluntary sector has gone though a very steep learning curve; I think also the Benefits Agency has gone through a very steep learning curse. And the medical profession? Will they have learned by their huge mistakes that have devastated people's lives? I don't really know. I still feel there is an over-reliance on the use of HAART medication and I think we will see proof of that."

In spite of Richard's most deep regrets concerning work-related matters, he told me of how he had learned so much from his involvement in the HIV field. He recounted:

"For me, the real gain has been that I have been able to get some additional education. I am not the brightest academic in the world and I am neither a numpty. There are some things that I wasn't particularly familiar with before my diagnosis; but the fact that I have had the opportunity to get involved, to volunteer and work in HIV organisations... to get opportunities to travel and to work with other people has given me a broader perspective and opened up avenues for me that wouldn't have been there before HIV... I have come across people who are newly diagnosed with HIV and I think many of the same issues are still there for people: fear, prejudice, stigma, fear of prejudice, lack of knowledge, the need for education and a need for an understanding of equal rights... yet there are different choices today. People live longer, you can take HAART, the Government are quite keen to promote career changes for people... but HIV is still more than just a chronic illness, so young people: BE AWARE."

To be sure, Richard did have an impact on people's lives; in particular he impacted on my life and was the initial driving force for this HIV study. He gave many talks to groups of people outlining what it was like to live with HIV and was involved in sexual health training. Richard often felt that working in HIV was a little too close for comfort but still he persisted in his work.

PERRY

Perry, aged 40, describes himself as a middle class gay man who no longer has a sex life; he works part-time and previously worked in the finance sector. He was diagnosed in 1990 and the route of transmission was sexual. His religious affiliation is Church of England (non-practising) and describes his ethnicity as Anglo-Saxon UK. Perry is single and lives alone; he was relatively healthy at the time of our interview. I asked Perry about how HIV had affected him and if he was involved in any networks of support for HIV, he told me:

"I don't really know that many people where I live and the ones that I do know, know about my HIV anyway... I have told people in the past and I had a bad reaction so I tend to be a bit more cautious nowadays... I find that if you tell one person you are effectively telling 10 other people because no matter what you do eventually it gets broadcast... this was at the hospital anyway... I have a mental illness and so I don't really know how HIV impacts on who I am... I think people generally are quite accepting of people with mental illness in the community, so I guess I am OK really... I don't feel resentful anymore; I accept the situation and I am quite even-minded about things. I think there have been a lot of resources put into HIV and HIV organisations are supportive... I read Positive Nation and access the Internet but I don't bother with support groups for HIV... I read articles and make up my own mind on HIV matters, that's it really!"

Perry's relationship with members of his family is improving yet according to Perry he leads a rather solitary life. He is relieved that effective HIV treatments have been developed and is happy to go along with advice on treatment issues from the medical profession.

RICK

Rick, aged 32, described himself as a working class gay man and is medically retired; he previously worked in the music industry. He was diagnosed in 1990 and the route of transmission was sexual. Rick described his religion as Baptist (non-practising) and his ethnicity as White and British. He was in a long-term relationship and lived alone. Rick was experiencing ill health and was awaiting salvage therapy at the time of our interview due to complications with previous HIV medicines. I asked Rick how HIV had impacted on social aspects of his life since diagnosis and he initially spoke about work matters, he told me:

"I had to stop work because of it. They needed a few people to take voluntary redundancy so I took it because I had to have quite a bit of time off work so it seemed appropriate seeing as they wanted some people to leave...well, since then I could have gone back to work and I wish I had gone back to work by doing something that wasn't as demanding or as many hours... but I never did because you get out of the routine of work. So the one thing I regret is not going back to work or to college... you end up at a loose end all the time. It has just been a waste of time... whereas now I can't go back to work... after I had had my operation I could have done another 4 or 5 years full time... but then my partner got poorly so I would have had to give work up again to look after him. I have many qualifications in music including a lower and higher national diploma in musical instrument technology which was quite good because there were 400 applicants from Europe and only 4 places per year...I did get offered to go work in an orchestra, which I had done before but my partner who gave me HIV didn't want me to because I would have had to travel a lot, so I ended up losing a lot of my music and I enjoyed my music."

I asked Rick whether he considered HIV to be a small or large part of his life and what networks of support he relied on for HIV, he told me:

"At the moment HIV is a very large part of my life because I've got a lot of appointments and there are a lot of different things wrong with me because of all the treatments I have had...all my family know this and most of my friends know too...I told my best friend in London and it was no problem for her and her husband. I told a few other friends with no problems... my very good friends, and I have got a lot of very good friends sit with me when I go to Bingo... they'll drink from my glass, they will use my knife and fork if I don't eat all my food, and my family are the same... they'll drink my water and my pop...my family and friends are supportive and know about my HIV...other networks of support I use are things like iBase and I am a member of a local voluntary HIV organisation here which gives fabulous support and I use the AIDS manuals there... you've got your AIDS helpline which is helpful and Simon at iBase is very helpful; London Free have been very helpful and ISIS are good, so you can access these if you want...I think I might rely on my local HIV organisation here too much, they took me to hospital when I couldn't drive. They have been very, very good and they gave me a grant to help me out... you have got Terrence Higgins Trust but they only help people in Leeds even though it is THT Yorkshire.. people know about iBase and National Aids Line and there are smaller charities around in towns and things...computers are great for accessing support too...and NAM is free to everybody, so I have access to a huge source of support if I want it, goodness me!"

Rick had always taken an active role in making decisions centred on HIV matters and had acquired a sound knowledge base around HIV matters; he was familiar with many networks of support for HIV which is understandable considering HIV was becoming an even larger part of life due to medical complications.

WOODY

Woody, aged 45, describes himself as a middle class gay man who works full time in Information Technology. He was diagnosed in 1992 and the route of transmission was sexual. He is Church of England and Spiritualist (non-practising) and describes his ethnicity as White and English. Woody was not in a relationship and lived alone. He is extremely healthy but has recently experienced weight loss which is a cause for concern. I asked Woody how HIV impacted on his sense of who he is and whether it was a small or large part of his life, he told me:

"At first it was a large part, yes... I thought of myself as a person with HIV. I suddenly felt as though I'd got a disease and thought about what would happen if I told people, like at the Gym or at work and how people would view me. I suddenly became a different person and it affected everything I used to do; you know, like going out meeting people... a different person is not quite right. I was the same person but I was a person with a transmittable disease if you like, so I had to look at everything differently...well that was ten years ago and I'm still alive...I haven't been ill as such... so I suppose I've carried on living roughly the same life, so my life hasn't changed drastically if at all...I probably resist HIV as a label... it doesn't take over my life because I haven't changed anything... the only thing that's sort of changed is my social life but that might be my age. As time goes by you tend to change anyway...it's at the back of my mind all the time... I've got round to thinking that it hasn't had a huge effect on my life and I'm still working. I haven't had any AIDS-type of illnesses...As time goes on there's a bit of denial because I haven't told anybody apart from one or two close friends...most of my family have died apart from I have two sisters who I haven't told."

I asked Woody about networks of support he might access and his perceptions on the HIV community. He recounted:

"I don't have a sense of belonging to the gay community or the HIV community... not that I would want to necessarily belong to the HIV community but I suppose the option of having it there would be nice if I wanted to access it... I suppose in London there are the Terrence Higgins Trust and London Lighthouse and hospices for the terminally ill... I think there are communities there but it's been couple of years since I've been to

London... communities have been built up and there are various drop-ins and people will naturally be drawn together at some point as they run into each other at local clinics... by design or by accident or there might be support groups but I don't know if there is an HIV community... I don't know anybody in my local area... I did sort of try to go to a local HIV support group which was set up by AIDS action... and I went to a couple of meetings where there were a handful of people from different backgrounds and different scenarios...the group was in the throes of lots of stuff, getting bogged down with politics really.. the support group was controlled by the City Council so it got very political and really it wasn't a group of people that I could identify with...if there is anything locally it might have changed now but I don't know, I am not aware of networks of support here. I don't get involved... I'm aware of people who were HIV-positive and I found this out basically by people gossiping in the local gay pub... this is about ten years ago."

Woody raised a point about volunteers, non-professionals and non-medical personnel working in HIV networks of support. He told me:

"I've got a problem with non-professionals being involved with support and advice or whatever, non-medical personnel who aren't bound by confidentiality. I am uncomfortable with that and with volunteers who volunteer to do whatever... it's not their job and although they should be bound by confidentiality, they won't lose their jobs, I am uncomfortable with volunteers really... it's not the end of their career and an example of this is a person I knew, this is going back 10 years, who worked on this AIDS helpline...this person used to come across people who were HIV-positive and then used to spread it around the local gay pub...I found out about a friend of mine who I knew about twenty or thirty years ago who's since died of AIDS.. But I never knew he was HIV-positive via any sort of proper channels, like his ex-lover or whatever... I found out about it through gossip on the grapevine...I can think of two or three examples of people who have officially died of cancer yet everybody knows they were HIV-positive...so I want to sort of stay away from the voluntary sector. I am quite happy dealing with the medical profession and associates but no-one else."

Woody did not have support of his family or close friends as he had not told them of his HIV-positive status. He is secretive about his status and is suspicious of voluntary HIV organisations and volunteers who might learn of his HIV and reveal his positive status to others on the 'grapevine'.

LARRY

Larry, aged 56, describes himself as a middle class gay man and is medically retired: he previously worked in the public sector. He was diagnosed in 1992 and the route of transmission is unknown but he believes it may have been via contaminated blood from a transfusion. Larry describes his religion as Jewish Methodist and his ethnicity as White UK. He was in a relationship and lives alone. Larry had recently started taking combination therapy and was experiencing good heath at the time of our interview. Prior to diagnosis, Larry was already a volunteer in a local HIV organisation. When I asked him how HIV had impacted on daily life, he told me:

"I actually wake up every morning and think, 'Larry you've woken up!'... whether I feel ill or whether I feel well, whether the sun is shining or whether it's snowing, I say 'thank you'…It's another gift, a new day. It's another chance. It's life and I try to make the best of each day as it comes and that's how I live with HIV. I try not to make too many plans for the future… I've never felt sorry for myself… that's sort of self-defeating…What a shame that someone has to have something like HIV in their lives to come to their senses… in many ways it does make you a better person."

Larry continued to talk about his family and in particular his relationship with his mother, he told me:

"…my wife had already died and I thought who do I tell? I tell the person that I love and trust the most… that was my mother. Now my mother at that time was 70 odd, so I thought I'd better tell her. I don't know what her reaction is gonna be but I don't really mind… I gave it some thought before I actually did tell her…I invited her over; I wanted to tell her in my own home… she came over and I invited my friend who used to be the facilitator at the HIV voluntary organisation I worked for because I felt I needed some support… I actually thought my mother might need support so I had a lady here from the same organisation because I thought my Mum might need another female… I didn't beat about the bush… I must admit I burst into tears telling her but after a few seconds I said, 'Now Mother I've shared this with you. I will understand that you will probably need to share it further.' I didn't want to pass on this awful news and leave her with the burden of it because that would have been criminal… I trust her explicitly… she was wonderful… she's now 87 bless her! Bless her! She even considered going on a course to learn more about HIV. She's been a rock. I couldn't have asked for more. She's my adoptive mother, she's not my real mother. I was adopted when I was about three and a half. She's wonderful...I consequently told my sister who thought I'd be dead in a week...she burst into tears. I've actually been far more open with far more people... some other relatives now know from my own mouth... more of my friends are now aware that I'm HIV-positive because I've shared it with them... as years go by I'm finding it actually a lot easier to share it and discovering that people are taking it very well. They're not treating me any differently... that's wonderful, for me that's wonderful."

Larry was still the same old Larry. He was no different than before yet he hid for many years following his diagnosis and he hated it. Larry had a good sense of who he was as he told me:

"HIV is neither a large or small part of who I am... it's an integral part of me. It's part of the whole. Sometimes it's more important than others, sometimes it's completely irrelevant. It depends on who I am talking to and what we are talking about, it's just part of me... it's like what size is your penis? Sometimes it is relevant, sometimes it is not. I used to hibernate... I used to hide away and now I've learned not to hide or suppress my feelings...I embrace it because I listen to it. In fact my body tells me I don't need consultants... most people are probably not aware that their body still governs everything but we don't listen; we haven't taught ourselves to listen to our bodies. HIV has taught me that it's imperative to listen to your body and don't ignore it... do what it's telling you because it helps... Life is not just about living it's about having a meaningful life."

Larry describes himself as a 'mad man' who has spent most of his personal and working life trying to help others who he feels 'were hard done by society'. HIV is an integral part of who he is but it is not a badge or label. Larry recounted:

"Being gay means we're not different to anyone else just because our sexual preferences might be different in bed; being HIV-positive doesn't mean we're different and therefore not part of society. Segregation in my opinion never worked for anybody. Integration. Integration. Integration. Let's all get on with each other. We're all the same... I was heavily involved with the HIV-side of things before I was even diagnosed...I'm heavily involved in the gay scene. I just love being involved. My involvement with people is my network of support."

Larry used the Internet for HIV information and as a network of support. He shifted from being a volunteer in an HIV organisation to being a client. At the time of our conversation, there was no local HIV organisation in place for support; this had been closed down due to changes in funding. Larry felt he had a good sense of belonging where he currently lived and believed his personality and character was part of being socially included.

RACHEL

Rachel, aged 39, describes herself as a middle class heterosexual woman who is a Mum and a housewife. She was diagnosed in 1993 and the route of transmission was sexual from her HIV-positive husband. She is a practising Christian who affiliates with the Church of England and Anglican Church. Rachel describes her ethnicity as White and British UK. She is married and lives with her husband and two children. Rachel recently started on combination therapy due to a decline in her CD4 count. She had already acquired an interest in AIDS and HIV matters due to her living overseas in Africa. I asked her to what extent HIV had initially impacted on her life, she told me:

"Well obviously it has… because of things like I had to give up work to look after my husband. We thought he was going to die in 18 months and he is still with me…So I gave up work to look after him because he was very ill at that time; he was having difficulty even going up and down stairs and walking 20 yards and that sort of thing…obviously this had an enormous effect on me because I loved my job… and we had so little information. We started providing information locally to anybody through health systems; for anyone who might be newly diagnosed to make sure that there was just a basic information pack including a newsletter and so on…so that people didn't feel isolated… because we felt very isolated… we picked up on that and we wanted to be positive about our experiences… we wanted to make something out of it rather than go and sit at home, with your head in your hands and cry. It is a very practical way of behaving quite honestly… we had been around the world; we had seen a lot worse than that and we knew that you win some, you lose some… and we picked ourselves up and we were quite happy. We faced up to the situation, we got ourselves sorted out… we were reasonably well adjusted."

Rachel went on to discuss HIV as a label which she resisted and how HIV impacted on her sense of who she is; she recounted:

"It is one of the things I get quite cross about, because there is a tendency to see HIV and nothing else… I mean people who have HIV do it as well, but doctors do it, health workers do it, many people do it… they see HIV and they don't see the person behind this label…they don't see you as a wife, a mother, a sister, a cousin, an aunt or whatever... you know they don't see all the other things you are; they just see HIV, they call you HIV, you are HIV and it has actually become the name. You know, I am HIV: No, no I am not...I am a human being actually. This is first and foremost; I am all sorts of other things and actually for me HIV comes pretty way down the line. That is something I have become more and more aware of as time has gone on, really. I have actually heard people saying, 'I am HIV' and I have pulled them up and I have said, 'Stop, you are letting people label you. You are not HIV; HIV is a part of you but there is so much more; it is not the whole of you.' It is something that I get a bit worked up about...Initially HIV was huge, it did take over. Drastically took over my life but as time has gone on, it is a large part of what we do because it is the area that we work in; so in that sense it still takes quite a lot of our time. But, as far as identity is concerned, for me, I have come to the point where I actually feel that it is something that I don't actually want to have at the forefront the whole time. I don't want it being there all the time any more...it is not an important thing for me anymore. I don't want to be working in the HIV field so much anymore. I want to be doing my own thing... I am starting an Open University course with a view to going back to work in public health not just HIV but general health. It is less important for me than it was at the start...I am hoping to go back to work and I am registered disabled. I do have a disability; I can't stand on my feet for too long so I couldn't go back to full time work doing what I used to do... I find that hard because that is what I always wanted to do and I loved doing what I was doing...I am aware that there are other options open and I can still use what I have done and what I have learned...I can plan on that level."

Rachel spoke about how HIV had impacted on family and friendship relationships, she recalled:

"I suppose if anything my friends have become closer, particularly the ones that know about HIV. Very, very supportive! I wouldn't say that I make friends very easily in a sense of having very close friends. But those friends that I have got are very close; I've know them a long time and I knew that I didn't need to worry about telling them. Do you know what I mean?...within my own family, funnily enough I had experienced not cruelty or them being malicious or anything like that... my brother without realising it had assumed that because we were HIV-positive and because we were going to have a family, we might die early, he was very supportive... fine... but when we said that we were going to have more than one child, his immediate reaction was 'you can't do that!' and I said why not? He said he and his wife could not look after more than one: 'we can't bank on taking on more than one child, we won't be able to look after more than one of your children'... I was absolutely astounded that he should think that he was even going to be expected to look after my children and I found a very tactful way of saying 'sorry mate you're not in the running'...it wasn't nasty prejudice but a misunderstanding... I suppose a lack of understanding, really...It is something I hadn't thought about... down here I have got my own circle of friends, there is the Church community, all my neighbours; we know each other and their children come round to play with ours; our children go round and play with theirs, things like that... it is a local community in a sense of a small town...I very much feel part of this community and the Church community... I am getting involved with the school side of things with the children; and I am hoping to go back to work and that will be different experiences for me."

I asked Rachel about her perceptions of the HIV community and networks of support around HIV matters, she told me:

"No there isn't an HIV community... I want to qualify it because there isn't a community and yet there is a sort of sense of brotherhood if you like... because people have faced similar fears and worries and concerns whether they are Black or White; whether they are drug takers or gay, they face other prejudices quite often. So in a sense there is a sense of kinship, so I suppose there is a community thing for those that are able to connect... but then there is a huge number of people who are very isolated, who don't know about that kinship, who don't know how to access it or who are afraid to access it, you know, for various reasons...I would hope certainly for most people that I know they would find an awful lot of support and fellowship but if they don't or can't connect, does that make them automatically part of the community? I don't know...most of the time people are too busy carrying on with their own lives; more and more recently with people who are in work, then there are asylum seekers who, by their very nature, are having a tremendous amount of prejudice and problems anyway. They're scared silly, there are illegal immigrants who daren't come forward and are very afraid that if they did come forward they would be thrown out or sent back from where they came from... I think people like myself are failing in some way in getting to them but I don't know how we can gain access to them...if you have got the right contacts for example in refugee camps and asylum seekers camps, you might get one or two if they then feel safe to talk to you...I mean there is a prison community as well and there is a huge amount of that goes on... the prejudice in there is enormous and the things that they face are far worse than anything that the gay community could possibly relate to...more bullying, you can't get away from the people and you don't really have your own space in prison, so it's a very difficult situation...I'm involved with a lot of people who are already active in the areas, in the community if you like, we are working together, so in that sense there is a community... but it is a very, very, very small number of people when you think about the whole...I think sometimes people feel alienated too... there are some women in Brighton for example who are positive and feel very alienated from support services that are available... because they are gay orientated or Black orientated or drug user orientated and if you don't fit within these categories, well tough!."

At the onset of diagnosis, Rachel and her husband faced up to the reality that premature death was a possibility; they subsequently sorted out financial matters in relation to Wills and so on. Neither of them was particularly afraid of the actual event of death but the fear of prolonged illness was an issue. Rachel and her husband both worked in the HIV field and Rachel was looking forward to moving away and following her own career.

TONY

Tony, aged 40, describes himself as a poor working class gay/queer man who is medically retired. He is a wonderfully talented artist and poet. Tony was diagnosed in 1994 after many years in denial and the route of transmission is sexual. He is a non-believer in religion but is optimistic and defines his ethnicity as a White Irish European. He was in a new intimate relationship and had recently moved in with his partner. Tony is fairly healthy but lacks energy which is a cause for concern. When I asked him how HIV had impacted on his life and his sense of who he is, he told me:

"There is a lot of stigma because the worst people around HIV are actually gay people, this is my belief. I had worked in this environment so I know what the 'queens' are like and how the gay scene works...HIV is a big part of my life, because when you're HIV-positive you always have doubt in your brain. You hear so many stories about life expectancy and as you get older and the years go by you let the illness rule your life...I'm tired and lethargic and have no energy; I am slowing down. ..going to the bus stop, meeting people and I am thinking that people are pointing the finger...your whole self-esteem goes...Paranoia is a big thing in HIV especially for those who are very self-conscious of themselves, like me... body image is a big thing that scares HIV-positive men. I had loads of ambitions and they've gone. I haven't got any now, it just knocks your self-esteem and self-worth. You feel dirty. I feel like I have been raped of everything. It is draining. My thoughts keep chopping and changing... people used to say I was a 'slow train'... my Mum used to say I never listened but I don't think so... when I am talking to someone I will be talking about something and then all of a sudden I'll go into another story… so I am absent-minded… I live inside this cocoon, this shell. I feel I'm in a shell… I can't see myself in the mirror and I don't see what people see in me… I keep getting black shadows over my eyes and there's a sharp pain in the back of my head… why do people like me? I think I'm nice and I'm kind and I do listen. I'm not tactile. My mother describes me as being cruel… I am tactile if somebody is genuinely in the shit and really down and crying. I am not frightened of that. I'm a lost cause, or a lost soul, I'm very lost."

Tony spoke about having no sense of belonging and how he was better living in his own place. He had previously lived alone for ten years and he needed his own space. He recalled how he got involved in HIV organisations over the years and experienced networks of support, he recounted:

"I've always had my own space…I have never had a sense of belonging but London I loved London when I lived in London. I could live in London and people just say it is because of the club scene. It's not like that for me, it's just the culture. I like that cosmopolitan feel and I am very relaxed with that…I got involved in a local HIV organisation here and I have decorated for them and everything… they were helping me with my forms but they were helping the wrong people on the basis of them being their friends; they help the wrong people instead of those who need help…and the thing is money is very important when you're HIV-positive… you start to become ostracised because you don't go out because you have no money…I have been on HIV committees and been actively involved in HIV organisations in Manchester, London, Birmingham and so forth… this one I am with now, I have helped them and given them ideas to make money which they used and didn't even say 'thank you'…people were there doing all this shit-stirring on the committee… I used to sit and listen to people… they were banning people from the HIV centre for the wrong reasons and excluding people… for me it has all been such a negative experience I excluded myself from them in the end…people coming in off the street gossiping and sitting in little groups tearing people apart…I've yet to see an HIV community really, so introduce me to one, I'd love to see it."

Tony was disillusioned with HIV networks of support because of his experiences and earlier involvement. His family relationships were, at times, strained but that was not because of his HIV status. He had told his Mum, his Aunt and nieces but they do not offer any support. Tony has changed his friendship relationships because he found them tiresome and depressing.

A forgotten generation: Long-term survivors' experiences of HIV and AIDS

SANDRA

Sandra, aged 37, describes herself as a working class heterosexual woman who is medically retired; she previously worked as a technician. She was diagnosed in 1994 and the route of transmission was sexual. Sandra is a practising Christian and describes her ethnicity as a Black African. She is not in a relationship, is divorced and lives alone. Her health is considered as reasonable; she has days of good health and days of complete tiredness and exhaustion. I asked Sandra how HIV had impacted on her life, she told me:

"At the time of my son's death I was just finishing my second year at University… I just dropped out…I changed a hell of a lot and became a different person. I felt guilty enough that I'd passed it on to my child and I couldn't cope with the possibility that I could infect my husband because I loved him; I still do love him… I decided the thing for me… was to leave so he could have a life…I think I have lost my status in society…I cut all my friends off…the physical effects of HIV are difficult to live with…constant exhaustion…I see it as an alien part of me and it's going to be there for life…I think sometimes I am in denial."

Sandra did not feel there was an HIV community as a heterosexual woman. She does access a couple of HIV support groups and gets together with other people but has no sense of belonging to these groups. Her family live far away from her and she misses them. Sandra does believe that she is slowly coming to terms with her positive status and it is a slow process.

National Long Term Survivors Group: self-help, empowerment and support

This final collection of quotes has been compiled to illustrate the personal experiences and perceptions of those story-tellers who identified with and were members of the National Long Term Survivors Group (hereinafter referred to as: NLTSG). The comments you are about to read have been made by story-tellers who had attended at least one residential weekend at the NLTSG; these were spontaneous conversations that emerged whilst exploring HIV networks of support. None of our conversations were directly linked to questions I asked about the NLTSG as part of any particular theme of enquiry. In order to maintain confidentiality and preserve anonymity I am going to present only quotes without putting names to personal experiences. As part of my research journey, I was fortunate enough to be allowed to attend two residential weekends at the NLTSG; I am honoured to have been an observer and facilitator at these events. I remain eternally grateful to those who organised and sanctioned my involvement.

The NLTSG is a self-help organisation set up in the 1990s, which seeks to empower women and men who have lived for over 5 years with an HIV-positive diagnosis. It involves the social integration of people from across the UK who come together and share personal experiences of learning how to live positively with HIV. The residential weekends include: workshops for self-help; open and closed meetings; counselling sessions; focus groups and access to complementary therapies in a safe and relaxed social space. The NLTSG offers practical help and information on financial matters, welfare benefits and current information on effective drug treatments; it further allows its members to meet other long-term survivors and share personal experiences face-to-face. There is no obligation to take part in any of the sessions throughout the weekend, the choice is yours. I will let the quotations speak for themselves.

NLTSG: an essential network of support

For many story-tellers the NLTSG is very much a valued community and being involved in this support network has, for many, been a life-changing experience:

"I go to the NLTSG which has been a major turning point in my life… it was my road to Damascus… I came away from there after my first meeting and it changed my life… I think what has changed for me is meeting other people who are in the same boat; meeting other people who have had a longer diagnosis than me, and have not been ill and are not on any medication. I meet other people who have been diagnosed a lot later than me and they are very ill… meeting other people that have been diagnosed the same time as me and are finding new partners… loads of stuff like that…I see the NLTSG as a community and I think that is key really because there are things you want to share. You know fears and doubts; the good stuff as well, you know, how well you have been. It is for people to understand what it means to live with HIV… so when I got told my CD4 count was 430 I was absolutely over the moon and other people with HIV will understand that. My family won't, my friends won't and actually some of my friends have openly said, 'and is that good?' or 'so what does that mean to you? I am *living proof,* we came up with that at NLTSG because it is more appropriate than long-term survival because I don't believe I am surviving, I believe I am living and living life very much to the full. The community of long-term survivors is very important to me; it is inspirational, it is a deep-seeded love; going to the weekends for me is also being allowed to be totally who you are and what you are... there is absolutely no judgement there and that comes from the people. It is nothing to do with the venue, we have proved that. You get this transient body of people, yes you have got people who are always there like the Trustees and some of the facilitators but you have got this transient community and it doesn't matter whether somebody comes just once: that feeling is there every time, every time. I am very passionate about it."

"I value the NLTSG and I go once every three months to that if I can and I learn a lot from those more newly diagnosed and long-term diagnosed...you know, not newly diagnosed but people relative to my own diagnosis. When you come to meet them you are going to be amazed how such a diverse group of people are just *one* when they are together really... people that you wouldn't talk to in the street or in the pub, are all friends and loving and it is just a beautiful group to be around...the long-term survivors group is for me because it is my contact with my people or my club because I have made a lot of genuine friends from all over the country, but they are not the kind of people who you see regularly so I go to a local support group too..."

"The only community that I have experienced is the long-term survivors group; that is my community that is my peer group, it's magical. Years have gone by now since we needed to talk about ground rules. Friday nights used to be horrendous without ground rules...other organisations don't have the same value, you don't get anything from them like this. I realised there is only one place I ever come back feeling great and that is the NLTSG... They are the people I feel totally 'at one' with and I find it frustrating to think that with a little bit more effort from a few people, that community could be so much larger...in some respects it is kind of a well-kept secret but it's not because we intend it to be... it is because of the lack of resources to make more people aware of it... I try to promote it. There is no one answer to the lack of awareness of the group nationally... the indifference of some people who say, 'what is the value of people coming together?' I know it's not everybody's thing but I would like everybody to have the opportunity of trying it and seeing for themselves... About 1200 people have attended residential weekends over the last 10 years and it is really heartening to know that it's still got a purpose. It's really, really heartening but as I say I just think with a little bit more effort from a few people this community could be so much larger."

"The closest I have come to a community is the NLTSG. I feel as though it is like a family."

"I can only mention one or two things about being part of an HIV community...I'm not asking you to agree with my perception. For instance, I spent many years trying to find out about the NLTSG in the UK, which I would consider to be an HIV community in itself. Now then, I couldn't make contact with them until very recently. Now I've been on one weekend, which I loved for various reasons. I actually had a good laugh and I also actually got an awful lot of information from it. A lot of sharing, a lot of caring, a lot of loving and a lot of laughing and those were the important four things I got from it. Now because I've only been on one, I wouldn't regard myself as being a proper part of the HIV community or whatever... Hopefully, if I can get the *funding* from Social Services, you know my Borough, Oh! Bugger them! If I can go more often then this would give me more of a feel of belonging...I don't want to actually feel different to other people it's self defeating."

NLTSG – not quite a community

Here I believe story-tellers do have a sense of community but would like to see the NLTSG grow larger as living long-term with HIV becomes even more of a reality:

"I think that the long-term survivors group could be a community. I don't see it as that now. As years go by I think it will become a community because more and more people are going to be living a lot longer and as time goes by there'll be more combination therapies on the market and there will be more and more people and it will become bigger. As time goes by they will probably have to get bigger premises. We also need to do a bit more about letting people know about the NLTSG."

"There's a certain understanding when you meet people that have also been long-term diagnosed as opposed to perhaps people who have been newly diagnosed. I do think there's empathy... but it doesn't necessarily mean that you get on with everybody but I do think it is easier to make friends because there's a kind of realisation that you pick up through the bullshit... I can go through this rigmarole of getting to know you over a long period of time or we can just cut the bullshit and be friends now and I personally think that's a far better idea... you probably don't pick any different friends than you would have done before either. I still have a problem with the idea of a community though."

"If you go to the NLTSG, that's a community when you are there for the weekend, but it's only every now and again, isn't it? I mean it's not an everyday community... I mean the NLTSG have all these intense meetings and things and to be quite honest I think they're more 'head fucks' than anything else. If you can handle that kind of thing then fine... I can't handle it."

We have now reached the end of this extensive chapter exploring how living long-term with HIV has impacted on social lives in terms of reshaping identities. How does HIV affect my sense of who I am? How have I changed since I learned of my HIV-positive diagnosis? We have exposed how networks of support and relationships with family and friends are essential in terms of promoting self-esteem and giving us a sense of belonging; we all, from time to time, need the encouragement of significant others so we feel cared for and valued. For some long-term survivors, personal experiences of social isolation and varying degrees of loss had led to support networks becoming 'off limits' due to problems of secrecy, disclosure and openness. For a few, family relationships had already been stretched to the limits due to issues of sexuality, on being gay and 'coming out: a double edged sword.

To be sure, the range of personal experiences and perceptions of living with HIV has been far-reaching and diverse. Have family and close friends been a good source of support? In some cases, absolutely! Have HIV organisations been an effective network of support? In contemporary times, we have seen the closure of many voluntary HIV organisations and many smaller HIV centres have been swallowed up by larger organisations, such as THT. Our story-tellers have revealed how they perceive the notion of an HIV community and we have explored other 'communities of support' along the way, such as the valuable self-help organisation known as the NLTSG.

Living with HIV has undoubtedly taken away a great deal from our story-tellers; and for those diagnosed in earlier times, many had been coerced into leaving employment and became medically retired in spite of experiencing good health. This, in turn, creates problems associated with social roles, the notion of self-worth as well as negotiating money and financial matters, pensions and future prosperity. We have explored a kaleidoscope of emotions, experiences and perceptions of living long-term with HIV. Again, as we approach the end of this story-of-stories, I ask you to reflect on the personal experiences presented and think how you might have managed and negotiated these experiences if it had have been you.

How would your family react to an HIV-positive diagnosis? What would you have done in terms of your career? Would you have told your employer and work colleagues? How would you access networks of support for HIV? Who do you relate to in terms of each story-teller? Who do you feel empathy for? Do you agree with any of the issues that have emerged? Why do you agree with them? What do you not agree with? Think for a moment before we move on and ask yourself if your views, opinions and beliefs have changed since you started reading this story-of-stories. Have your opinions and beliefs changed in any way?

A forgotten generation: Long-term survivors' experiences of HIV and AIDS

CHAPTER NINE

Living long-term with HIV: positive and negative elements

∞

"When one door closes, another opens; but we often look so long and so regretfully upon the closed door that we do not see the one that has opened for us."

Alexander Graham Bell

"Anyone who has never made a mistake has never tried anything new."

Albert Einstein

Introduction

It is more than thirty years since we became aware of an apparently new condition known as *Acquired Immune Deficiency Syndrome* (AIDS) which led to the scientific discovery of its causative agent: the retrovirus we know as *Human Immunodeficiency Virus* (HIV). Just over ten years ago in 2002, I was privileged to have recorded conversations with twenty eight women and men living in the UK who spoke out about their personal experiences of living long-term with an HIV-positive or AIDS diagnosis. At least five of our story-tellers, to the best of my knowledge, have sadly died. The memories of our departed story-tellers will, I trust, always live on. Without exception, every one of our long-term survivors who have told us their story ought to be recognised as truly extraordinary human beings.

Before we explore how each story-teller reflected on the positive and negative elements of living long-term with HIV, we shall examine how AIDS and HIV has had a notable effect on social aspects in our society both within and outside of the UK. In many ways these were largely unanticipated and often go unrecognised yet most certainly do require our attention. First of all, we must appreciate the links between vulnerability to HIV and poverty, deprivation and social inequalities as these have been firmly established across the globe. Access to HAART and other medicines is dependent on wealth; the most marginalised people in the poorest of countries who are likely to contract HIV will inevitably die of AIDS. Without the access to HIV treatment in Central Africa and developing countries, it is difficult to see any positive social effects of HIV; apart from those continents like Uganda who have negotiated and maintained successful community AIDS projects. Across parts of Europe and in more tolerant cultures we might glean a positive light, however dim this light might be.

At a public level, HIV has undoubtedly raised the visibility of the UK's gay community in terms of opening out gay-centred spaces in large cities, such as Manchester, Birmingham and London. We no longer see the blacked-out or smoked windows of gay bars and clubs as once was the case in the early 1980s. Gay 'hot spots' in large towns are, by and large, now frequented by not only people who identify as gay, bisexual or 'queer'; we see a huge eclectic mix of sub-cultural groups in bars, clubs and restaurants, for example, in Manchester's Canal Street.

During the initial AIDS epidemic particularly in the UK and United States, lesbians and gays experienced a backlash of public opinion because of the label of the syndrome known as the 'gay plague'. The struggle to get appropriate health care for an already marginalised and stigmatised sub-culture, led to an upsurge in community-based activism. The speed with which some communities responded to this crisis has been incredible. 'Action for AIDS' groups have been prevalent in many countries since the onset of the AIDS epidemic. It must be appreciated that these rapid responses and community-based activism could not have existed without the previous decade of organising gay men and lesbians which had continued after the student riots in France in 1968 and the US Stonewall Riots in 1969. In 1999 gay pride marches took place in 38 countries of which 13 of them were in the developing world. Across Europe in 2010, gay pride marches took place in 29 countries. To name and shame the countries where sexual diversity is not tolerated included: the Czech Republic; Cyprus; Bosnia and Herzegovina; Albania; Estonia; Georgia; Latvia; Ukraine; Montenegro; Moldova and Macedonia.

At a level for future HIV activism, we have learned from our predecessors to be flexible, tactical and strategic when participating in direct action. We must be prepared to familiarise ourselves with the discourse of science and medicine in order to effectively engage in research programmes and clinical trials. Future treatment activists cannot demand more from scientific accomplishments than can be realistically provided. Science is not magical. Unreflective and dogmatic activism can impede scientific advancement and activists need to be prepared to renegotiate proactive programmes for changing policies when required. How have we come to learn these skills for more effective strategies?

We have learned how previous AIDS treatment activism in the United States and parts of Europe focussed strategic direct action towards monitoring, lobbying and fighting governments, the Food and Drug Administration (FDA), the Centers for Disease Control and Prevention (CDC) and the pharmaceutical industry for drug treatments; this was at a time when Governmental complacency and indifference was prevalent. An assortment of unique circumstances played a pivotal role in the explosion of AIDS treatment activism; this incorporated six years of pioneering AIDS activism in the US. The growth of HIV service providers in the US such as Gay Men's Health Crisis (GMHC) in 1981 and the establishment of the People with AIDS (PWA) self-empowerment movement in 1983 all contributed towards some of the victories of social change across the world.

AIDS Coalition to Unleash Power [ACT UP] was founded in March 1987. It was built on 'a diverse, non-partisan group of people who united in anger and was committed to direct action to end the AIDS crisis'. Other independent ACT UP groups subsequently materialised in large and small cities across the United States and in London, Berlin and Paris. The emergence of ACT UP groups brought human beings a collective power and promoted a new sense of cultural and political community. Whilst this was occurring, other AIDS activists were developing a more long-term strategic focus on direct action towards research on AIDS treatments. AIDS treatment activism was born and had many successes and victories which have extended health for people living with HIV in Western societies. One such victory was to put pressure on the US Federal Drug Agency [FDA] to be more responsive and flexible to AIDS matters which instigated the accelerated approval of HIV drugs in the late 1980s. AIDS treatment activism has had less success within the developing world.

At a public health level, HIV has changed the way we talk about sex, sexual health and sexual practices. As research and epidemiological data materialised on AIDS and HIV within other countries at a global level, we learned that the affects on both individuals and communities were apparent in a multiplicity of different ways. In particular, we have seen in a number of African countries an almost equal number of men and women infected with HIV; this led to claims that *heterosexual intercourse* is the most common route for transmission of HIV. How we come to understand and talk about divergent practices of heterosexual intercourse across cultures is nevertheless ambiguous. Global patterns of HIV transmission challenged the western view of HIV as a 'homosexual disease' and thus forced us to re-examine patterns of sexual behaviour. As a consequence, this required that we come to recognise the complexities of sexual identity and diverse sexual practices. From the late 1980s, health education policies in the UK underwent a number of important changes to promote more effective HIV education campaigns. Yet matters of sexual health and sexual practices remain a problematic in many cultures globally.

One particular shift in focus led us towards the identification of risk behaviours as opposed to concentrating on 'risk groups' for strategies of HIV prevention in relation to sexual transmission. On matters of HIV and sexual health, we have concentrated our gaze towards sexual acts, such as anal and vaginal penetrative intercourse as 'high risk' behaviours rather than having to contend with the ambiguities of who might or might not identify with certain 'high risk' groups. This is a particularly significant shift in focus which has the potential to be more advantageous in terms of successful outcomes.

Whilst we are nowhere near open and honest enough about speaking publicly on matters relating to sex and sexual behaviours, we have moved forward in terms of promoting more constructive prevention campaigns for safer sex. Within the context of HIV, the notion of an individual's responsibility for their own sexual health during sexual encounters has attempted to remove the burden of responsibility away from individuals who are aware of their HIV-positive status. It is not a realistic expectation that an HIV-positive person should automatically disclose their status to others in every sexual context. Unquestionably, taking personal responsibility for your own sexual health is recognised as not always attainable in some sexual contexts across cultures.

At a medical level, HIV-positive women and men have helped shape the way in which we as patients interact with more self-confidence, self-awareness and assertion during medical consultations with the medical community; this has evidently spread across other communities living with chronic illness conditions. The emergence of patient-led self-help groups has challenged dominant medical practices within and outside of an HIV context and the 'empowered patient' has influenced how doctors interact and negotiate with patients living with chronic illness over time. HIV patients became the 'experts' in their disease and took on an active role in managing their health and negotiating decisions in terms of HIV combination therapies.

We have observed momentous changes in how HIV medicines have now been tailored to fit in around an individual's social lifestyle rather than the 'patient' having to adapt their everyday lives to accommodate complex and highly toxic combination regimes. Confronting issues of adherence and compliance has forced changes in the way the medical profession typically expect HIV-positive patients to strictly adhere to complex drug regimes; widespread failures to comply and adhere to HAART has now led to significant modifications and variations in terms of how medicines are manufactured and prescribed. We are now coming to recognise the extent to which doctor-patient relationships are being transformed; the balance of power is shifting towards the patient in terms of mutual participation in medical consultations within a chronic illness context. Dependent upon the individual, as patients we are now able to adopt shared roles and responsibilities and negotiate medical matters if this is the desired outcome.

These powerful and constructive transformations do not necessarily point towards the eradication of personal and social challenges and uncertainties in relation to living long-term with an HIV-positive diagnosis. The expectation of a more optimistic future is not solely dependent on effective medicine in the management of HIV. Hope and optimism is largely dependent on each human being and their personal and social circumstances, in conjunction with health, illness and psychological well-being. Having to take highly toxic and complex combination therapies long-term can impact on other aspects of our health and affect quality of life issues if adverse side effects continue to be persistent. Medical treatments are extremely costly and as budgets are depleted year-on-year we are already experiencing rapid changes and transformations in health care provision.

Links previously made between AIDS activists and the medical community have undoubtedly promoted an encouraging relationship in the attempt to combat HIV health-related matters. Yet despite the determined efforts of gay and other activist groups, we must not view HIV as something from the past or yesterday's disease. HIV is not simply a matter of the biological, as stated in previous chapters; effective HIV medicine does not eradicate the public and social issues that still prevail within cultures. At a social level, if we become complacent with HIV matters and fail to acknowledge the diverse social consequences of living long-term with this disease, we will undoubtedly have to confront new challenges and uncertainties in the not-too-distant future. Martin Luther King Junior once said, *'our lives begin to end the day we become silent about the things that matter'*. How much of your free time or financial support would you give to an HIV charity as opposed to say a cancer charity or the British Heart Foundation? Statistics suggest that public support for HIV is diminishing rapidly - Does HIV still matter in 2013? I believe so!

A forgotten generation: Long-term survivors' experiences of HIV and AIDS

The social and psychological effects of living long-term with HIV and AIDS have, to some extent, been silenced and overshadowed since the time when effective HIV medicines became accessible in the UK. Funding is a scarce resource and has a tendency to only find its way into medical and clinical research. Where are the voices that speak of personal experiences of living with HIV since 1996? If the social and psychological aspects of living with HIV are ignored and become obscured, perhaps effective prevention campaigns will not be heard or taken seriously. How are we to appreciate the impact of effective medical treatments on the lives of HIV-positive people if we no longer enquire? Just because people are no longer reported as dying from AIDS, are we to believe HIV is no longer seen as a medical or social problem? The medical community have almost discarded the term AIDS as out of date; yet HIV is the retrovirus which attacks and damages the immune system, our body's defence against invading diseases. HIV is still out there even if we accept AIDS as an outdated term.

Reported cases of sexually transmitted diseases are on the rise in the UK and elsewhere. The consequences associated with rising cases of sexually transmitted diseases are extensive and transcend beyond matters associated with HIV. Yet it begs the question as to whether or not sexual health and safer sex educational campaigns are actually reaching our sexually active populations in an effective way. How will HIV-negative human beings stay HIV-negative? I am left wondering if HIV has become a problem of the past now it is medically defined as just another chronic illness condition. I still consider long-term survivors of HIV and AIDS as the experts who can further enhance our understanding of crucial matters that still exist; as a collective voice it is one that requires our particular attention. Social research need to refocus its gaze towards the community of long-term survivors to improve and extend our limited knowledge.

There can be no conclusion to this story-of-stories of a forgotten generation. Living long-term with an HIV or AIDS diagnosis is an everyday experience and is an on-going enterprise. In previous chapters we explored and gained valuable insight into the everyday lived experiences of our story-tellers from the onset of diagnosis to the time of our conversations. We are approaching the end of this exploratory journey into understanding and appreciating how HIV impacts on the lives of human beings long-term. This chapter presents a valuable space for our story-tellers to reflect on the positive and the negative elements of living with HIV over a great number of years. The layout of this chapter is straightforward: we start with Minnie who was diagnosed the earliest in 1981 and conclude with Sandra diagnosed later in 1994. Using the voices and personal experiences of all our story-tellers we now discover how living long-term HIV has positively and negatively impacted on their personal lives.

MINNIE

Minnie was diagnosed with HTLV III in 1981 and when we met face-to-face to discuss living with HIV he told me that it was 'hard work being unwell'. At a time when information was extremely limited, Minnie learned about HIV along the way and carried on with his usual life until 1996 when he became ill. He believed he was 'lucky' in terms of the timing of his illness and how this coincided with the promise of new treatments within a few months. Minnie took AZT for a number of months until a time when he could access HAART. He was reliant upon a wheelchair for mobility purposes because of problems associated with vasculitis and peripheral neuropathy. When I asked Minnie about the positive and negative elements of living long-term with HIV, he recounted:

"Well, the positive elements are I suppose having the last laugh because according to the professionals I shouldn't be here…it's had a positive effect on my life and certainly on friendships; it has strengthened friendships and made me see life in a completely different way…I can appreciate things that are under our noses which can be easily overlooked…but then I think that comes from facing one's own mortality. I suspect any one diagnosed with a terminal condition must at some stage feel like this. As I said to you before, I found this rather empowering and it's a nice feeling; it's a warm, comfortable feeling I find…The negative aspects I suppose, as I've said so many times to people, is when I am ill. You know isn't it fucking hard work being ill? And it is…I don't see it as a constant fight every day of my life but I am reminded of what's wrong with me when I have to take my drugs…so the real negative things I would say comes from the long-term side effects that I have endured… it has taken its toll down the line. It is so wearing and it is hard bloody work… but the positive thing that comes out of a negative is that I know that I have got a complete and utter right and ability to say when I've had enough… that's down to me and no-one else. And I will do it when it's necessary. When I don't think I can fight any more or take any more tablets or do any of whatever I was doing and I've had enough, I will say 'I've had enough!' and that will be it. My long-term survival is something to be proud of… I feel very proud and that's something you get from others who are the same, you know the pride that people feel as long-term survivors…you know to me, the Red Ribbon lost its meaning a year or so after it was invented. Everybody jumped on the band wagon with ribbons and who knows what they are for? No, I think living long-term is about being

A forgotten generation: Long-term survivors' experiences of HIV and AIDS

proud and yes, sure I have got through what I've got through and still come out of the other side all right... More to the point, for those that died, they never had the chance to live... whereas I got a chance but for them it was for the sake of a few months but there were no drugs available... I think long-term it is about the people that come from behind of you, which was something my Grandmother used to say... Always think about the people that come behind you... whatever you do in life, clean up, wash up, make sure you leave things the way you want people to find them, or the way you would like to find them. My idea is if I don't take part in this whole big exercise which is what it is... an experimental exercise because they're still dabbling with the medicines. Nobody knows what they do yet. We only know by juggling. You know, it's a big juggling act of which has been going on for the last twenty years and I'm still here... The juggling act might come to an end soon but at least I would know that through my longevity I'd have done my bit for the people that come behind me. That's what it's about, I think."

As a long-term survivor Minnie believed he had made many personal achievements, particularly in assisting those people who are likely to be following; the newly diagnosed population living with HIV. He was, unsurprisingly, proud of living long-term with HIV and had faced many adversities in the face of HIV medicine and side effects. His notion of helping others who might follow, especially whilst enduring periods of illness as a result of side effects of HIV medicine, is rather remarkable, commendable and not uncommon. Minnie's hospitality was overwhelming and his fish pie was truly the best I have ever tasted. It is now his time to rest in peace.

JO

Jo was diagnosed with HTLV III in 1982 and when we met face-to-face to explore HIV issues, he told me how he believed life is for living. In the mid 1970s, Jo had lived in New York for a number of months and had friends in Los Angeles; he reflected on how these were 'steamy times'. Following his positive diagnosis, he became socially isolated and extremely depressed and during the Christmas period attempted suicide. Jo could not bear the thought of someone clearing up after him, so decided that if he was to live he must piece his life together. Whilst he continued to work until he medically retired on the grounds of ill health, he also became active in the gay community and the fight against AIDS. I asked Jo about the positive and negative elements of living long-term with HIV, he told me:

A forgotten generation: Long-term survivors' experiences of HIV and AIDS

"Oh, God! I don't know what the sort of positive things are. Sometimes I think there's nothing positive [*laughing*] about it because all that one sees is a lot of change and it's not necessarily a change for the better…I have had a really amazing experience but then that was I suppose because I was fortunate in that I sort of got myself out and met someone and we started a relationship and that relationship is still on-going and my whole life in a way changed. So I can almost have the 'before HIV' and the 'after HIV'… my life after HIV is incredibly rich and has been but a lot of that is due to meeting my partner and then all the interactions that have come from that. The fact of my re-training which enabled me to do things that I might never have done… In those terms it's been hugely rich but I have no sense of where it's going. I still don't see that I'm going to get to dotage… in a way that doesn't matter. I don't value my existence that highly but I hope that in some way it means something, even if it's only as a cautionary tale, that it can have an impact… that's why I wanted to do the poster campaign. It was as a cautionary tale if that just made people stop and think momentarily then that was something."

Like Minnie, there is a motivating force to help others which is not uncommon amongst our story-tellers; this substantiates my claim that long-term survivors as a collective voice must continue to be heard. Jo continued to reflect:

"I mean sometimes I think about it and I think that not enough has been made of it nowadays and used…and there is survivor guilt I mean just the fact that I'm still around and others aren't; and you know there were a lot of people that once did amazing things and I don't feel like I've done amazing things with my life…the poster campaign it was a moment… and maybe that's much more to do with my own self-worth which is a whole other issue. I used to feel that it was good to be a long-term survivor if only to just disprove aspects…but where does it go? I'm not sure that I have got much to say… I couldn't say to someone this is how you need to live your life to survive, right? It's difficult because I have housing and I mean if you don't have housing that's a real problem… I've got a decent rent. I'm really fortunate in terms of having benefits so that one has got DLA and housing benefit and Income Support… OK it's a fixed income but is it secure? I can eat and I can pay the rent and the electricity bill and gas bill but you can't go and say to people 'well you've gotta get all that sorted out and then you'll be all right… it's a difficult area…I think perhaps the only thing that I do think is important about being positive is that for me the one saving grace is to be able to be positive in one's aspect to living. What is important, as difficult as it may be, is that once you get that diagnosis is to just live absolutely every day to its fullest, whatever you do. That is the bottom line."

Jo was concerned with the uncertainty of HIV yet believes he is lucky and fortunate to have what he has in terms of his relationship with his partner and close friends and a reasonably comfortable lifestyle. He has no desire for people to become complacent about HIV matters. I too hope that complacency does not overshadow the importance of HIV. I will never forget the beauty and tranquillity of Jo's garden.

SPIKE

Spike is the youngest story-teller and was diagnosed with HTLV III between 1981 and 1983 when he was a small child. We met face-to-face to discuss HIV issues in conjunction with Haemophilia and Hepatitis C Virus (HCV). Whilst HIV is a big part of his life, it does not prevent him doing things he wants to do any more or less than his other conditions. Spike believes HCV is likely to be more of a problem than HIV. I asked him about the positive and negative elements of living long-term with HIV, he told me:

"I am still alive and I'm the person I am, to a large extent, because of what's happened and it's made me the person I am. I think I wouldn't be the same if it hadn't have been for HIV… because a lot of people my age tend to get lost in trivial, frivolous things which don't really mean much…I have really never known anything else. So speaking to other people who are probably in their late 30s or 40s, they are sort of more acutely aware of what they had before HIV and what happened to them when they first got diagnosed; they probably have more issues of stigma because they were older and experienced social exclusion and stuff…I was still a kid when I was diagnosed…I was probably allowed to do more things because I was going to die. I wasn't wrapped in cotton wool at all by any stretch of the imagination, which I think is good…the positive is that I wouldn't be the person I am without HIV. I have learned a lot; I have experienced a lot and I wouldn't have it any other way because I am ME and I am happy with that. So there are always more positives to pull out of it… I was speaking to someone the other day and he was saying how he's happy with his way of life. I said I wouldn't have had my experiences and I wouldn't have my knowledge and I wouldn't be the same person without being HIV-positive… so I should be happy about life more than thinking it's all negative. It's never really been a negative experience for me having HIV because I have never been really badly ill… I mean it's a pain in the arse sometimes and I'm still alive… Good old Nietzsche quoted something like 'what doesn't kill you makes you stronger' so I think that's important."

A forgotten generation: Long-term survivors' experiences of HIV and AIDS

In spite of Spike's positive mental attitude towards living long-term with HIV I did press him on any negative elements he might have. He reflected:

"Well, the fact that I probably will die from HIV or Hep C eventually which is probably negative…and the fact that all this crap happens with blood products in the early 80s and nothing changes at all…it's even worse. It's all down to money… they are still pumping us full of blood products and even though they are heat-treated they don't know whether they are safe or not. But I don't know if that is negative; it is negative what they are doing but is it negative that I think it is wrong that they are still doing this now? It is a positive thing that I think like this, but it's negative that they are still doing this. It is negative that they don't learn from their experiences and that they are overlooking this, even though our community is quite small… the Haemophilia community living with HIV. It's negative that we get overlooked and forgotten about to some extent."

Spike is referring to the medical community not learning from previous experiences with HIV and contaminated blood products. As already mentioned by our story-tellers living with Haemophilia, they are now vulnerable to contracting new variant CJD via contaminated blood products and have already contracted Hepatitis C Virus (HCV) through the same process. Spike continued to reflect on what it meant to be a long-term survivor:

"Erm, it's quite important. I do think sometimes like when I get up in the morning and I take the dog for a walk and I think it's good to be alive. I'm still alive basically and survivorship is a good thing. I think it teaches you a lot and you can learn a lot of things from it. I was reading Lawrence Armstrong's book, he is a cyclist by the way, and he had cancer and he fought back and beat his cancer… then he went on to win the Tour de France which is a big cycling event and he talks about survivorship and hope. You only know about survivorship when you can be part of that so-called group and reading his book was quite interesting. Even though it was a stupid Yankee book his thoughts on survivorship were interesting… I think it's important for me to be a survivor with the rest of the Haemophiliacs more than the rest of the HIV community… I can relate to those things…I mean watching people die around you is quite something… it never really upset me because there's only been a couple of people like me and they're still alive but seeing kids in hospital… because when I was a kid growing up, the consultants' method of treating us was to put us in hospital and stick us in a bed basically… I have seen kids all the time and they've been in hospital and they obviously had AIDS-related complications and I didn't realise… and then I would get up there in the next couple of weeks and they would be dead... it's not frightening it just makes you think and that's obviously made me think over the years...I think sometimes I should have gone to more funerals than I did because I knew one or two of the young kids... perhaps to pay my respects to the fact that survivorship means I am still alive and they are not."

Spike enjoys extremely good health in spite of his CD4 count being low. He struggled to search for any negative elements of living with HIV and survivorship is an extremely important aspect of his life. Spike is still unsurprisingly sceptical of the medical profession in terms how he contracted HIV and HCV; he believes there is a reluctance to learn from previous lessons as viruses are still being passed via blood products, which is clearly unacceptable and improper medical practice. Thank you, Spike for taking me out for a delicious meal after our conversation.

GLYNN

Glynn was diagnosed with HTLV III in 1983 as part of a mass screening process for people living with Haemophilia. When we met face-to-face to talk about living with HIV, he told me how his Haemophilia had been severe in the past; this resulted in Glynn having an artificial knee in one leg whilst his other had been pinned straight due to serious bleeds. He walks with a visible gait and stated that his visible disability had, in the past, led to questions by others concerning the status of his health. Glynn has also contracted HCV from contaminated blood products. He was initially diagnosed with 65 other people who also tested positive and he is only one of three still surviving. I asked Glynn about the positive and negative elements of living long-term with HIV, he recounted:

"I don't know because I don't know where I would be if I didn't have it...and we have now gained this bloody Hep C haven't we? The positives of living with HIV is staying alive... the negatives I suppose is getting ill, feeling down and feeling depressed sometimes... not being able to do what you want to be able to do...whether you are capable or not of doing it or having it always there in the back of your mind...maybe you know just thinking one day I am going to die before I should do or for me, maybe never having your own family together and maybe having more children. I don't know, I suppose they are the negatives. Positives? [*long pause*] Can't think of any...Oh, well! We're not allowed to go to America are we? Which is a bloody laugh in itself, isn't it? I mean that's the pot calling the kettle black, isn't it? Sod it I don't want to go there anyway... They'll probably turn around and say we're not allowed to go to Africa next or something [*laughing*]."

Glynn is relatively healthy in terms of his HIV-positive status and had never taken combination therapy. His overwhelming desire to have more children was apparent but he felt it was too risky with HIV. Glynn only saw being alive as a positive element of living long-term with HIV and believed that he 'just went on with life really'. I wish Glynn the best of luck in everything he accomplishes.

TYLER

Tyler was diagnosed with HTLV III in 1984 and when we met face-to-face to discuss living with HIV he was experiencing ill health and having difficulty breathing due to emphysema. HIV was inevitably a big part of his everyday life and he lived each day at a time. Tyler spoke about knowing the time when he felt that life was no longer bearable; choosing the time of his own death was extremely important to him once pain had taken over and his quality of life was intolerable. Tyler was angry that he did not have the freedom or the necessary information available relating to successful ways of taking one's own life. His feelings were strong on these matters and he had made two failed attempts at taking his own life in the past. In the face of this great sadness, Tyler was a very spiritual and hopeful human being. I asked him about the positive and negative elements of living long-term with HIV, he told me:

"The positive side I would think are things like if you've tried to keep alive, you have to have certain objectives and certain challenges which overcome the illness; so you develop a strength that you might not otherwise have developed. I think my best example of that is the piano. Taking that up and going all the way and getting Grade 8 with a distinction…when I didn't think I had it in me… I didn't think I had the brainpower left and I proved I have despite the deterioration in my memory… you can still develop abilities and I think HIV has done that for me. The negative side is, as we've already discussed, losing your friends; instead of having a life where you can plan wonderful things, it's very much a case of getting up in the morning and surviving the day… I think it's very sad for anyone who has it but although it sounds an odd thing to say, it does give you challenges if you want to get up and face the challenges…I think many people can benefit from it…If HIV-positive people sat down and took stock, they would find they have accepted challenges that perhaps they might not have done had they not have been positive…life does not owe you something, if you work hard at it you can pull through with a positive attitude."

Whilst Tyler took each day at a time and had suffered great loss, he nevertheless was able to laugh about matters and certainly made me laugh during our conversation. He was not frightened of death and negotiated every day as a personal challenge. He played the piano beautifully and I am honoured to have been able to sit and listen to his amazing accomplishment. It was a great pleasure to have met this amazingly compassionate human being.

PAUL

Paul was diagnosed with HTLV III in 1985 as part of a mass screening process for people living with Haemophilia. Paul and I had met on previous occasions, yet due to the limits of time, we spoke about living with HIV over the telephone. He was a member of a support group for people living with Haemophilia and HIV and became the only surviving member of this group. HIV is a big part of his life and he would have liked to have had children and continued to work, but he believes HIV prevented this. When I asked him about the positive and negative elements of living long-term with HIV, he told me:

"Without a doubt, it has made me appreciate so many things I think other people just don't appreciate… like when I am feeling really good today. I feel really well when I go out and do some things. I think most people, I don't know… I don't moan about the things most people moan about in life because I put things into perspective. It has given me a pecking order to a problem; HIV is right at the top, so you know, worrying about little things in life is something I don't do…HIV has become detrimental in some respects because it has made me not very sympathetic to some of my friends' problems…If my friends had problems with their relationships or problems with the way they are living or problems with their jobs, sometimes I have not been very sympathetic because I have just probably said in my mind: 'there are other real things in life to worry about' and I may have said, 'don't worry about it!'… I suppose it is negative, sometimes. These are real problems in people's lives you know relationships, employment issues and stuff. I do feel sometimes I have not been as supportive to my friends because I have got a different agenda. But looking back on the positive side of things, yeah, I have had to push myself to do things, because I know that I might not be here next year… so I am going to do this. You know, I have done a lot of travelling. I have toured a lot of the world that I would never have dreamed of doing. I certainly would not have had the time to do it because I would probably still be in my job... Those sorts of things I have enjoyed and I appreciate things. I probably see these are the main positive elements."

Paul had a tendency to focus primarily on the positive elements of living with HIV, but did reflect on the negatives issues, he recounted:

"The biggest complication for me now, having lived with this for 17 years is this... It is better medication now and I have to now change my outlook on life; the fact that I now don't think I am going to die of AIDS. At one time I only gave myself six months to a year... every time someone died I would give myself six months to a year... that was how I lived my life, you know. I didn't have to think about what was going to happen after that, because I didn't think I had to. Every holiday I went on was my last holiday. Every time I went to a good gig, every time I did something was to be the last time I did this. I don't feel like that any more. I don't think like that because I think a lot further ahead. But what really, really annoys me is that so much of my adult life I have been preparing to die...I have given up the fact that I could have a really interesting career...I could have had a really interesting job that I really enjoyed. All those things that normal people do... I don't feel that I fit into my normal friends' society when, you know, all my non HIV-positive friends all have different outlooks on life. They all look towards the future, they talk about their pensions, their retirement, kids and what they are going to do when their kids leave home, you know, make a ten year plan. I find that I still can't fit into that because it's not part of me... it is very depressing that I have been preparing to die all my adult life, that I was going to die and I am still alive. I don't feel cheated, that is what I want. I still want to be alive but I just wish it were different. It is quite poignant my outlook on life. When I was younger because I thought I was going to die of AIDS, I just didn't think I could die of anything else. So I drank a lot, took a lot of recreational drugs and really did things like that because I thought: what was the point? I was going to die soon... and now I am a lot more sensitive about my life because I am still alive. I don't do reckless stuff now. I have stopped drinking because of my Hep C, although it has nothing to do with the HIV but it has a big impact on my HIV at the same time...I don't think that everything I do is the last time I am going to do it anymore. I don't do that. I used to do. "

Paul continued to reflect upon how in the early days he buried his head in the sand and compares this to current times since he has become actively involved in HIV, Haemophilia and HCV issues, he recounted:

"By becoming informed as well that helps a lot; it has become a conscious choice of mine to accept information and get involved with outside organisations; I physically go to conferences. It leads to a greater sense of empowerment, I feel like I have control, but I also feel because I know other people who don't have drug options, who are resistant to drugs, I know I am lucky...If someone said that I was resistant to drugs I think I would quickly revert back to panic mode. I know that when I had a difficult time and became ill, I thought I would be able to handle things and cope but I couldn't. I just... that huge black cloud of depression you just can't shake off. I know that part of me if the drugs stopped working, I don't think I would cope. I really don't. It's something I am able to think about, it is not something that I feel I don't want to think about. But if they stopped working I don't think I would have control over my life as much as I do when I am healthy. I eat healthily and sensibly...I had a lot more of a reckless attitude in the early days when I thought 'I am going to die'. I will do whatever I want to do. No-one is going to tell me that I can't do this or I can't do that... I was like that. Now it is because I have got older [*laughing*]...When you are young you follow a reckless lifestyle... But as far as HIV is concerned, I am more conscientious about my health. I am more sensible and because I have more of an education I know what to expect. I know when things go wrong, I know what they are and I know what goes with what drugs and so on...Knowledge empowers me; it scares me sometimes because obviously the more things you find out about, the more things can go wrong, well you know, ignorance is bliss! I am not saying that everybody should go out and educate themselves but if you don't have the support mechanisms and you don't have people to back you up with things, it can be very, very scary to find out about all the HIV illnesses and the things that can go wrong. You really have to have your head in the right place... Just being able to know you can get the information is important...if people want to bury their heads in the sand then ignorance is bliss! It is an individual thing, I did bury my head in the sand for a while and then I became ill. I mean this is what I am talking about. It is life of contradictions."

Paul believes HAART is a positive advancement as it saved his life. In spite of the great losses he has endured, he maintains a positive outlook on life and has become empowered with knowledge around HIV and HCV treatment issues. The most negative element of living long-term with HIV is based around him believing all his adult life that he would die prematurely. I hope Paul has still got his dazzling smile and I will remain eternally grateful for all his help and support.

A forgotten generation: Long-term survivors' experiences of HIV and AIDS

ELISABETH

Elisabeth was diagnosed with HTLV III in 1985 and was an injecting drug user for many years. She had previously viewed her addiction to heroin as far more of a problem than being HIV-positive. Elisabeth and I met on many occasions and because we had to cancel a number of scheduled meetings due to illness, we spoke about living with HIV over the telephone. A few years after diagnosis, she became actively involved in the field of HIV and held a deep mistrust of the pharmaceutical industry. When I asked her about the positive and negative elements of living long-term with HIV, she recounted:

"I think one of the good things about being diagnosed for a long time is that I have become so used to it that it's not an issue any more… that is definitely a very positive thing…it really isn't an issue. At the moment it's my liver that's an issue so while it is still my health, it is not HIV because it's pushed way into the background. Yet this was happening anyway, because when I was four years diagnosed and it was a part of me, apart from the odd thing that happened, you know, when somebody that I knew and loved had died, I was generally coping very well with it… It's a good thing that it's not in your mind every day as it used to be… you can allow yourself to just enjoy life on a day-to-day basis… but I think also that it works the other way as well… because when you are first diagnosed, although you are very, very frightened, it does give you a different perspective on life if you think you don't have long… it makes you look at things differently. A few negative things… I didn't take friendships and sexual relationships further than I may have done or I certainly haven't progressed in my career as quickly because of like, what is the point? I am very well aware of what is really important now because I'm sure on my death bed I'm not going to say, 'Jesus, I wish I spent more time in the office'… even now it's actually really important for me to build up my business again and I've got all these plans in twelve months… I want my own office because I don't really like working from home… I need to be out there with people and I need to know that I'm part of that community and I like to dress up and sometimes I need a reason. I like being part of that going to work and coming home routine… I don't get that here, so these are my plans. And there's a good old saying in Alcoholics Anonymous: 'if you want to make God laugh, just tell him your plans.' That keeps my feet on the ground and I think it is important to have plans and I know what I want to achieve… so I do know what is important."

Elisabeth went on to speak about her involvement in HIV organisations and self-help support groups as a positive feature of living with HIV. She told me:

"I think make the best of what is there. I am positive and so I joined an HIV organisation and it just so happens that it is international and they send me all over... I mean I've been to Russia, America, Geneva, South Africa, Barcelona and that's all in like three years... I'm sure in three years I would never have travelled to those places so... but maybe I'd rather not be HIV-positive."

To be a long-term survivor for Elisabeth meant a great deal, she reflected:

"It means being a winner and I don't really know where that came from...I know that when I had been diagnosed 10 years my doctor actually turned around and said, 'you are what we call a long-term survivor' and that was when I decided to tell the kids actually... I was ready to tell them as that was one thing that motivated me because I felt that I was able to say I was a long-term survivor, it is also called a non-progressor... so I felt that although I had bad news for them I had good news too and I really felt quite happy telling them that... of course it hasn't been true now with the HIV and this is the same with labels... when you don't fulfil them you feel a bit of a failure... which is why I am thinking 'what is it that I'm doing?' I have to take HIV medications and why has my liver suddenly decided to collapse? I wasn't so much of a drinker and I know other people who were absolute piss heads and their liver is fine... it just doesn't seem fair, and then I get to thinking that there is no fair and unfair: it's just pot luck...when I was in hospital with my collapsed liver the first time, I really did think I was gonna die... I knew it wasn't going to be that day or even that week or month, but I did think I was gonna die and I'd get really pissed off because I wasn't ready... but then you get to the point and you think OK, I think you must do as that's what I've found watching other people getting really sick and knowing they are gonna die, and you get to the point where you think, 'well you know you don't die angry'... I think most people I have seen have accepted death at the time...I want to get my old age pension and I would like to do a few more things...I think if I am honest I would rather have lived the last twenty years without being positive and without the knowledge of being positive just because I would have felt more a part of mainstream life... all I do know is that generally speaking I wish I'd never been diagnosed... I wish it had never fucking happened to me...I can see how addiction has given me the life that I have and I'm quite happy now. I regret a lot of things but the HIV I could have done without that, thank you very much. I'd much rather have done without the HIV."

A forgotten generation: Long-term survivors' experiences of HIV and AIDS

At the time of our conversation, Elisabeth had been experiencing acute illness with a serious liver condition and she had been hospitalised on three occasions: she required a liver transplant. She still maintains a positive approach to life and is an extremely determined long-term survivor. Hopes and aspirations for her business were paramount for Elisabeth and her strength and determination was extraordinary. I did enjoy the times we spent together and I got to see Stereo MCs live in concert. We recently spoke by telephone and she is doing just fine.

COLIN

Colin was diagnosed with HTLV III in 1985 and has, at times, barely escaped death as a direct consequence of AIDS-related illness. When we met face-to-face to discuss living with HIV, Colin was a paid worker in the HIV field and had acquired a vast amount of knowledge around treatment issues and new developments. He did suggest that he did not want to work in HIV forever and ever. I asked Colin about the positive and negative elements of living long-term with HIV and he told me:

"Over a long period of time, the negative elements are pretty much what everyone would imagine they were, I think. It makes you a little bit afraid to take bold steps in your life, which you might take otherwise and there are certain things I constantly cannot do… What happens if the NHS can't look after me, which is a real issue in our relationship because my partner doesn't understand it all and love doesn't always compensate… it makes you a bit afraid of taking certain steps you might otherwise take. I'm afraid of the side effects starting to affect me more than they do, for instance. My cholesterol's slowing creeping up and that is definitely due to the drugs. Will I start getting horrible things happening to my face because so many of my friends now have, which really marks them out. I have got this [*patting his stomach*] and this is not all middle-aged spread, some of this is from AIDS drugs and there is the fear of other people's prejudices, put it that way… so all those things affect you and make you feel a little bit erm… I feel sometimes put in a bit of a box by HIV…The positive side, I would say, is all the stuff I have been through… absolutely seeing life and death at close quarters, in a way that most people miss in this society of ours… they get shielded from it until they get really old. I think that is a really valuable experience and it makes you very strong psychologically… I am not really, on a sort of really basic fundamental level, I am not really scared of anything anymore for myself…I have almost braved the worst that luck can throw at me and I think, well if that's the worst… but obviously awful things could happen but I'd probably deal with those too… there is a certain kind of strength, yes… this stubbornness. My partner calls it my Taurian stubbornness, in fact it's what they all call it at work, as well…they call me Sergeant Major because I sort of stomp around the office issuing orders sometimes. I get a bit bad tempered. It is partially my ego because I wanted to be a pop star in my twenties and I still want to hang on to shreds of sort of dreaming of being famous now and again."

Colin has, in one sense, followed part of his dream as he has been a prominent figure in the HIV field. Because of his work commitment, HIV is a larger part of his life than he would like it to be. Colin worked hard to maintain a positive mental attitude to living long-term with an AIDS diagnosis and sees HAART as a positive advancement. Colin still remains hard working in his work commitments.

NEIL

Neil was diagnosed with HTLV III in 1985 and was working full time at this juncture. When we spoke face-to-face about matters of living with HIV, he told me that he felt like he needed a new challenge in his life. Neil described living with HIV as a 'battle' and believed that his long-term relationship of 20 years and family life was incredibly important to him. Neil came across as a quiet and thoughtful human being who had serious concerns about his changing body image because of lipodystrophy (the proper medical term is lipoatrophy) and rapid weight loss; this was as a result of the side effects of his HIV combination therapy. When I asked Neil about the positive and negative elements of living long-term with HIV, he reflected on the positive elements to start:

"I feel there must be something incredibly strong somewhere in me to still be here… somewhere in my own physical body to have kept the illness at bay and my immune system was so healthy for ten or eleven years…even now to have come through cancer relatively straight forwardly, I feel that there must be something very strong there. It does make me feel a bit indestructible [*laughing*] which is odd, compared to what I said before… I do feel a physically different person which is strange and a bit unnerving for me and I'm still getting used to that…I think since I have been ill I have been more business-like. I mean I am quite a kind and easy-going person. I can sit and chat and chat but I think I was going to say that I would certainly say that I am more assertive. I am more likely to say 'No, I don't want to do that!' rather than just going along with things…I had to make a very, very big change because of giving up work and I can remember when that first crossed my mind... I can actually remember back in 1996 when the doctor first suggested that I cut down the number of hours I worked; I researched all the financial side of it and in the process of doing that I remember actually going up to see my Head of Department who I didn't like, I didn't know how he would react to it, when I said to him what I was going to do...I think since having pushed that through, it's made me feel certainly more assertive and, at the same time, when we bought the house, there was a lot of pushing too to get that done...I think I was pushing because I thought, at that time, I did believe I had sort of finite time left...if I was going to die, I was going to die in the way or the circumstances that I wanted... they were big changes which involved a change in the way of life and a change in almost everything we did together. They were huge changes to go through and we did go through them fairly quickly, in a couple of years, in two or three years."

Neil continued to reflect on positive and negative elements since his medical retirement, he recounted:

"In a sense of being retired, it meant I have had time to do some special things; one is the relationship with my parents and my relationship in particular with my nephew. My partner's brother and sister both died of lung cancer over the last four or five years and I was able to spend a lot of time with them and do an awful lot of things with them and that has been important to us...The down sides have been, I remember being on the treatments for a couple of years and just the sheer grind of having diarrhoea every day and vomiting every day; just how wearing that is and how it can make you feel... you are so sort of ill and unclean a bit, because you know it is coming out of both ends...there were certain points and factors – shitting yourself is one of those things which is the last straw, especially in public, it is one of the last straws...Another negative element, I mean the cancer itself wasn't actually so bad because it was a specific illness with a specific treatment... it's when you get like that almost day-in, day-out kind of feeling; certainly the prospect of it being like that with no let-up. I have a strong sense of if I had felt like I feel now, all the way through then perhaps I wouldn't have given up work. I'm fairly sure I wouldn't have done that...I sense that there is another change coming up, but I'm much less sure about what I want to change to, because it was very clear that I wanted to get the house, sort out work and a pension...but there's something else. With my health I think the situation is that I am in control over my health rather than relying on the doctors to be in control of it... so there's just another bit of my life I want to take back control of but I don't know what it is...When I chat to some people on the Net, some people I talk to, particularly the ones who are still well and in work and some of them have been infected for a long, long time, they seem very anxious that their lives aren't defined by being HIV; I was in that situation for ten or eleven years and that changed... Now I feel that my life has been defined by HIV and I'm not comfortable with that... I am not sure if I can really articulate why, but I think a change is looming... HIV is much larger than I would like it to be."

Neil was, in part, relating to recent visible bodily changes in relation to weight loss and lipoatrophy in his facial features when he was talking about change. He was going to the gym in an attempt to change his body image, yet was concerned about his own reflection in the mirror. His desire to take control over aspects of his life was of extreme importance to him. I hope Neil remains in good spirits and still enjoys his close and loving relationships with those around him.

MARTIN

Martin was diagnosed with HTLV III in 1985 following a mass screening process for people living with Haemophilia. When we met face-to-face to discuss living with HIV, Martin told me of his interest in areas of studies concerning Delta 32, which is a genetic defect in his quest to learn why he is alive whilst others, particularly his younger brother, have died. He is very healthy and fit and has not taken HIV medication. Martin has also contracted HCV via contaminated blood products and was taking the drug Interferon for Hepatitis C-related complications. When I asked him about the positive and negative elements of living long-term with HIV, he told me:

"I will start with the negative and then hopefully we can end on a high note...the negative side is it is always there. It is always a worry and you live your life day by day which is great fun but long-term planning makes it very difficult. Now there is a pension up there somewhere, but I don't think I am going to reach that. So it has financial implications as well, because you are spending all the time. You know, well come on, let's live for today! That is a financial implication because I can't get life insurance, and you think you can't get that high paid job; maybe you could but do you really want to try and go out there and be rejected?... those aspects are the down side. And also, with the regular testing, it is like getting a lottery ticket. You know, what are the results going to be this week? If your CD4 count is down, the doctors always tell you... your count can always vary going up or going down, up and down...when you get a low one that really knocks you for one, you start thinking and every time you wake up with a runny nose or a cold, you think: 'this is it!' Those are the negative sides of living with HIV.

The positive side, I like to think it makes you a stronger person... you look at life in a different way. Taking each day as it comes, you think I am alive today. I am still alive and you go out and look at the trees and the flowers [*laughing*] It sounds so corny but it is great...when you have someone who stays with you with all these problems then you realise how lucky you are to have somebody who feels so strongly about you... then this isn't an issue. And it is great to be alive and I may never get ill, you may die of other causes or natural illness. But you do know that life is a precious thing. I consider myself to be lucky for what I have got and if I were to describe myself, then being HIV-positive would come pretty low down on the scale, it is not my first descriptor."

Martin's wife was present during our conversation and wanted to add the following:

"I don't think you do yourself justice... I think he is incredibly brave and I think a lot of people we know who are HIV-positive say, 'why me?' and he says, 'why not me? Why would I be so special that I shouldn't have this?' He is a very calm and accepting man... I think things like him not going for jobs... he can just say this in a sentence now. But beforehand it was like a huge issue for about 8 months and he actually wanted to go and try and earn more money in a different job. I think I was very selfish; I was like, 'No, you have got a good job, reasonably well paid."

Martin interjected 'Good death and service benefit' and his wife continued:

"Yes, the salary is not bad. I know it is horrible, isn't it? But I told you though [*all of us were laughing*] Well, I just thought I was terrible because he had made so many sacrifices and I know that I asked him to make another one... and yeah he made it and he works so incredibly hard and he has got a lot of coping mechanisms that he won't give himself credit for. I don't even think he realises because he won't get involved in petty things and squabbles and silly politics. I might worry what somebody said if they haven't liked something or if I had offended them or something. He says it is not our problem, it is not your problem it is their problem. He won't take on board anybody's crap but he has a great empathy and is very sensitive...I find him hugely inspirational whether it be personal or at work...he doesn't get angry about the deal that life has thrown him or the doors that have been closed, or that he might feel different and I think that comes with living with HIV for a long time."

Whilst Martin was blushing and laughing during this conversation, he added:

"I would like to say that I feel very lucky compared to other Haemophiliacs who are HIV-positive that I know... In terms of my physical fitness and also that I am well and not on treatment. I don't know of anybody else who is not on treatment, so I feel extremely lucky about that. I think that this gives me a different view of things and a different way of looking at life than they have...so perhaps my story is different to theirs, but still valid...I suppose because they are all on treatment, which makes it far worse for them than it does for me, perhaps, although I have never actually done this, perhaps it would be nice, at some stage, to try and find somebody else who is a Haemophiliac and not on treatment."

Martin's son was unaware of his HIV status because neither he nor his wife wanted to spoil his childhood. Martin did say that he would like, for example, to go on a reality TV show like Big Brother to see how far he got through the process. He would let the nation observe him and then he would like to come out and say, 'By the way, I am HIV-positive, I have Hepatitis C and I am a Haemophiliac'. Ideally he wanted to give the nation a chance to see somebody as an individual first before the attachment of labels were applied. An ambitious thought yet I doubt the media could stay quiet that long. I wish Martin and his lovely family all the very best in life.

TOM

Tom was diagnosed with HIV in 1986 and was working full-time at this juncture. When we met face-to-face to discuss living with HIV, he told me how he was slowing down possibly due to the ageing process rather than HIV. Tom frequently travels to San Francisco and shares HIV knowledge with his contacts in the United States. He tells me that uncertainty has been a dominant feature of living long-term with HIV; this impacts on planning for the future, yet Tom deals with the present by adopting a positive mental attitude. When I asked him about the positive and negative elements of living with HIV, he recounted:

"Well, the positive bit is certainly that it has allowed me to view my life much more objectively than I did before... it is looking at the 'now' and the value of things that I have, rather than coveting mythological things that I may never have had anyway... So it has allowed me to see through the bullshit. It has allowed me to have better relationships with other people because of the way I have lived with it, because of the openness that I have about HIV...I personally think I have experienced more from relationships rather than the former stuffiness when you only relate to people at a certain level…HIV has provided me with a much richer vein to tap into, in terms of relationships with people… it has forced me to confront a lot of my own prejudices about 'race' and about lesbians…I didn't have any prejudices about lesbians until I experienced this group up North and they scared the shit out of me, so you know you stay away. But after diagnosis, I finished up living here and most of the women I met happened to be lesbians and relationships changed and I wouldn't have had that if I hadn't been diagnosed… forced circumstances can change relationships for the better…I have two brilliant relationships with my two ex-partners which are better than they were when we were lovers, much better!... I wouldn't have left my first partner if I hadn't have been diagnosed, I would still be there…and I would never have met my second partner if I hadn't have left the first one. I still don't know the reason why the second relationship ended but it empowered me when I decided, 'No, I can't just give up' I have to go on and fight to get out of the relationship in order to establish a good friendship and it's become more than that really… so my views, my hang-ups and my previous prejudices, about a million and one things have been smashed and broken up because being HIV-positive has put me in situations I wouldn't have been in otherwise… I would have been a really narrow-minded prick really. I was never really positive about my sexuality and I would have finished up in a ghetto."

Tom reflected a great deal as to why his relationship with his second partner ended and he believed this was because of his status and the fact that he survived, he recounted:

"If I had died in the early 1990s I think the relationship would have been great, but I survived and I think… well it's partly from things he said and I overheard a telephone conversation [*laughing*] where I heard him saying to someone, 'it was never a relationship that was meant to last anyway'. At that point, I knew the direction of how he was thinking really…I don't regret any of it at all. There's nothing I wish to change. In a very uncomfortable way, it's been like being forced into a very powerful, intense learning curve, if you can call 15 or 16 years intense… I think there is much more to me now than there would have been if I hadn't been diagnosed. Internally, I am a much richer person and more useful to people."

Tom went on to talk about being a long-term survivor and reflected on the term 'survivor' before moving on to his fears around medication and pain. He told me:

"I was reading an article about long-term survivors and some people in this cohort didn't go for the word 'survivor' because they felt it was too close to the word 'victim'... this is an endless debate we'd had over the years but it's eased off in the last couple of years. At the end of the debate 'survival' and 'survivor' is I think usually a term more people are in favour of seeing; it is an empowering word rather than the opposite, the pejorative or negative word is 'victim'...In some ways it is a shock to find myself here in a way, now... it is pleasant but the key word for me around HIV is uncertainty, it is a word I use over and over again...living with uncertainty...it's strange I am not sure that I would want to live to be 70 but I would like the option...all it really needs is something to go wrong with my drug regime and like many thousands of other people I am right up shit creek without a paddle, even more so because of it being in my brain...So that's hard for me and I think that is one of the reasons why I got into this 'I will withdraw my medication' stage because I didn't have the confidence in the combination therapy... my friend in San Francisco was talking about Protease Inhibitors and how initially people who were like the 'walking dead' were all out of their beds, doing more things, they went back to work and da-di-dah. Two or three years later these people were in desperate states and awaiting new drugs to come out on trials because there was nothing else available for them...they'd tried everything. I had all this at the back of my mind and it's still there...I've got to put that to one side but I still have to admit that this is something that is still there...it makes it all so difficult to plan ahead in terms of going back to studying in higher education...education has taught me how ignorant I really am...My fear is being old and poor... yes, being old and poor and not being able to afford to have the heating on and stuff like that really... I have fears about pain too...I fear different forms of pain and wonder is it going to be more devastating than the one I have just experienced...I am always aware that there is potentially worse things to come and I don't welcome that...So... HIV allows you to create an opportunity to re-prioritise your values in life and move away from the materialist end. It has taught me to be more humanistic and less judgemental...treat people like they hope to be treated, and that's it."

Tom has concerns about dementia and as a consequence HIV has become a large feature in his everyday life. HIV is an integral part of his identity, his sense of who-he-is is formulated around being HIV-positive in an influential way. Tom has already previously experienced a brain seizure during the 1990s and has recurrent fears around future uncertainty, pain and poverty. In spite of this, he approaches life in a constructive way as he negotiates the challenges of uncertainty. Tom remains close to my heart and keeps in touch; he also ensures that I have good reading material for the winter months. Thanks, Tom!

A forgotten generation: Long-term survivors' experiences of HIV and AIDS

CLAIR

Clair was diagnosed in 1987 and remains cynical of the medical community, HAART and the pharmaceutical industry. When we met face-to-face to discuss living with HIV, she told me how, since the death of her husband, loneliness rather than HIV was a problematic in her life. Clair had not seen any HIV consultants in relation to her HIV-positive status for about 6 or 7 years and claimed that HIV science does not know enough; whilst she does not profess to be an AIDS dissident she does raise rather important questions and challenges many claims made about HIV. When I asked Clair about the positive and negative elements of living long-term with HIV, she recounted:

"I think you are forced to look at life and death as you see it... I mean you realise and acknowledge this and a good thing that did come out of this is, years ago I thought, you know, logically if I am going to die I might as well enjoy myself and if I think I have only got a year or something was going to happen to me in a year, then I might as well make the most of what it is I am going to do. And then I realised that once I had got that attitude, how do you know I'm not going to have this kind of attitude for fifty years? Life is a great gift if you have got even longer with that attitude, so what are you going to do about it anyway? And I was smoking at the time and I just thought well it's not a very good idea; if there is something that might make me ill then leading a healthy lifestyle might make it a little bit better so I stopped smoking. I had been smoking on and off for a few years and I had periods when I was a heavy smoker, but I was always sort of an odd smoker, then I stopped smoking. I just stopped... I got into doing things like Yoga...I had a terrible problem with my skin which started to get worse, and that shook me, that was a big mark for me when my skin got worse. Why is my skin bad? Even just dealing with that and the transformation in the last few months with my skin... and seeing the results of what happens when you let go and stop wallowing, you see the sort of positive thing and you realise what is important and how we are... I realised I was too influenced by what other people thought... how people patronise you, but again it is about me being too concerned about what other people think, it's their problem... my skin is so much better."

Clair moved on to reflect on the negative aspects of living long-term with an HIV-positive diagnosis, she recalled:

"The negative side has been basically the erosion of people's rights to choose...I've come into contact with people I really don't like; I have been shocked particularly by the medical profession and I think that goes across doctors and any person working in the health field. It's just their attitudes! To me the way people want to force their belief system, which is what it is, onto others is the negative side. To watch somebody who stood up to that die... you know she stood up and tried to fight the system and what it did to them, it crushed them, so that's why I stood back and am careful. You have to be, if you have got a view on things, then I manipulate it to my end, and this is what I say about why I don't actually see my consultant... because I just thought 'well if I get ill for whatever reason the last thing that I want is someone kicking and screaming in your ear' ... you know, saying well I don't think you really believe that the drugs are good. You don't want that! You need to have a good relationship that's all I need. I mean I'd like to have had a child...something happened last night at Yoga which is strange at the end of the day. During the last few minutes, the door opened and I heard someone creeping in and I thought 'somebody's coming into the class,' and I was a bit tense and I looked and I felt this presence at the side of me. I looked across and I saw this little baby and I could smell this baby and then we finished Yoga and what happened was this woman used to go to the class and she'd had a baby, it was five weeks old. She brought it in to see us and I just thought 'oh, it's a baby!' and it was just so bizarre. It was just the smell and she just sat there and all the women gathered around this baby and I felt really upset because the decisions you make about yourself are your own and are very different...the medics push for antenatal testing so that you can take drugs and stop breast feeding and have a caesarean and that's not an easy decision to make. I am getting older now. Anyway, I know that the Camden case set a precedent and now you have to have your baby tested... so I have looked at all the things and what if I did get pregnant, actually they could treat me, but I wouldn't go. I wouldn't actually let people know, so it's almost going back to the negative side. I also realise that you can actually overcome things by just being wise to it and don't let the anger which has gone on in the past, take over, particularly with the medical system. The negative side was having let me GP know. I wouldn't advise anybody to take the test. Ask yourself why you would want to have the test. And if you do take the test, take it anonymously because once you are in the system that is the negative side. When I was applying for a job and I went to the GP and I asked her not to mention my HIV and she said that she had to. But I said they want to know if I am capable of doing the job, there is no evidence. I am not sick so why on earth mention it? Don't be part of the system! I mean test anonymously if you really want to, and there are good reasons why people want to take the test, but you must ensure that you do have choices."

Clair made reference to the 'Camden case' which set a legal UK precedent and received widespread coverage in the national press from 1999 onwards. AN HIV-positive mother and her HIV-negative husband living in the London borough of Camden had a baby and refused to have the child tested. Both parents believed that antiretroviral drugs to treat HIV were toxic and damaging to the immune system and resisted all modern medical opinion. Both believed in alternative medicine and the father was a practitioner of holistic medicine including massage and reflexology. The child's mother had lived healthily with HIV for many years and was licensed to administer shiatsu massage; she also believed she had taken control over her own immune system with alternative therapies. In 1999 there was a high court ruling that the child had to be tested. Both parents, feeling persecuted and isolated defied the court ruling and fled to Australia with their 5 month old child; they believed in the right not to have the child tested.

In February 2000 it was reported that the 'HIV baby case' was to go to the European Court of Human Rights in Strasbourg. The case ruling went against the absent parents and it is believed they might still have been in hiding in Australia if the mother of the child had not died in a Melbourne hospital in October 2001. Days after the mother's death, the child was taken into protective custody and after medical examinations, an Australian doctor proclaimed that the child needed HIV medical treatment; it was perceived that the girl would only have a 50 per cent chance of survival for one year without HIV medical treatment. Again, the father broke a court order demanding the child was to be treated and absconded once more with his daughter to Sydney. It is alleged that he went to Sidney in an attempt to obtain his passport to return to the UK; the father believed that UK doctors would not enforce HIV medicine on his daughter. In May 2002, after being on the run for 3 years, the child was again made a ward of court and was escorted to a London hospital by British court officials to assess her medical condition. The child's father was at her bedside after agreeing for her to be medically examined.

Unsurprisingly, Clair's belief in 'the system' being too restricting and controlling is understandable. As she states, HIV erodes human rights and further reduces individual choices; she was therefore extremely reluctant to become part of the system in relation to her own HIV-positive status. Clair continues to remain healthy and is now taking medication and is happily involved in an intimate relationship.

PETER

Peter was diagnosed with HTLV III in 1985 and had been involved in a clinical trial called the Forty Trial when new combination treatments were being tested. When we met face-to-face to talk about living with HIV, he told me of his overwhelming desire to help others as much as he possibly can. Peter was experiencing sexual dysfunction and believed the medical profession was reluctant to help him overcome this problem. He no longer engaged in sexual activities and this situation did not pose a problem. When I asked him about the positive and negative elements of living long-term with HIV, he recounted:

"When you are faced with something that is potentially life-threatening as HIV certainly is, then decision processes speed up quite a lot and you come to make quite important decisions much more rapidly than you would if you thought you had another thirty or forty years to deal with these things…it brings about life changes and you make decisions about what you really want to do and where you want to live and it enriches your quality of life…I can't agree with those people who have said that HIV is the best thing that's ever happened to them… especially at a time when there was little in way of treatments. I can identify in part with coming to make decisions that enrich the quality of your life which gives it a different dimension and a feeling of purpose that wasn't there previously…I have passed all the markers that I thought I would not reach with age and other things, like I used to think wouldn't it be great to see the new Millennium in… that was a couple of years ago so I have done that one, what's next? There is not a great deal that one can do in respect to death because nobody knows when; and also as horrendous as death with HIV can be and all its implications of dying before one's time and all those feelings, tomorrow isn't a promise to anybody…it is about quality of life that really matters…I suppose my worst fears and darkest moments would be that I would become increasingly unwell and at some point would be hospitalised and that care would be given so that I could die comfortably…being in a hospital bed and being cared for and treated by people in the caring profession in an AIDS ward beats getting knifed to death or murdered simply as a result of appearing to be a gay man and attacked by some of these homophobic bastards that we have to share this planet with…It's a shame the world is like this."

Peter went on to discuss his experiences of loss as a negative element of living with HIV before moving on to more positive aspects, he reflected:

A forgotten generation: Long-term survivors' experiences of HIV and AIDS

"People that have died...people not just known to me of which there have been many over the years, partly as friends that I have come to know being involved in HIV organisations and people I have known from the gay scene... I mean the tragic loss of all those lives (*Peter is crying now*)... I mean who would have thought that AIDS could happen at the end of the twentieth century? But then I suppose there are probably many things like AIDS that have happened in different countries around the world that people who are fortunate enough to live in the West haven't got a clue about. It is absolutely tragic...The positive side of it is the love that has shone through in so many people in so many unexpected ways. When people held and nursed and looked after other people who were not always close to them personally... people who were dying of AIDS... before it was even known about the routes of transmission and the possible risks in the early days...it wasn't known whether perhaps you could get it from being in the same room, breathing in the same air and people were brave enough to care more for fellow human beings and potentially risk their own life... there's no greater love than that, and it did happen...and one of the best examples really of that love was Princess Diana... I feel that I have been fortunate to make friends with people that I perhaps would never have come across in my happy-go-lucky previous boozy, cruisey younger life and in a peculiar way, as devastating as HIV has been there has been a peculiar quality of enrichment and value given to lives in spite of it being amongst us."

Peter has acquired a vast amount of knowledge about HIV matters and has worked in the HIV voluntary sector for many years helping others as much as possible. His positive attitude towards living long-term with HIV has encouraged him to see life as a challenge as opposed to a threat in his own personal crusade in the fight against AIDS. Peter is a very warm and caring human being.

CHRISTOPHER

Christopher was diagnosed with HIV in 1988 and was very healthy and fit and worked full time. When we met face-to-face to discuss living with HIV, he told me how he is dying to live, rather than living to die. Christopher firmly believes he is lucky in terms of not experiencing any adverse side effects of HAART or problems associated with being HIV-positive. He has previously had two strokes and he uses this and his on-going arthritic condition as a smoke screen for hospital appointments for HIV health checks. When I asked him about the positive and negative elements of living long-term with HIV, he recalled:

"From the start and more so in latter years, I have become more selfish or self-centred, these are probably the wrong words. I don't take the shite anymore. I don't give a shit! I have become more assertive, definitely. And I have got rid of people who have used and abused me, so I have ended quite a few relationships with people. I may have done that anyway, but I think well to become more assertive makes you wise and I am not taken as a fool anymore by some people…My outlook has changed since my diagnosis and I think, well I don't know how long I have got on this earth and though none of us do, I have got this thing hanging over me; I have got this diagnosis, this virus living within me and I don't need to take this shit from anyone anymore. You know, if you don't like the way I am, if you can't handle it, you know… this is how I want to be and if you don't like it then you are not my friends and therefore I don't need you in my life…one person has tried to make contact with me again through my mother and I have just been very cold. No, I have made my decision and I have not missed them so why I would want to go there, with them giving me grief and adding to my stress… it's called getting rid of the wastage…The only thing is that I won't tolerate and suffer fools anymore…and I did do that before and I was probably not comfortable doing that if I am honest…I think my status has something to do with it because I don't want to waste what energies I have on people that don't really matter to me."

Being assertive and not 'tolerating shit' from other people was something Christopher was very proud of; he saw this as a positive element of living with HIV. He continued to reflect:

"I think the negative is you wonder when your luck is going to run out and I think the positive of this is the longer you go on being reasonably healthy generally, why won't I live to be an old-aged pensioner? So there is always hope and you can see that in others too…I believe I am living and living life very much to the full…this is quite unusual for me to speak about my positive status and to really think about these matters. I think we all have our 'highs' and 'lows' and there are times when I do feel sorry for myself…I think the only thing that I am a bit concerned about is when I cut myself, if I ever cut myself or injure myself where blood is concerned, I have a little panic usually only if there is someone around…do you know what I mean? I think I am mainly fine about it all."

Christopher has an amazingly upbeat and cheerful personality and enjoyed many active leisure time outside of the HIV arena. He is optimistic about his health and is a very open and sincere human being; he wishes, however, that he could be more open and honest about his HIV-positive status. It is perhaps the prevailing social prejudices in conjunction with the desire not to burden others with the knowledge of his status that prevents him being as open as he would like to be. Always keep your dazzling smile and quirky sense of humour, Christopher.

JOHN

John was diagnosed with HIV in 1989 and is still healthy and working full time. When we met face-to-face to talk about living with HIV, he told me of how he had paid for private medical treatment for a diagnosed hernia which turned out to be a malignant tumour in his groin; if he had not decided to go private he would have been dead. John is not totally absorbed in learning about HIV issues and has a positive outlook on life with HIV. When I asked him about the positive and negative elements of living long-term with HIV, he recalled:

"I suppose the negative thing is the unpredictability and the fact that it is all very new and therefore it is all still evolving. As I said earlier, I was told I was going to die within 5 years and then 10 years later I am still working and perfectly fine. So, when was it? About 4 years ago I actually took out a private pension scheme…I suppose certain things in life became less important like material possessions and social status… you become more aware of the other people and their problems and perhaps become a little more caring about other people. I have certainly done some voluntary work… if I weren't positive I probably wouldn't have done that much volunteering…HIV is not desirable, it makes life uncertain… well I know life is uncertain anyway but you don't really think about that sort of thing… I never thought I might be run over by a bus tomorrow so therefore I am not going to take out a pension or get a mortgage or whatever…so it changes things in that way. I suppose as time has gone on and I don't think people die as quickly and as dramatically, it has become less of an issue. I think it would be good if somehow the whole thing was less hidden…if people felt that they didn't have to hide it."

John has never experienced adverse side effects from previous combination therapies and was not taking HIV medication at the time of our interview. He lives well with HIV, is asymptomatic and yet does admit to being frightened by the prospects of future chronic illness associated with HIV. I hope life remains as good as it was when we met and I apologise for spilling my wine.

A forgotten generation: Long-term survivors' experiences of HIV and AIDS

MARC

Marc was diagnosed with HIV in 1990, has never taken medical treatment and was working part-time. When we met face-to-face to discuss living with HIV, he told me how he was currently pursuing sexual relationships with women as he believed 'men are dogs'. Marc believes he is lucky in terms of being healthy and asymptomatic and will only consider medication when he becomes ill. At first he lived 'as if he was going to die' but after a couple of years decided to opt for a healthier lifestyle. I asked him about the positive and negative elements of living long-term with HIV, he told me:

"Well I suppose the advantages in my case have been that it has given me a way into a career that I really enjoy doing now. I am also behaving like an adult at last, which is nice…so it has been good professionally and thanks to HIV I have got a pad which is also nice… the rent is cheaper than the private sector. What else? I suppose the only negative side is I feel that it has impeded my voyage of discovery into heterosexual land which is becoming quite interesting for me… because of my HIV I have been a bit hesitant because I would want to tell someone I was HIV-positive before I had sex with them…I do think women do more in their head compared to men… I would like to have a relationship with a woman… and I realise I don't really understand how women think; I don't really know how to explain it… I don't know, anyway…I think HIV only changes something if you are sick and everything else is just in your head…HIV is as big a problem as you let it be…it is a choice really as to how much you let it affect you, and whether you let it affect you a lot or a little depends if you act like a victim or a survivor…it is a choice and it depends on how you react or respond to it…I think that I treat it differently today than I used to do… I eat properly, I sleep properly and try to do exercise, but it is important to try and keep that all in perspective and that is what I calmly try to do."

Marc has not experienced prejudice or discrimination on the basis of his HIV-positive status and puts this down to his ability to manage situations and read people. He is currently finding his ability to read people a little ineffective in relation to his pursuit of sexual relationships with women. His approach might be more successful if he focused his attention away from trying to 'understand how women think'. Good luck, Marc!

PABLO

Pablo was diagnosed in 1990, is medically retired and enjoys extremely good health. When we met face-to-face to talk about living with HIV, he told me he was lucky in terms of his health and did not dwell on his medical condition; yet he believes HIV does impact on his life despite his positive mental attitude. Pablo has acquired enough information on HIV matters to 'get him by' and is able to access information from HIV organisations and other published sources if necessary. When I asked him about the positive and negative elements of living long-term with HIV, he recounted:

"To be honest I actually do more now than I did before. I suppose it's about enjoying life more and appreciating stuff…I have begun to appreciate life more because I think…what's the word I am looking for? I think I value life more and while you're here appreciate what you've got…one day the inevitable is going to happen… it's like going abroad, I mean before I was diagnosed I never dreamt of going abroad but now I go here, there and everywhere, I am always going on holiday. It's strange you know because I think why haven't I done this before now? It's really weird. I suppose for me it's changed my life a lot because I'm helping other people more. I mean at one time I used to be a really selfish pig. I used to just think about myself and not about anybody else. It was all me at one time and now I've changed that around. I am helping people all the time and you know doing all the voluntary work. I wouldn't want to sit back 24 hours a day in here it would drive me bloody mad. I think this is why I am going out and doing what I am doing, the voluntary work… getting out and getting on with my life. I mean as far as I am concerned very little has changed in my life, very little. Sometimes I wish that everybody could be like me and be as positive but everybody reacts in different ways."

Like other story-tellers, Pablo believes being HIV-positive has prompted changes in how he relates to other people and how he appreciates life. He continues to reflect on the positive and negative elements and told me:

"It's a difficult question…I suppose a positive side of it is, like I said, it does change your life. Sometimes for the better and sometimes it knocks you back. For me it has changed my life for the better. It's made me grow up actually to be honest and it's made me think about other people more. I also do not fear things too much now; I always used to fear things all the time. It's quite strange because before I was diagnosed I used to worry about death all the time. It really sounds strange but since I have been diagnosed I don't worry about it at all…I was petrified before. Even things like going into hospital for an operation and you know going under the anaesthetic you know, I was thinking that I am not going to come out of this…having really severe panic attacks about it but now I think, 'sod it' if I don't come out of it, I don't come out of it and my time has come, sort of thing…I have made a Will and I have spoken to my sister about things, I am quite close to her… What's negative? I suppose there is a negative side to taking medications…as I was saying earlier about hiding medications and I mean some of that is a bit paranoid… obviously if people see my tablets in the cupboards they are not necessarily going to know whether they are for HIV or not, unless they are medically minded, so that is negative…erm, my lack of sexual drive does get a bit annoying sometimes, it can be negative but it's not really a big issue because I've got my life still at the end of the day…my long-term survival means I am a fighter and regardless of what someone has got, they can beat it. They can! Obviously one day, if it's terminal it will take over but you just keep fighting until that time comes…I think if you are positive in mind and in body then you shouldn't have a problem. Take a grip of it and don't let it beat you."

Like Marc stated earlier, Pablo feels that living long-term with HIV has made him grow up and not be as self-centred and self-absorbed. Interestingly both story-tellers are asymptomatic and are enjoying long periods of extremely good health; yet Pablo is taking combination therapy as a preventative measure whereas Marc is not. Pablo reveals that he is not a planner because he likes spontaneity and maintains a positive mental attitude which he believes is attributable to his good health and well-being. Keep on being spontaneous, Pablo!

LISETTE

Lisette was diagnosed in 1990 and described her health as reasonable; she was medically retired. She had a problem with her back which presented a few difficulties at times with mobility. When we spoke face-to-face about living with HIV, Lisette told me how she had given up injecting drugs in 1979 and had never taken HIV medicine. She believed biomedical treatment could not answer all her questions and she was therefore unwilling to take risks whilst she remained asymptomatic. Lisette told me that uncertainty was a paramount feature of living with HIV; for her there was no certainty, no wonder drug and not a lot of plausible answers to her questions. When I asked her about the positive and negative elements of living long-term with HIV, she recalled:

"I don't like all this having to be a secret. The idea that someone would be ashamed of me, like I've done something wrong, I hate all that. I hate the fact that, you know, I remember talking to a friend of mine who is also positive on a train going to London… this is a few years ago now, and I think it would still be the same today; the train was packed with people and we were standing up in a carriage with people all around us…we'd been having this conversation at the train station about HIV drugs and that, and I just remember us getting on the train, resuming our conversation for about 2 seconds and then both of us looking at each other and kind of going, 'Oh, no! Better not carry this on'…I do wonder about people who don't have HIV, or don't know whether they have it, or those who work in HIV. Surely they must go home at night and talk on the train, don't you think? I remember being horrified a few weeks ago when they took my blood because my arm was black and blue and I wouldn't go out until it was no longer bruised because I was thinking people will be talking about it or asking me, 'what have you done there?'… and also another negative is the not knowing what's going to happen. I think that perhaps a lot of illnesses have this in common. Nobody can really tell you what's gonna happen and I think the unknown is always the most scariest. It would be great if they could map it all out and say, you know, in five years this and ten years that… but it doesn't work like this."

Secrecy and having to hide one's HIV-positive diagnosis from those around us, is a reoccurring problematic theme amid our story-tellers. Lisette, like others, would much prefer to be open about her positive status yet she perceived the burden of social pressures and prejudice prevented this from taking place. Lisette continued to reflect on more positive elements, she recounted:

"I think initially it's just a freak out and I think that the longer it goes on there is an opportunity to confront mortality, which is definitely something everybody should do but not many people get the chance until it's too late. I do think that it's easy to drift through life and do nothing and achieve nothing and that's fine if that's the way you want your life to be…I think the sad thing is that once you reach 70, 80 or even 90 and you still didn't do much, you know… I'm a great believer now in 'don't really put it off'… in reality it's so easy to say but quite hard to live out…the way we all live really is we say leave it until tomorrow…for a while after you are diagnosed it is a really big thing to do important stuff because of the time factor. If you think you have only got six months to live then you probably have to cram everything you can into it or at least all those things you promised for yourself. I remember doing a couple of things but I never went mad. I know people who went absolutely crazy."

Lisette moved on to reflect on her family and their needs before she spoke about equality of opportunity and the negativities of accessing social support as a woman, she told me:

"The thing is my family, there is always something else for me to do…I always had a kid either in crisis or something… You know one kid had no money and was starving and my Grandchildren weren't getting fed and the other was having a baby…so I had to fly out there to be with them. So, for me if you like, there was always so much going on and there wasn't time to dwell on things or have great fancy ideas for yourself. Every time I would go to do something for me, some family member would come up with some better thing that they needed the money for [laughing]…from day one you see it's not just about you…I think again that may be a really big thing that is different for a woman with HIV, I don't know but I've always felt that right from the day I was diagnosed, it was never just gonna be about me…it's the same with offering HIV services for women and things being equal, nothing is equal…I used to say to them at the support group, what do you have to do as a man if you want to go out to the support group tonight? And I am talking to a guy and he would say 'put my jacket on, right? And what do you have to do as a woman?' A woman might say 'bath the kids, do the laundry, make the tea, do this and that' so unless you're prepared to make it as easy for the woman to go to the support group, nothing is equal…it's not just about putting stuff on; service providers used to think that because they offered services to everybody that was equality, but being equal is about having equal access and equality of opportunity…we used to always have this argument about why I couldn't be allowed to have therapies at home because they couldn't provide transport for me to get to their premises… but I couldn't have therapies at home, but surely if they're not prepared to get me to the organisation's premises, then they have to get the therapy out to me…the silly thing is that the therapists have to drive past my door practically to get to the support organisation."

For Lisette equal access and equality of opportunity is something she fought hard for as a woman living with HIV, and often she failed to win these battles. She told me what long-term survival meant for her:

"My long-term survival is just more of the same really…just keep going, more grandchildren [*laughing*]…I suppose one changing skill is, I mean it all depends on other people really but I used to have this thing about if I could just live to see my kids growing up…you know I had more or less done this by the time I was diagnosed and then it was, if I could just live to this or just live to that… but in reality I don't do that anymore. I remember being really angry when I had the first Grandchild, because in reality I could be that one person who didn't have to care about anybody else; and that went out of the window because there was a grandchild… it was like everybody expects you to be around now you know [*laughing*]… if you didn't have a purpose before well you've got one now…and five grandchildren later, your whole life is consumed by it really, because it is always somebody's birthday…or one going back to school, or one changing school or somebody's Sports Day…What is really important is this! I just wonder what on earth it is that we're gonna have to do to get people away from the idea that having HIV is something to be ashamed of…or it being stuck in the closet, because I don't know…I've wracked my brain and I've done training and I've done all sorts of stuff in the hope of helping…I did a talk to a bunch of college students and asked them about using condoms…Oh yes, we use condoms! They said but only when they got new girlfriends…I asked them about the decisions to stop using them and they told me that when they had visited the girlfriends' house and found out they lived in a nice house, they would stop using condoms…so I summed it up by saying 'so you would use condoms to protect yourselves from HIV! Lovely…but the minute you find out that the girl you are going out with has Laura Ashley curtains, you would stop using them?' This is scary…And I don't think we as a nation have got any better about talking about sex, it's not moved on at all."

Lisette had acquired a vast amount of knowledge about HIV matters and was conscious that earlier knowledge around AIDS and treatments was largely centred on men. She had never taken HIV medicine but did not rule out taking HAART in the future when it became necessary. Lisette was a woman who knew what she wanted and was firmly in charge of managing her HIV-positive diagnosis; she was assertive and not afraid of taking control of any situation. I still have the tobacco tin she bought for me and it is Lisette's time to rest, now. Bless her!

DAVID

David was diagnosed in 1990 and took early retirement from his full-time employment a few years later. He had a positive mental attitude, had never taken HIV medicine and used complementary therapy to maintain his immune system and his extremely healthy state. When we met face-to-face to talk about living with HIV, David told me of his attempt to get the medical profession to acknowledge the importance of using complementary and alternative therapies for the treatment of HIV. He believed that if the Primary Care Trusts (PCTs) can budget for biomedical treatment for people living with HIV, they should also budget for those individuals who prefer to follow alternative or holistic medicinal therapies. When I asked David about the positive and negative elements of living long-term with HIV, he recounted:

"Well if I say negative I really can't think of anything that is of importance perhaps because of my age. I don't really see there is anything negative…We are hoping to go to Australia later this year and I am now a

A forgotten generation: Long-term survivors' experiences of HIV and AIDS

little bit concerned about the health risks of travelling long distances on an aircraft but, you know, what greater risk is there crossing the road and being hit by a bus? It does make me think about things but it might be age. Do I really want to go and sit on a plane for that long? So, I think that is the negative side really…The positive side is the joy of life and meeting other people and helping other people and being there for other people. And, of course, setting an example because I can say to so many people that I have done it, surely you will be able to do it too…Quite often when someone is newly diagnosed, our local support group will ask if people can come and talk to me and my partner; and the people have come over and then we have not seen them again…So they either rejected our way of life or otherwise…But there are one or two people I know who have just been able to talk to us about us because they were scared and they want to see what life has been like…we would be available if younger people who were diagnosed wanted some kind of parental guidance… we would be there to do it… I don't meet older people, there is nobody older than me, my dear [*laughing*]…let's face it, a lot of my contemporaries have died of…well not died of HIV… you have road accidents and all sorts of other things that take your friends away… and of course I lost a lot who did have AIDS in the early days…I was dreadfully upset because we couldn't talk to people about it, you've got to respect that people didn't want to discuss it and didn't want to admit it…It is difficult to remember the emotions… because each death was a separate thing. I did get a little bit tired of going to funerals… at that time I went to seven in one month… but then I was very involved with HIV groups and I think, at one stage, this is going back to my guilt I was starting to forget people's names that had died. I made a list and I got to about 70 something…I've got rid of that list now but again it was… somehow I had this kind of feeling I shouldn't lose respect for those people who's lives had touched mine and mine had touched theirs…that seemed so sad…I went into hospital on St. Valentine's day one year and I took everybody I knew in there a red rose…I got round seven beds and I just couldn't cope with any more…it just drags you down… I was going there to cheer them up and honestly it was a bit of love leaving a red rose, but it was having a negative effect on me."

David's extraordinary approach to life made it difficult for him to reflect on his own personal experiences as negative elements. He told me:

"I am quite happy with my situation…you have got to put the whole thing into context. I have got my partner, I have got a home and I have got these lovely cats…a nice garden and I enjoy every day… sometimes it is circumstance and sometimes it is the individual and I want to be friends with people and I don't want cross words between friends; I would try to immediately put that right and not let it build up before it got out of hand and just let people go...it must be something in my character...the other couple that I told when I was first diagnosed, I had known them for forty years and we see each other regularly. I must have the ability to stay friendly with people and keep them, if you know what I mean? It is not something that suddenly became so because I had been diagnosed with something life-threatening...I really do treasure this, I want to be supportive to you because you are doing this for us; you are not doing this for yourself, this is obvious my dear."

David is a wonderful gentle man with a big heart who has an astonishingly remarkable approach to life and all the people around him. It was a massive pleasure to meet him in his home and share his personal environment for the day. Over time, David has helped many other people and has always made himself available to assist those who require support. He had never taken HAART for HIV and believed his healthy diet and alternative therapies maintained his good health. He did enjoy a healthy approach and it saddens me to have learned that in October 2013 he died of an unrelated HIV-illness. May you rest in peace, David and I know I will see you on the other side. Bless you!

RICHARD

Richard was diagnosed in 1990 and was working at the time but soon afterwards lost his job. He was relatively healthy but struggled to maintain a healthy diet and found it difficult to sometimes look after himself. When we met face-to-face to talk about living with HIV, Richard told me how he was initially frightened about the effectiveness of HAART because it presented different challenges in relation to uncertainty and was constantly 'changing the goal posts' in terms of its potential to successfully manage HIV. He reflected on the positive and negative aspects of living long-term with HIV, he told me:

"I have changed massively for the better I think [*laughing*] but I think we all aspire to changing for the better, changing who we are, what we are and moving on in life...It became clear with HAART that HIV could be manageable...that people could go back to work and people could start taking more responsibility for their own lives...I had become comfortable with my own life of not having to take responsibility of my own life...I could use other people to get things done that I wanted doing, I suppose to my own advantage...it became clear that eventually I would have to take responsibility all over again and that was quite frightening really...it was a

A forgotten generation: Long-term survivors' experiences of HIV and AIDS

daunting thought because I had been labelled… it put me in a blind panic…it was more about if this works then all the things I had accepted was about to change… I had become comfortable…knowing that I would never have to work again. Not having to put up with that stress and knowing my lack of education. I won't have to go to college, I can't go to college because I am on benefits and I am benefits because I am HIV-positive and am probably going to die…it frightened me really…I had lost my future, my career, my life. It had gone. It was the doctors who told me that my life had gone…now I am back at work."

Richard was frightened and angry to a certain extent about the AIDS rollercoaster ride from the onset of his diagnosis. HIV equals AIDS equals imminent death. He reflected on being a long-term survivor and recounted:

"To me it means that I am really glad that I am here but I am also clearly aware that the parameters and those goal posts are just going to keep on moving… because when I have lived for 15 years then to be a long-term survivor is going to move to 20 years and then you will have to live for 30 years. You are never going to be a long-term survivor. You see, I was a long-term survivor in 1995. I was an official long-term survivor in 1997 and then the goal posts were moved and it is now 12 years, this is my twelfth year. I am a long-term survivor but I bet my life it will go up. I am a survivor. Full stop. Having to basically live and learn as you go along means the situation is constantly changing, in relation to living, in relation to treatment and so on…I shouldn't worry so much whether I would or would not be here because I am here…I will be here until I am gone. That is the only thing I can be certain of."

Richard did, at times, struggle to survive alone especially in relation to taking his medication; he was not always fully compliant with his drug treatments and special dietary requirements associated with these complex regimes. He further believed that his poor diet and his difficulty in looking after himself was down to his personality and not a consequence of his HIV-positive status. Whilst Richard was open about his inability to sometimes cope with the management of his illness condition, he never gave up his fight to survive. I think of you every single day, Tricky Dicky!

PERRY

Perry was diagnosed in 1990 and had recently given up his full-time career prior to this discovery. Later he was diagnosed with mental health problems which led to him receiving psychiatric treatment as an in-patient within the mental health system. When we spoke about living with HIV we did this over the telephone due to the limits of time, as Perry was working part-time. He told me of his difficulty in separating out his experiences of living with HIV and his experiences of living with mental health problems. Perry reflected on the positive elements of living long-term with HIV, he told me:

"Well, I don't know really. It's part of life's experiences and every experience in life is something to build on. I think I have got a better perspective on other people nowadays than I used to have. I used to be very emotional and used to get excited and upset very easily…you know during the days in 1990 when people weren't very accepting of HIV, I think you learn quite a lot about other people from their reactions…I think I take more responsibility for myself now. It is difficult to explain but I think you become more responsible for what happens in your own life. You become more empowered in your own mind by saying to yourself, 'well, this is what I really want to do and this is what I am going to do, and I don't want to do that because I don't like it'… you don't get pushed around by people quite as much because you are more forthright because the anger has been there in your mind about the situation that you are in. So I think it gives me a sort of empowerment in myself that I never had before. I think that is something positive…It brings home your mortality and though you may have over-reacted at the time, like I did, it nevertheless brings back the memory of what it was like at the time and that stays with you for the rest of your life. I suppose it is a similar effect to being in a war, except much, much milder. I am sure that people in the Second World War that were sent to Burma thought they were going to get shot and killed at any moment…in a way it allows you to judge things in a better perspective if you do survive. Those soldiers in those days who lived through that and came back home and they lived a calm and peaceful life for the rest of their lives. I think the rest of their lives are probably more focussed perhaps… but I am not saying that having HIV is in any way as bad as living through front-line action… but it was certainly life-threatening at the time. I mean we are talking about the situation in England and if we were talking about Africa then that is terrible… each country will have different experiences and different challenges."

I asked Perry about the negative elements of living long-term with HIV, he told me:

"Negative aspects, well yes at the time of my diagnosis I was just shunted off and left in a corner sort of thing…it isn't as bad nowadays perhaps and I mean you have got to take pills morning and night…it is not too bad but it really depends on what regime you are on. As I said before, I was on quite an intrusive regime before but this one that I am taking at the moment is not too bad...it was all very upsetting at first, as I said before, it brings the idea of your own mortality into greater focus and you tend to sit down and mull over things...I just sat for a week in my living room drinking alcohol and generally getting more and more morose... That's what I did when I discovered my status...It made me dwell on things an awful lot... the worst thing for me is the effect it has had on my mental health as it was the catalyst that really brought it all out...Because I was only expecting to live for a few years when I first found out I think I am a long-term survivor...it makes me feel like I shouldn't have got so worked up about things...I hope I have matured a lot."

Perry is a very thoughtful, honest and considerate human being with an outstanding sense of humour; we had many bouts of laughter throughout our conversation. In spite of his traumatic experiences after the discovery of his HIV-positive status he maintains a very calm and positive approach to life. Perry is thankful and relieved that effective HIV treatment is now available and is happy with his current combination therapy. I wish him all the best in life.

RICK

Rick was diagnosed in 1990 after previously testing positive back in 1987 when he used a different name. He was awaiting salvage therapy due to resistance issues when we met face-to-face to discuss living with HIV; he was also experiencing high levels of stress as a result of constant changes in medical practitioners at his HIV clinic. Rick told me how he had stopped taking treatment six weeks previously to go to the United States for private treatment for facial injections to fill out his face as a result of lipoatrophy. This had been successful. When I asked him about the positive and negative elements of living long-term with HIV, he recalled:

"The negative things are that now they realise they shouldn't use the drugs like they did in the first place...as new drugs came out they tried them out on you, they blast you with one drug and then take you off them and put you back on them again and then you can't use them at all...the drugs don't work as effectively the second time around... the positive side is that there are new drugs coming out but we just can't get our hands on them...like the London Free can get hold of a lot of drugs but if you are in a small town you can't get them...other negative things are the side effects seem to get worse as the drugs change. I get nausea and my peripheral neuropathy is getting worse and some days I just feel dreadful...I feel better about myself because my face looks good after the treatment and people have noticed a change in my appearance…that really makes my day even if some days I feel so poorly…I have never regretted a thing I just occasionally get a bit miffed with things… I don't blame anybody for it but myself… the amount of appointments I have are difficult especially when I am feeling unwell…I am waiting for new drugs and playing the waiting game, waiting for the doctor to make a decision about new treatments and I am waiting for a gastroscopy down my oesophagus to see if I have developed any tumours because I am coughing up blood…research suggests that after 10 years you can be prone to getting tumours but I am trying not to worry about it…I found a very good article which suggests that people living with HIV for over 10 years often develop cancerous tumours…I am trying to look on the positive side."

Rick had acquired a vast amount of knowledge of HIV matters as it developed and took an active role in medical treatment. Unsurprising, because of his situation at the time of our interview he was preoccupied with hospital appointments and waiting for new drugs to become available. Rick had experienced many adverse side effects of previous treatments and had developed resistance to almost all combination therapies. In spite of all his health problems, he maintained a positive approach to life until the very end. Bless him!

WOODY

Woody was diagnosed in 1992 and was still in full time employment. He lived in New York for 5 years during the early 1980s before returning to the UK. When we met face-to-face to discuss living with HIV, he told me he had recently experienced rapid weight loss which was a cause for concern. People had started noticing this bodily change. Woody was finding it difficult to separate whether changes in his life was due to the ageing process or was HIV-related. He considers himself lucky not to have experienced HIV-related illness since diagnosis. When I asked him about the positive and negative elements of living long-term with HIV, he told me:

"Well whether or not this is positive or negative, I don't know but it's made me more impatient and slightly selfish in a way. I can't explain other than that…well I've not really voiced it but if somebody has been talking about their terrible problems they've been having I sort of think, 'well so what, I'm HIV-positive'…it's made me, erm…if I don't want to do something and I don't feel like meeting somebody or going to dinner with somebody then I don't do it, just so as to keep another person happy or risk upsetting another person, no I wouldn't do something just to make somebody else happy...I just don't worry about it. I mean I don't go out of my way to upset somebody and I wouldn't sort of do this, you know the interview, just because I didn't want to offend you...If I don't want to do something I just say 'No sorry I don't want to do it'...It is more honest and straightforward...I wouldn't do something I didn't want to do purely because I fear it might offend another person...do you understand that? It's also made me more impatient because I haven't time I suppose...I don't have time to spend my life worrying about what other people will feel or think...and yeah I've got to put what I want to do first because of the lack of time...I still think of myself, in a way, as having a terminal illness although I suppose I don't think like it's next year or the year after...it's made me impatient definitely especially with people who are concerned or worried or talk about what seems to me to be sort of petty problems. You know what might seem to me petty but to them something major... Oh, I don't know like getting a few spots of something...so I'm impatient and it has made me more honest and straightforward with people...not suffering fools gladly, I mean I never did but it's increased...So I think the major thing is if I didn't want to do something I am more inclined to say 'No, I don't want to'. It makes me generally more selfish and I think about my own needs a lot of the time...I am sure this is a positive thing... it makes you look at life in broader terms and ask what is it all about? You know deeper issues... It makes you think about the type of person you are and whether you are being punished. And then whether you decide you have or have not been punished for your lifestyle, it makes you think about life, the world, war, famine, disease and poverty. All the big social things which wasn't really one of my big concerns before...it makes you think about life I don't dwell on them but all the big stuff in general."

Woody found it difficult to separate the negative and positive elements of living long-term with HIV, but his assertive, honest and straightforward approach to life was something he considered as positive. He continued:

"It makes you think about immortality and the after-life... it makes you think about bigger things in life, you know the big picture as well as the everyday sort of picture...you draw conclusions from your thoughts. Are they negative things? I think they're all positive because it makes you think about being a better person and doing things for the right reasons and not doing things for the wrong reasons...For me the negative things are it makes you dishonest, either dishonest or less open with other people about yourself, I mean you don't disclose everything about yourself because I don't want to disclose that I have HIV...it makes you dishonest if you are not completely open about yourself...I sort of quite like to tell I mean I don't wear my heart on my sleeve but I decided with HIV not to tell...you can't throw yourself headlong into personal relationships and social situations as much as you would otherwise want to…so that's negative because I am always holding back because I am HIV-positive…I don't know whether to mix with HIV-positive people and if this would be supportive and positive or would it be negative and depressing?…I'm lost as to what I am trying to say…would you get support and understanding from other like-minded people who you could share issues with or would it be negative and would you dwell on the negative things like illness…I just don't know."

Woody, I believe, was contemplating whether or not it would be valuable to be involved with other long-term survivors living with HIV for the purpose of shared understanding and social support. He continues to reflect on the positive and negative elements before moving on to long-term survival issues:

"One negative thing is that it affects your whole sexuality as it affects everything that you want to do inasmuch as you've got to view everything in terms of being HIV-positive…it takes away a lot of freedom of choice, it restricts your freedom and this is brought on purely by having the virus…because it is something you can pass on to other people…it also means you can be exposed to other viruses or conditions which could result in the deterioration of your health…I suppose long-term survival is about…it is difficult because not only am I a long-term survivor but I happen not to have had any major illnesses and I know others who have been very ill…so they must have a different viewpoint to me…it goes back to this thing about different people are affected in different ways…I have moments of thinking that I am one of the lucky ones that isn't going to get ill…I am certainly one of the lucky ones who didn't die after five years because I didn't…although you might have to spend the rest of your life on medication and living with this thing of being somebody who is HIV-positive is it actually something that is seriously going to affect your life? Everybody should be having safe sex with condoms whether HIV-positive or not…in some respects can I say it might do me good if I had a good bout of pneumonia or a serious illness so I will take it seriously again because you run the risk of complacency…I am not taking it seriously because I have not had anything serious for the last ten years now…you always have it in the back of your mind but the longer it is, you know, I have not had any disastrous problems."

Ultimately for Woody, lying and secrecy about his HIV-positive status has been a negative element, as he feels partially dishonest in particular social contexts. He has not been as open as he would like to be about his status and has disclosed to only a few friends. Woody regards being more selfish, honest and straightforward as a consequence of living long-term with HIV and sees this as a positive element. His ability to deeply reflect on matters is not, I believe, a sign of complacency. Thank you for cooking me a lovely meal and I wish you all the very best in the future.

LARRY

Larry was diagnosed in 1992 and the route of his HIV transmission is unknown. He was medically retired and had recently started taking combination therapy due to illness. When we met face-to-face to talk about living with HIV, he told me that his treatment was like '*someone or something has breathed the life back into my body again*'. Larry has acquired of lot of information about HIV along the way and believes that he knows as much, if not more, than most health professionals. He describes himself as a 'softie' who had spent his whole life trying to help others. When I asked him about the positive and negative elements of living long-term with HIV, he told me:

"The negative elements I have got to mention them because although at the moment I don't feel they're high on my priority, they were recently very high on my list…the negative aspect of living long-term with HIV is the worry of becoming unable to cope anymore. These are personal to me, not being able to cope with things that I want and need to do every day like keeping the house going, doing the shopping, getting to the doctor, getting to the hospital and all the practical things…they're purely practical because when I wasn't well I couldn't do them all and there was no one to do any of it and I really suffered. Now that's the negative bit…the positive bit is actually, I don't know…It's being thankful that you're here today and really being aware that every day is a new gift, I've said this before haven't I? Every morning that you wake up, that's the good bit about it all. You don't take things for granted and you're responsible for yourself and other people are responsible for themselves…I certainly won't take on other people's responsibilities…I'm responsible for enough things already for myself."

Larry continued to reflect on what it meant to be a long-term survivor before going on to talk about other things he would like to do, he recounted:

"Strangely being a long-term survivor is something to be proud of, I must say that… it might be hurtful to friends and relatives of those who have gone, who have left, who have died quickly with HIV, and I know enough people whose sons and relatives died quickly because of HIV… erm, I do feel proud that I've lasted as long as I have and I feel even more proud that I seem to be, well I feel human again now because I wasn't feeling human

A forgotten generation: Long-term survivors' experiences of HIV and AIDS

before, as you know...so I am also lucky. There is an element of luck in everything we do in life. Now it's a mixture of emotions and when the medics say that each one of us living with HIV is living with a slightly different strain of the virus, is that why I am a long-term survivor? If someone's unfortunate enough to have a strain which might be more severe and affect them quickly, it's a shame, a terrible shame...I have obviously been lucky that I've managed to live a long time, in my opinion, with HIV for all this time without any bloody combination therapy and I've only just started taking it...In fact I intend to die of old age. I do and I will...I'm not gonna die as a result of living with HIV. Oh, no! I'm not gonna let it, no way...long-term survival has become a natural phenomenon and I am proud... I'm very lucky and I have more control now than I ever had...more now because it was ultimately my choice to go on to combination therapy. No one actually said you have got to...the choices have been mine...I am not only coping with everything I am actually dealing with things fairly well as far as I'm concerned. One thing I would like to say is I wish I could actually be totally open about my status because I would love to share my experiences, the good and the bad bits on a much wider scale than I feel I have been able to do...I have shared experiences and I think spoken twice now on the local BBC radio but I've actually hidden my own identity which I didn't feel good about...my voice is apparently a fairly unique camp voice, I don't know what you would call it dear...I think one or two people did recognise my voice who bothered to listen...I'd love to do something on a much bigger scale...I now feel well enough and there are no support services here where I live, like I told you and what I'd like to do is start a self-help group but it's got to be started by the clients themselves, it is no good expecting a third party to run it...it's not going to work. There's a lot of people living here with no support...that's what I would like to do but I haven't got a crystal ball or a magic wand and I think I would need to get permission...I don't have a crystal ball and my magic wand hasn't worked for ages darling [*we are both in fits of laughter*]."

Larry, like other story-tellers, had an overwhelming yearning or aspiration to be much more open and honest about their positive status at a social level. Why is it that so many people living with an HIV-positive diagnosis do not feel free to disclose their status publicly? It is a great shame! Whilst Larry had a brilliant sense of humour he was, at the same time, a very sensitive and thoughtful character with a positive mental attitude. As promised, Larry, I did not throw the Gladioli. Over and out!

A forgotten generation: Long-term survivors' experiences of HIV and AIDS

JAY

Jay was diagnosed in 1992 and describes himself as a *one hundred per cent poof*. He was medically retired and extremely healthy and held a magnificent attitude and outlook on life. When we met face-to-face to talk about living with HIV, Jay told me of his previous involvement in an abusive and violent relationship which affected him taking his treatment and subsequently made him ill. He was now taking his second regime of combination therapy which he considered was effective with no adverse side affects. Jay had an aspiration to move back to London as he did not have any sense of belonging where he was currently living. He was, however, happily living with HIV and believed that one should always try everything once and if you don't like it, so be it. When I asked him about the positive and negative elements of living long-term with HIV, he recalled:

"I think living with something like this makes you a better person; I don't know how can I put it? It just makes you realise obviously you've got a terminal or chronic illness whichever way you want to put it…your life is sort of restricted, as you never know when it's going to come to an end, whenever…so you do tend to just care more. It makes *me* a more caring person, not so much for myself but for others…well there is a certain amount of uncertainty with it. I just think…the way I meant there was like things are being taken away from me so I try to do as much as I can, you know…when I am at home I try to get up really early in the morning, about three of four times a week like 6 am or 7 am because I hate missing out on that part of the day…It's just things that I like to do and there are things that I still want to do and I know that I am going to go out and do them…You know living here means I am not going to do what I want…It's hell here and I want to go back to London…if something is going to be taken away from you, you've just got to get everything done because you don't want to deteriorate to a degree where you can't do these things."

Jay believed that the threat of uncertainty hanging over him was something he could not ignore because of how many other people had died and it would be like denying their experiences and existence. In a positive way, Jay believed this drove him on to do things he wanted to do. He continued to reflect about negative aspects of living with HIV, he told me:

"Probably the most negative element is not being as honest with my family as I should really be but… I just don't want them to feel any more hurt or upset and I have always sort of had a bit of a pretty shit life, so it's negative for not being able to tell them… I mean I can tell them, there is nothing stopping me from telling them, it's just that I don't want to see them hurt any more than they already have been. I don't think there is anything else that is a negative point…Most of my friends will just say that I'm probably loopier now than I was before I was diagnosed. So I am just me and I mean I am a better person when I am in London as well I think…Since living here I have had more bad moods and miserable times in the last nine months than I have probably had in the last five years…you know if you go into a bad mood it puts you in that frame of mind for a day or something and that doesn't help you. I mean if I feel bad it is a horrible thing…stress is a big part of living with HIV. A major factor probably only when I'm in my bad moods because it comes to the forefront of your mind…I mean I'm just Jay and I just get on with life and I try not to wallow in it. If you are going to get down, you are going to get stressed and if you are going to get stressed you're HIV is going to kick in. If you have a good outlook on life and just go about life and do what you want to do within boundaries of course, then you are happier. You will live longer…That's it so put the kettle on!"

Jay did not particularly consider himself a long-term survivor, as many of his friends had lived with HIV for 15 years and more. He believed as time moved on with the advancement of more effective medication there would hopefully come a point when you could just take one pill per day. Time was a precious thing for Jay and his kind and caring personality was clearly evident. Jay had an amazingly wicked sense of humour and was extremely positive about being positive. The kettle is still on, Jay!

RACHEL

Rachel was diagnosed in 1993 and went on to have two children with her HIV-positive husband. She has a medical background and was not earning a wage but was planning to return to work perhaps in the field of health. When we spoke about living with HIV we did this over the telephone. We had met previously at a conference and had spoken many times before our conversation. Rachel told me how HIV was a small part of her life and she totally disliked being labelled. First and foremost she is a human being and looks forward to seeing her children growing up. When I asked her about the positive and negative elements of living long-term with HIV, she told me:

"There are a huge number of things; there are so many things I wouldn't have done. I know it sounds daft! You don't choose to have something dreadful happen to you but you have a choice in how you react to it. I wouldn't have chosen it but of all the things I have gotten out of it. I have been to Canada, to Australia. I have been invited to all sorts of meetings that I wouldn't have been invited to otherwise. I have met huge numbers of people that I wouldn't have met otherwise. I have been involved in areas of work that I find fascinating and I have been able to help people that I probably would never have come into contact with, let alone been able to help otherwise...these are all positive experiences...On the negative side, I mean not being as healthy as I would like to be. Not being as fit as I would like to be. I have minor niggles about worrying about if I do cut myself, worrying about making sure that I take care of the cut if the children want to help and I am saying, no you mustn't help. Things like that, but these are relatively minor, quite honestly...I want people to be more HIV aware, I suppose I take care of that by being willing to go and talk to midwives, nurses and social workers...going out and trying to involve myself with their education and I do talks in schools, so that they can see an ordinary face. It is not something to be frightened of but it is something to be aware of and be sensible about. It is a caution. If I am involved in an accident, hopefully people will be sensible enough to take precautions; paramedics ought to know better than to take risks... you can be very destructive if you are not careful. I have come across people who are incredibly destructive about the way they think about things. They are the ones that suffer the most, yes and their families and they probably lose an awful lot of friends that way as well. You have to enhance the way you live your life...I can use it in a way that is useful but it doesn't mean that I have to be responsible for other people it means that I can help them make more sensible decisions."

Rachel is extremely assertive and will not be brow beaten into making decisions about health matters. In a bizarre way, she is relieved that she is HIV-positive as her husband is also positive and to be in a discordant relationship would have been difficult to negotiate. Rachel told me how her Mother had told her 'Life is a sexually transmitted disease and it is invariably fatal' and she believes this is very, very true. I wish you and your lovely family only the best in life.

TONY

Tony was diagnosed in 1994 after spending many years in denial about the possibility of being HIV-positive. When we met face-to-face to discuss living with HIV, he told me that life was like a light bulb when you go out, you go out. There is no after-life! Tony had recently embarked upon a new intimate relationship and had moved further south to be with his partner. He firmly believes his self-esteem and self-confidence has been affected as a result

A forgotten generation: Long-term survivors' experiences of HIV and AIDS

of being HIV-positive. When I asked him about the positive and negative elements of living with HIV, he recounted:

"HIV has affected everything. There is nothing positive about being HIV-positive... It has killed all my ambitions and my dreams...it has changed my body image and it's not nice being invisible on the gay scene...there is finger pointing and nasty stuff and I am disgusted at the people I see who have the audacity to point their finger at anybody...I have less friends but I don't blame that on HIV, it's me I have grown up...in terms of long-term survival I still question every year, you know and I don't see a future. Yes, you live day by day and I don't make plans...It has limited my opportunities in many ways being labelled as HIV and my gay friends would go on and on about my positive status when I was out. It made me feel uncomfortable but it interested me I was intrigued and wanted to get into a debate about it but they didn't want to talk...I am at a stage in my life now I'm 40 where things are just completely slowing, I don't know... I get frightened and am conscious about my eyes. I feel I need to get my eyes sorted. I keep getting black spots in front of my eyes...If this was a lot clearer my brain would be more in function... I don't feel like my brain's in function, it is slowing down."

Tony did wander off down different pathways when he was talking about HIV matters. He struggled to think about positive and negative elements of living with HIV, but he continued:

"HIV is very challenging as the numbers of years grow. You start looking at your medication and you start to programme yourself...It's the years that start to become a challenge for me...you start to look at yourself differently but I don't want to grow old. I think I'm ready to, well I'm quite ready to die and I'm not frightened of death. So I reckon when I'm about 44 that will be me...I suppose it's actually quite sad to think this way but I would be comfortable with that, I know it kind of sounds a bit sick, but you know...I have got osteoporosis because of the side effects and that is not nice and I don't know if these tablets that I am on is making me lack energy. If I didn't take them would I have more energy? I want to tell my doctor if I could please stop taking my medication for a bit but I don't think they would like it...I'm all talked out now."

Lethargy and a distinct lack of energy was a major cause of concern for Tony. He did reach the age of 44 and beyond and is still reflecting on life using his own special approach to the many wonders of our world. As he grows older he remains an extraordinary and very talented human being. Whilst HIV has killed many of his ambitions he is still able to dream and carry out some of the activities he likes to do. Keep the camera clicking, Tony! Your artwork still stands in pride of place in my home, thank you.

SANDRA

Sandra was diagnosed in 1994 and lost her five month old son to AIDS soon after this discovery. She is reasonably healthy and has days of good health and days of sheer exhaustion and tiredness; she is now diabetic as a result of the side effects of taking protease inhibitors. When we met face-to-face to discuss living with HIV, she told me how she was currently embarking on a new intimate relationship with an HIV-positive man. This sadly did not work out and turned into yet another horrible experience for her. Sandra's life is full of secrecy and she feels that her social standing has been lost as a result of her positive status. When I asked her about the positive and negative elements of living with HIV, she told me:

"The positive things for me have been that I have begun to take care of my health, well my physical health and my emotional health and well-being…I take life at a slower pace and I am quite discriminating in what is important in life. I don't spend time on what I consider as useless things…The negative aspect of living with HIV is the uncertainty of life. The funny thing is life is uncertain for everybody regardless of the diagnosis of an HIV-positive status… but for us I think our mortality has been brought into question and we have been brought face-to-face with it, I am talking about positive people generally… but long-term survivors even more so because the body can only take so much and there is going to be a time when you can't take any more drugs. So, you are very aware that your time is precious. I suppose that is a negative and a positive thing…One of the negative things for me is that I have lost my social status in life, this is my feeling… I don't feel as though I can hold my head up and say who I am because we are judged on our occupation, or your job and social role and most people with HIV aren't in work and so it becomes *the* most dreaded question: 'Oh, so what do you do?' and then you get, 'well you look healthy'. It is frustrating to have to keep explaining all this stuff to other people; we are always having to explain ourselves. And you know people put you in boxes… I mean we all do it, don't we? I would finally like to say that I think it is a constant struggle, an emotional and physical struggle. The drugs help you cope with the virus, suppressing it but it does not eliminate the personal struggles in life…There is a tendency for some of us to attribute everything to HIV, but this is not always the case, quality of life is important and in most of our experiences we have to struggle."

A forgotten generation: Long-term survivors' experiences of HIV and AIDS

Sandra has experienced many problems associated with social rejection from previous friendships in relation to being HIV-positive. Sexual relationships have also suffered and she will only consider having relationships with HIV-positive men in the future. Sandra tries to maintain a positive outlook on life and is now a stronger human being but she still does not wish to disclose her positive status to others. I wish her all the very best for a peaceful and happy life ahead!

We have now reached the end of our journey of discovery into how our long-term survivors have experienced every day life living with an HIV-positive diagnosis. The final chapter reflects on my own personal experiences of *being there* during our conversations and reveals how I initially designed and implemented the original small-scale qualitative research project for a PhD programme of study. Whilst it is a huge relief to have finally completed this story-of-stories it is also strangely poignant to think that I have now reached the end of this long and winding road. My heart feels heavy yet I know not why this should be. The lessons that might have been learned throughout our journey, I hope will teach us how important life really is and greatly influence how we behave towards other people we might know who live with an HIV-positive diagnosis.
Throughout this chapter we have revealed quite convincingly how most story-tellers have attempted to help others around them in the face of their own adversity. The love, warmth and friendship and the overwhelming desire to have a purpose in life is beyond any doubt. We have heard our long-term survivors speak of: survivorship, assertiveness and empowerment; valuable experiences that made them stronger psychologically and more appreciative as human beings; being proud to still be alive and having the opportunity of facing mortality. A valuable lesson we have learned is that we must never put off until tomorrow what we might achieve today.

Perhaps 'having the last laugh' at the medical community in terms of still being alive, at the time of our conversations and beyond, might teach those in the profession a valuable lesson; our long-term survivors are living proof of the mistakes and errors made by the medical community although we appreciate some story-tellers have sadly since died. We have learned how our story-tellers have put significant matters into perspective in terms of seeing life and death at such close quarters. Many story-tellers are no longer fearful of anything life may throw at them since diagnosis day. Friendships have grown and blossomed in most cases; family and friends are to be seen as an important and valuable source of support for many of our story-tellers. Confronting one's own prejudices and acknowledging that materialistic things in life are no longer important can teach us all a lesson in life. Every day is a new gift and the transformations in terms of our story-tellers becoming more compassionate and caring human beings has to be a gift that benefits us all at a social level.

The negative elements of coping with HIV-related uncertainty are indeed multifaceted and potentially devastating. Not knowing what is around the corner is a feature of everyday life; yet when something like HIV threatens: your mortality; your 'sense of self' and, dramatically affects your health this is a different kind of uncertainty. Having to be secretive about being HIV-positive is a burden that should not exist; our story-tellers' anxieties concerning lying and secrecy are stressful and can impact on psychological health and well-being. HIV has eroded people's rights to make decisions of their choice and this should be acknowledged and resolved. When we feel ill, experience bouts of depression, feel socially isolated or rejected or when we might be experiencing adverse side effects of toxic drug treatments, immediately we start to question the quality of our life. Surely the quality of our lives should surpass quantity.

The huge losses in terms of lives lost to AIDS and HIV has been a disturbing feature of this disease. HIV presents life as an unpredictable challenge. Having to give up work, losing social status, and having no sense of where you are going in life is stressful and causes anxiety which can further comprise our health and psychological well-being. When will your luck run out? HIV brings with it uncertainty, more uncertainty than in our general lives. HIV affects our sexuality as sexual beings and brings with it a burden of responsibility towards others in terms of disclosure which is totally unrealistic. Some story-tellers feel guilty about surviving when others have died. Must we always value our existence in the face of illness and adversity? Why should HIV affect our self-confidence, self-worth and self-esteem at a personal and public level? Poverty and financial insecurity can be a feature of living long-term with HIV, as is the case with other chronic illness conditions. Because HIV has no defining structure in terms of disease progression, it affects different people differently. We must never become complacent towards HIV because it is still a major public and private concern.

The idea that any human being should be ashamed of someone who is HIV-positive is beyond my own comprehension. Nevertheless it still exists. A great number of story-tellers have accomplished so much in life living long-term with HIV and have attempted to help others along their journey. Why is this you must ask yourself! This is the last time I ask you, the reader, to reflect on these personal experiences to understand how these stories have impacted on your established beliefs and opinions. Could you construct a negative element into a positive feature in life? If you came face-to-face with your own mortality how might you negotiate everyday life? How much do you appreciate in your everyday life that makes you feel glad that you are alive and well? How honest and straightforward any of us are when we interact with others is something we can all reflect on. I sincerely hope that your views, opinions and beliefs have been greatly influenced by reading and engaging with our story-tellers throughout this journey. We must at all times attempt to embrace a hopeful and optimistic view in our journey of life. I ask you to reflect on what you have learned and I hope that this story-of-stories will transform us all into more compassionate and tolerant human beings. Good luck!

A forgotten generation: Long-term survivors' experiences of HIV and AIDS

CHAPTER TEN

On being there: a researcher's tale

∞

"Histories are arguments created by people in particular conditions. These conditions include the very social worlds in which they live, and which, by their telling, they model and sometimes seek to alter."

Tonkin, E (1990)

Introduction

This closing chapter reveals my own personal experiences and critical reflections of the putting together of this story-of-stories and incorporates various stages of the design and implementation of a small-scale qualitative research project for a PhD programme of study. It is difficult to know where to start as this journey has taken so long and the finished project is something quite different from what was originally intended. However, I believe the intended political aim of writing this book in this format has not lost its original aim; to enrich our knowledge and develop and enhance the understanding of how people manage and personally experience living with HIV from a long-term survivors' perspective. It was always my intention to ensure that the findings of this explorative study be accessible to everyone, and not simply remain in the realms of academia. My biggest regret is that it has taken so long to complete.

To start I briefly discuss why I believe it is essential to incorporate my own story to complete this story-of-stories. Afterwards, we explore how the rigour of the PhD process and specific academic demands proved somewhat challenging and, at times, an overwhelming enterprise. In particular I reflect upon aspects of my research training based on prevailing expectations of 'proper proceedings' for the researcher; this led to thought-provoking and complex decision-making strategies affecting many stages of the design of the HIV study. Here we delve into some of the necessary deliberations, expectations and multiple tasks required for the purpose of a PhD programme of study. Following on, I share some of my personal experiences and critical reflections of the interview process including arranging meetings and talking to the story-tellers [the makers of meaning].

I use my reflective diary and notes taken during each interview to aide these memories. I also recount a number of shared experiences with several women and men outside of the interview process which significantly shaped and maintained genuine, meaningful and long-lasting personal relationships between ourselves. Even now, to this day, I enjoy friendships with many of the women and men who took the time to speak about their personal experiences of living long-term and managing an HIV-positive diagnosis. I am extremely privileged and blessed to be part of their lives. And finally, I briefly reflect on how writing this book in this particular format presented a few unexpected challenges which were substantively different from previous academic writing.

The telling of stories: why should I tell mine?

Everywhere in life there is an interest in stories; we gather other people's stories and often use them as social commentary to construct pathways leading us to a more meaningful understanding in terms of the many ways of being in our social world. Repeatedly we tell stories about our pasts, our present and our futures. Stories are crucial to create and make meaning and allow us to understand our social situation. We all live in a kind of story-world. We experience our own bodies, thoughts and feelings; we act out behaviours and talk about ourselves and situate ourselves both within and outside of our own social milieu. We give meaning to our selves in relation to the world around us; a world that is not fixed or permanent but is changeable and can always be contested.

Traditionally, in earlier academic and empirical research the subjective or personal experiences and emotions of the researcher or story-teller have often been excluded within a number of [positivist] disciplines from around the nineteenth and early twentieth centuries; the inclusion of subjective experiences was not considered 'proper procedure'. Yet over time such notions have, to some extent, been essentially challenged and we are able to contest these standpoints with considerable and vociferous debate. I appreciate the ways in which research approaches within disciplinary perspectives are historically grounded and situational; yet to follow any procedure blindly without critical consideration will almost always have a dramatic and direct impact on the planning, the flow and interpretations of any research process. By excluding this chapter and ignoring my own personal emotions, reflections and research experiences, it would only serve to obscure a more comprehensive depiction of the complete research journey.

Why should we leave insufficient space for the experiences and subjectivities of those *doing* the research or telling the story? How are we to become acquainted with who is behind the work, why they are doing the research, and how they experienced the research process if we do not hear their voices? Surely, we should include ourselves in the narrative; we are the story-tellers and the experiences of 'being there' must unquestionably count for something. By removing the person(s) behind the research, this initiates an almost authoritative and magical creation. This is most certainly something I do not wish to conjure here. I was the person who constructed the research proposal to explore HIV-related matters which subsequently resulted in the coming together of all of whom participated in this journey. I was *there* when each story was told and I am telling this story-of-stories founded upon the numerous personal and everyday lived experiences of our long-term survivors concerned. I truly believe my own story must be integrated into this story-of-stories to present a more holistic picture; there is nothing magical or authoritative about this creation. So here is my tale...

Research design, personal experiences and critical reflections prior to interviews

The PhD journey: a long and winding road

One of the drawbacks of undertaking a PhD programme of study, funded by the Economic and Social Research Council [ESRC] or otherwise, is having copious amounts of tasks to contemplate and execute in addition to the actual design of the research study, and having very little time to accomplish them. For instance, within my first year besides fulfilling mandatory research training, I had to intensively prepare for an academic upgrade from M.Phil to PhD which was a terrifying experience. For sure, the research training is an absolute imperative for anyone embarking upon any social research activities. The academic upgrade was extremely time-consuming and pretty fearsome for me although I do acknowledge it was a necessary progression and ultimately rewarding. It was rather like being pulled from many different directions which, in part, produced even more confusion, frustration and an overwhelming desire to quit before I had even started. I did, nonetheless, successfully complete the upgrade to PhD; it might have been more appropriate, however, to have featured in the early part of the second year of the programme of study.

Within this same year I had to attend regular meetings with my supervisors to make sure my research plan, theoretical and disciplinary approaches and schedule of work remained on target and were consistent. At times I considered these meetings rather bewildering, sometimes awkward and often frustrating. I was attempting to construct a tangible and credible HIV-centred explorative study; I therefore had to build up authentic and meaningful relationships with people in the HIV field from the onset due to the sensitive nature of my enquiry. My schedule of work was often at odds with academic expectations. I felt I was being bombarded with too many theoretical approaches that appeared to be unconnected and, dare I say insignificant, to my chosen topic. It was impossible to realistically consider a few of those brought to my attention until I had completed my interviews and critically examined our conversations.

Having said this, there were times when meetings were useful and constructive, especially in relation to the academic upgrade and those meetings that were spontaneous without appointment. I must say I was always grateful to my supervisors for their time and enthusiasm; I never felt neglected in terms of access and support over the years. Nonetheless preparing for, attending and writing up notes of frequent scheduled meetings in the first year generally-speaking were unnecessarily time-consuming, troublesome and on occasions uncomfortably like a battlefield. It might have been more prudent to have scheduled fewer meetings at the start and steadily increased these at a time when they were considered more essential.

On a more positive note, it was obligatory to regularly attend postgraduate seminars and conferences and submit a paper relating to our own research. I thoroughly enjoyed listening to and commenting upon other postgraduate students' experiences and research projects; these productive events were extremely constructive and thought-provoking and proved to be a valuable and creative arena. I was fortunate enough to enjoy a positive response to my own paper. I presented a candid and unrestrained version of my HIV-related research proposal, in addition to a what-to-do list for the fear-provoking academic upgrade looming ahead and then shared some experiences of the treacherous life of a postgraduate student. It was a warts-and-all academic account of my HIV study and personal experiences to date.

Also during my first year, at the suggestion of one of my supervisors, I attended an HIV conference in Brighton which turned out to be a lonely, costly and forbidding experience. Whilst this conference did prove informative and a good networking site, it was a huge expense which came out of an extremely limited budget and therefore created problems in the second year when it came to travel expenses for the purpose of interviews. If I had my time again, I would not have attended this conference. Perhaps if there had been money left over after the interview stage, and during the write-up stage of the research, I would have considered this more of a fruitful endeavour.

Finally, I had to conjure up enough time to sit in on relevant subject-specific modules, for example Sociology of Health and Illness and Medical Sociology to help develop and enhance theoretical approaches for my HIV study. I considered this a valuable use of my time as it was beneficial and essential to the theoretical progression of the study. Lest I forget, I also had to undertake compulsory part-time assistant teaching as part of the requirements of the PhD programme. This was all incorporated in the first year of the PhD programme in addition to planning and designing the HIV-centred research; the wide range of activities was indeed plentiful and therefore time-consuming. For me, not all activities were constructive in terms of my time. My primary concern was to clearly focus on my research design and gain access to volunteers who, by telling their stories, would become the makers of meaning in this sensitive enquiry.

As with all postgraduate students doing empirical and social research, we had to develop, organise and maintain a strict regime to adhere to our own timetables and planned schedules of work for the purpose of the study .I had to maintain a rigid focus on my research question. For me the construction of the research question itself took an absolute age to conceptualise:

> *How are we to understand the experiences and social implications of changing scientific knowledge and medical treatment in the management of HIV for long-term survivors in the UK?*

I had to design a credible research stratagem that would seek to effectively address this question. There was a huge gap in our understanding of what it meant to live long-term with HIV or AIDS-related illness since scientific developments of more effective medical treatments took shape from 1996 onwards. How should we understand the social implications and changing experiences of living long-term with HIV and AIDS-related illness? I had to think about the most effective way to accomplish this as I did not claim to know the answers to my research enquiry.

I was particularly determined to engage with only significant themes that were pertinent and relevant to the people who were going to take part in this enquiry. I did not want to give way to academic pressures of focussing on dominant studies and/or theoretical perspectives that had gone before. This was difficult to sustain at times but I remained unyielding and stayed focussed. My research study was, after all, supposed to be innovative and original. Without a doubt, I could find few studies that claimed to explore long-term personal experiences of living with HIV since more effective medical treatment and scientific advancements had changed HIV from a medical 'death sentence' into a manageable chronic illness condition. My research proposal, therefore, was certainly original or as original as it could be within the constraints of a PhD programme of study; yet, how should I successfully design the research?

As mentioned previously, few empirical studies were concerned with the psychological and social experiences of people living with HIV and AIDS post 1996 since medical advancements with Highly Active Antiretroviral Therapy (HAART) dominated our lives. This raised significant problems in the writing of the literature review. There was an abundance of studies reviewing the clinical aspects of living with HIV and AIDS; sadly, these studies revealed very little about individual women and men's experiences on a day-to-day basis within an HIV context. In particular, there were few that turned their gaze towards *long-term survivors* who had lived with an HIV-positive diagnosis prior to the advancement of HIV medicine and, in some cases, prior to medical health checks in terms of the CD4 count and the viral load test.

All the same, I had to maintain and keep afloat with the relevant and changing theoretical perspectives I had chosen to work with for this HIV study. I had opted for a multi-disciplinary approach. I believed issues relating to HIV and AIDS were not simply a matter purely for the psychological, or the sociological, or the cultural or indeed the economic. Living with HIV and AIDS-related illness permeated all of these spheres and I had to leave room to incorporate them all where appropriate.

Reflections on designing the research study

How I was to conduct the research was equally of considerable importance from a methodological standpoint. Methodology quite literally means the study of method and also incorporates [research] practices and techniques used to obtain information. The principal concern of methodology comprises philosophical debates based on underlying assumptions we might have about our social world and how we theorise knowledge; this is dependent upon a range of perspectives and viewpoints within social science. How do we know what is true and false? It requires rigorous thought and in-depth discussion, as a method is not in itself a methodology. In other words, I needed to clearly justify and defend, using a methodical and logical argument, why I had chosen the specific research strategy, methods and techniques to conduct my qualitative research at the expense of other methods: How do we view our social world? How do we know what we know? How will I conduct the research and for what purpose? Why have I chosen the interview method to gather data? I needed to clearly argue how and why the research question would be best addressed using my chosen exploratory approach.

Accordingly, I opted for an in-depth, semi-structured interview technique to gather personal narratives in order to construct knowledge. This type of interview, often regarded as a guided conversation or 'conversation with a purpose', is a useful way to collect large amounts of information and ensures the focus remains on relevant themes under discussion. Most importantly, it allows social interaction and co-operation between the researcher and the people telling their stories. During the interview process the story-teller is able to clarify and elaborate on central themes particular to their own specific personal experiences; each person can tell their own story at their own pace and within their own time frame. This was to be my chosen pathway.

For me, the principal justification for this particular research strategy was that it:
   a) facilitated women and men living with HIV to construct their own individual experiences of illness;
   b) enabled people to reconstruct their own life histories and
   c) made HIV and AIDS-related health and illness matters more comprehensible by the telling of these stories.

This then allowed me to thematically assemble and collectivise personal narratives using a cross-sectional indexing system. I could then critically analyse individual narratives to formulate knowledge and understanding pertaining to health and illness experiences from a long-term survivors' perspective within the context of HIV. From this, we can see the emergence of a collective voice.

Broad themes and research questions: an overview

Certainly, I wanted to explore specific themes within a semi-structured interview format but, at the same time, I wanted to create space for other themes/issues that might emerge from individual personal experiences within a broader context. I chose therefore to ask chiefly open-ended questions that did not potentially lead or confuse the story-teller. The dominant themes I set out to explore were: how people discovered they were HIV-positive and the subsequent impact this had on everyday life following diagnosis; if there were any personal issues around death and dying both prior to and/or after diagnosis; specific matters which centred around perceptions and/or personal experiences of taking HIV medicine before and after the advent of HAART; differing personal relationships with HIV and other medical professions; the types of decision-making processes involved in managing an HIV-positive diagnosis; how people practiced intimate relationships as positive sexual beings, and to what extent, if any, had HIV impacted on everyday life and personal relationships with others. I believed using an open-ended strategy would create space for story-tellers to speak about their own personal experiences peculiar to their own social situation. And undeniably it most certainly did…

At the start of each interview I asked: *How and when did you discover your HIV-positive status?* And usually I went on to ask about a person's knowledge and awareness of HIV at this time and what medical treatment might have been available. Because many people had discovered their HIV-positive status in the early to mid 1980s, it could not be assumed that there was an abundance of knowledge around HIV at this time. I regularly steered our conversational flow towards how the diagnosis might have impacted on daily life and to what extent HIV influenced any lifestyle changes if at all. Typically matters relating to death and dying were raised or touched upon without my intrusion, but in case this had not been raised or was an oversight, I asked: *can you tell me of any death and dying issues prior to and/or after diagnosis?* In earlier times a medical 'death sentence' was regularly synonymous with an HIV-positive diagnosis, as we discovered in chapter two.

At an appropriate point during the interview, I guided our conversational flow towards the medical profession and medical treatment by asking: *has anything changed for you since more effective treatment became available?* Frequently I would ask those taking or had previously taken combination therapy if they considered their medication intrusive in everyday life. After a few interviews, it soon became evident that side effects were problematic for many, so questions relating to side effects were incorporated within this theme. During each conversation, I asked: *How would you describe your relationship with the medical profession?* This enquiry teased out how relationships were managed and experienced within a medical or clinical setting over time and was extremely illuminating as we have seen.

Often during our conversations, we moved from one theme back to another dependent upon the personal experiences under discussion or how the story- teller was remembering events; this was not a problem. Once we felt we had exhausted matters pertaining to the health profession and medicine

A forgotten generation: Long-term survivors' experiences of HIV and AIDS

I would ask: *Have sexual relationships been affected by your HIV-positive status?* This theme, when I first started, was the most apprehensive section of the interview. I would become uneasy, anxious, dry mouthed and extremely hesitant before we broached this topic. As I had built up a good working relationship with many of the women and men who took part, the theme soon became easier to openly discuss and in some instances, it was quite humorous.

In many earlier publications in relation to social aspects of AIDS, terms like 'stigma', 'discrimination' and 'prejudice' have often been connected with matters concerning HIV and AIDS; yet for me it has always been rather vague and unclear as to how such behaviours have been enacted and, equally, where these might have emanated. I thought it was particularly worthy and valuable to locate the sources of any HIV-related discriminatory practices, perceived prejudice and stigma-related experiences so I could understand how such behaviours were enacted and how these impacted on the lives of long-term survivors. To this end, I asked all story-tellers: *Can you tell me of any discriminatory practices, prejudice or stigma-related experiences you might have encountered on the basis of being HIV-positive?* I can say that many experiences of discriminatory practices exposed in this study based on being HIV-positive was a surprising and, in some ways, unanticipated finding.

We concluded each interview with the question below, as I thought it enabled each story-teller to encapsulate their own personal and lived experiences, whilst, simultaneously giving space for new issues to come to mind. The concluding question was: *can you tell me what are the positive and negative elements of living with an HIV-positive diagnosis?* This final question revealed some illuminating and informative characteristics of the women and men who took part in this study. Some positive and negative elements, for example, included:

- It has changed my life for the better; I am more honest and I think about other people more often. I am less selfish.
- I have lost a lot of my friends over time.
- Every day is a new gift and I am thankful I am still here.
- I am constantly tired and lack energy.
- Taking life at a slower pace and identifying what is important in life.
- I have always wished I could be open about my HIV-positive status because I would love to share my experiences.
- As a long-term survivor I feel like I am a *winner*.
- I feel guilty for surviving when others have lost their lives. I don't value my existence that highly.

All of the above open-ended questions were the basic semi-structured arrangement I employed to explore the central themes of the enquiry.

On researching 'sensitive' topics: still more considerations

Notions of sensitivity surrounding women and men living with HIV and AIDS-related illness affected almost each stage of the research from formulation and design right through to implementation and application. Just the idea of putting together and planning this research proposal impinged on the personal, emotional, ethical and political spheres of life which required significant thought and deliberation. No-one can argue that the topic of HIV is not sensitive at a variety of levels and from divergent perspectives. Yet what do we actually mean by a sensitive research topic and how do we understand the term 'sensitive' in a given context? All these matters required significant thought and debate prior to the design and execution of the interview process.

In the main, any study in which there are *potential consequences or implications* for those directly involved in the research or indeed as a group of individuals represented by that research can be regarded as sensitive. However this is exceptionally broad and one could argue all research has potential consequences or implications by the very nature of doing the research in the first instance. Similarly, research endeavours that have the potential to pose a *substantial threat* for any individual involved can be perceived as sensitive; be it the researched or the researcher. Any threatening features of a research venture and its potential consequences and costs should therefore be approached with caution. This exploration was no exception.

The sensitive nature of exploring HIV and AIDS-related matters based on long-term survivors' personal experiences had to be appreciated and, at all times, respected. One substantial threat I duly acknowledged was how this study might possibly present problems leading to potential costs to certain individuals as a result of my making frequent demands during our conversation. Of course, all research involves potential costs to those who participate, if only in terms of time, effort and inconvenience; however actively participating in any research should not involve substantial threats for any person. What I mean here is the possible substantial threat in terms of bringing into play emotional or psychological costs based on the internalisation of negative public beliefs and HIV stigma and prejudice. I did not wish to unleash any feelings of fear or embarrassment, guilt, shame, painful memories of social rejection or general awkwardness during our conversation. A risk assessment of particular themes which might stimulate unwelcome or unpleasant consequences for each story-teller had to be considered. I was, however, unable to realistically assess every personal outcome prior to exploring every theme during each conversation. To the best of my knowledge there were no unpleasant or negative outcomes experienced during our interviews, yet the potential threat or risk was always there in my mind beforehand.

For that reason, the welfare and integrity of the women and men taking part had to prevail over the advancement of knowledge at all times. I consequently adhered to the principle of 'no harm' to ensure the physical, social and psychological well being of all story-tellers. Our relationships were founded on a mutual commitment of trust and openness therefore the interests of us all were considered at all times. Equally, I was always prepared to listen to the dominant themes relevant to the story-tellers (the makers of meaning) rather than hear only what I might want to hear. In other words, I did not wish to be guided by my own intellectual enquiry and the imposed academic considerations solely for the purpose of the PhD. This was why I specifically chose this particular research strategy. In effect the relationship between the women and men taking part in the study and myself was one of teacher and student, respectively. The group of long-term survivors became the teachers in this social context and I was, rather pertinently, the student.

Ethical considerations: confidentiality, privacy and anonymity

Confidentiality, privacy and anonymity have to be vigorously maintained throughout any research process. Confidentiality was mutually agreed and assumed for each interview on a one-to-one basis. Nevertheless, a few people who took part in the study knew of others who were also taking part. This came about because several individuals accessed support from the same HIV organisations or social groups and, as a consequence, deliberately chose to speak of their own personal involvement with the research. By no means did I divulge confidential or personal information regarding persons involved to any other individual. I became the 'keeper of secrets'.

It is usually assumed as a fundamental right to expect and uphold privacy, anonymity and confidentiality throughout the research process. This is occasionally more difficult to put into practice when people engage in discussions about other individuals particularly within the HIV community.

Numerous women and men living with HIV, particularly those who work in the HIV field are often in the public eye and open about their positive status. Nevertheless they still have a right to privacy and anonymity and are no different to those who are not in the public eye, or indeed those who actively choose not to disclose their HIV-positive status to others around them.

From time to time, issues of confidentiality and privacy become problematic and unintentional disclosures can and do occur. This is not to say, however, that deliberate and intentional disclosures never occur because unfortunately they do; we are not discussing these matters here. Unintentional breaches of confidentiality can often be due to human error and the essence of being human: accidents do happen! Often if it is well-known that you work in the field of HIV, and say Jack knows Jill and knows that you also know Jill, Jack might let something slip unintentionally. "Hey, did Jill tell you how *she* discovered she was HIV-positive?" Of course it might never occur to Jack that perhaps I do not know Jill's HIV status. There you have it! It is out in the open and it cannot be unsaid. Announcements such as these and the manner in which they are said are clearly not deliberate but accidental breaches of confidence.

I can truthfully declare that I myself have never made such an error. This has, however, happened to me on one occasion. Let us go back to Jack who knew I had close contact with Jill. Jack made certain assumptions based on his awareness of my relationship with Jill and his own knowledge and involvement with my research. Jill was kindly helping me negotiate access to people living long-term with HIV within her own work environment; she was not participating in the research and we had never discussed her HIV status. Jack asked me if I knew how Jill had discovered her HIV-positive status. As our working relationship was outside of the HIV study, I was unaware that Jill was HIV-positive. I was kind enough, incidentally, not to disclose to Jack my ignorance of Jill's HIV status which would alert him to his unintentional breach of confidentiality. I merely replied, "No, Jill hasn't told me her story and therefore we had better change the subject." Disclosing someone's HIV-positive status by accident can be as easy and unintended as this. There was no harm done.

On the matter of anonymity, it is prudent to briefly mention whilst it is considered a fundamental right to uphold anonymity throughout the research process, it is not always a fundamental desire for those who participate. I asked each person prior to our interview whether or not they wished to adopt their own chosen pseudonym for self-identification purposes. Not everyone involved in the study had a desire to remain anonymous and therefore chose their Christian name wherever possible. Every person involved chose a specific name to be known by, be it their own or a chosen pseudonym for the purpose of the study.

This aside, I had to later approach as many women and men as possible to seek assurances that our previous agreement continued to be appropriate for the purpose of this story-of-stories as opposed to the PhD research study. For those I contacted it most certainly remained the case, as the burning desire for their stories to be heard had not altered. For the few I was unable to contact I have used either their chosen pseudonym where applicable or allocated a different name to preserve anonymity. For those who have sadly since died but had stayed in contact with me prior to their death and expressed a desire to keep their real names for the purpose of this book, I have of course granted their wish. As mentioned earlier, I remain truly regretful that I did not complete this story-of-stories sooner.

Locating long-term survivors living with HIV: negotiating access

After vigorously addressing many academic considerations, as well as sweeping some under the carpet until a later date, and fulfilling relevant requirements for designing a robust and defensible research project, I then had to locate women and men at the centre of the HIV and AIDS phenomenon; namely *long term survivors* who had endured living with and managing an HIV-positive diagnosis prior to 1996 and the advent of HAART. The real experts who, in my mind, could fill the widening gaps in our knowledge, and further enrich our understanding. How could I gain access to a group of long-term survivors who might be willing to tell me their stories?

As one would anticipate, there is a distinct lack of statistical data on matters with reference to long-term survival and the research findings were never going to be representative of [the sub-population] of people living with HIV and AIDS-related illness. Nevertheless, I had to attempt to gain access to women and men living with an HIV-positive diagnosis in a society where stigma, prejudice and social rejection still prevailed. How will I be granted access to a group of people that is largely socially invisible due to the secretive and sensitive nature of HIV and AIDS? I had little option but to choose to adopt a mixture of non-probability sampling methods and techniques for practical and strategic purposes. There were few choices available in real terms

In other words, I opted for opportunistic and purposive sampling techniques to locate individuals who might be willing to take part in this exploratory HIV study as and when I came across them. For example I approached women and men at various networking locations including: HIV-related conferences; Haemophilia & Co-infection seminars and local and national HIV organisations to spread the word about my HIV research focusing specifically on long-term survival. In addition I advertised in a newsletter for people living with Haemophilia and also in the HIV press, such as Positive Nation and +ve magazine, calling for volunteers to come forward to tell me their stories. I used the internet and identified HIV-specific websites to access message boards to publicise and raise awareness of my research focussing on long-term survival. I made contact with members of the National Long Term Survivors Group which was pivotal in situating the research to my targeted audience.

The HIV-related conferences, co-infection seminars, local and national HIV organisations and related websites all played an enormous role in gaining access to voluntary participants, thus creating an effective networking strategy, commonly referred to as a 'snowball effect'. At times, however, it was quite nerve-wracking and intimidating to have to confront people face-to-face at conferences and seminars about my exploratory enquiry. The fear of indifference or personal rejection was always a possibility. There were a couple of instances when I was told *'I'm sure someone who is HIV-positive could do this research better than someone who is not'* or comments like *'Not another university bod jumping on the AIDS bandwagon. We can do this work ourselves'*. I had to learn to rise above such comments, as in the main, the positive responses far outweighed the negatives. Undeniably, I had an enormous response from adverts placed in the HIV-press, which I must add, were free-of-charge and key members of these organisations were so accommodating and creative.

Whilst negotiating access to women and men living long-term with HIV and AIDS-related illness, I was constantly mindful many individuals might have personally experienced: levels of social rejection; discrimination and social exclusion; prejudice and stigma in relation to lifestyle choices, and perhaps marginalisation as a result of being HIV-positive. To be granted access to voluntary participants, whether directly or indirectly in terms of approaching HIV organisations was not always easy due to the sensitive nature of the enquiry and matters associated with service providers shielding members of their organisation from research projects.

Often key workers at HIV organisations acted as 'gate-keepers' and were incredibly protective of HIV-positive people who accessed their services, and quite rightly so. I also worked in the HIV voluntary sector and we were frequently inundated with questionnaires and surveys on HIV-related matters; at times we became 'research fatigued'. Yet these studies were never concealed from individuals who accessed our organisation, just in case they wished to take part. They were always included in our newsletter or placed on the notice board. Surprisingly, I did encounter a few workers in HIV organisations who were overly protective and refused categorically to inform people accessing their services about my HIV study. Ultimately they were denying people knowledge and the opportunity of taking part should they so desire. I was dismayed and, at times, appalled as my study did not involve questionnaires or surveys and there were few HIV-centred studies that offered the chance for story-tellers to share their personal experiences within an interview setting.

There were a few occasions when I had to decline kind offers of involvement in the study because of my thematic criterion. The main focus of the study was to explore HIV-related issues with women and men who were diagnosed several years before the advent of HAART in 1996. I was unable to include women and men who had discovered their HIV-positive status after 1994 and this had to be the cut-off point. This was a great shame and I do know that a few people were disappointed.

During my journey, it was paramount to demonstrate sensitivity and have appropriate knowledge and awareness of the dominant issues within an HIV context. As a voluntary worker immersed in the field, I strongly believe that this assisted me to overcome some of the major challenges I encountered. I consider that had I only been informed and guided at an academic level in relation to HIV knowledge, many of the research achievements would not have been successfully accomplished. Why do I believe this? Because I was conscious of very real diverse lifestyles, attitudes and beliefs and differing habits, needs, fears and potential risks linked to HIV and AIDS-related matters from a more grounded and grass-roots perspective.

To be sure, I was told on more than one occasion by participating long-term survivors that I demonstrated very high levels of awareness of relevant and dominant issues associated with living with HIV. Often I was asked in a humorous way '*Are you sure you are not HIV-positive yourself?*' and I would answer: '*No, I am not HIV-positive as I would say if this were true*'. Such exchanges gave me the confidence I initially lacked to talk to and build up trusting relationships with all the story-tellers involved. For that I am eternally grateful – thank you all as it eradicated the negative comments.

Matters of relationships: emotion, attachment and rapport

In research training, it is often an expectation to remain emotionally detached during the research process when exploring 'sensitive topics'. Such emotional detachment might transcend the interview process and data collection, the analysis, the writing up and the reporting of findings and might be considered as 'proper procedure'. How can I possibly be emotionally detached from my own research and, more importantly, the people who tell me their stories? It was not my intention to gather information using an impersonal and standardised questionnaire for this HIV-related enquiry. The study had been designed to incorporate conversations with real people, often in their own homes, about sensitive and intimate matters of living with HIV in everyday life. How is it possible to be detached emotionally within this context?

Throughout previous chapters, we have heard stories depicting incredibly highly emotive personal accounts of lived experiences from long-term survivors during our explorations of specific themes. The emotions expressed and displayed by women and men whilst sharing their personal stories have implications both for themselves in the telling of their stories and for me, the listener who has taped and later transcribed each individual narrative. A kaleidoscope of feelings and emotions radiated throughout the entire research journey for us all. These included: laughter, tears, sadness, happiness, love, grief, anger, disgust, loss, fear, anxiety and sheer determination. I became and remain very much attached to all the women and men involved and indeed the prevailing matters we explored during our conversations. Any notion of personal and/or emotional detachment within this research study has to be considered unworkable, unfeasible and totally impracticable.

During our conversations, the mixture of emotions expressed and experienced often merged with another. Some were intense, whilst others were carefree. An assortment of memories was deeply sad, entrenched in grief and loss, whereas other recollections were happy memories recounted as treasured moments of love, fondness and pride. Many of the narratives of lived experiences were intensely personal and gave way to powerful emotions which should be acknowledge as being expressed in an essentially public way within each guided conversation. As researchers certainly we should be aware of our own perceptions and emotions, and, to some extent, we must regulate and control these for our own personal protection and those of our story-tellers. However a high level of personal and emotional detachment can not be considered an option in this given context.

Prior to interviewing, I developed and subsequently maintained a significant rapport and built up degrees of mutual trust with *almost* all of the women and men who told me their stories. For me, it was considered crucial to establish an authentic relationship between ourselves for this exploration to flourish. I had to be as open and honest as practicably possible about myself, about my own personal goals, interests and ambitions in doing this research. People asked: Why did I want to do this research study? Was it simply to further my own academic career? How genuinely interested was I in crucial matters relating to HIV? How will I help address issues that unfold from the research? On a personal basis, I was asked about my own sexuality, my personal and intimate experiences and my HIV status on a regular basis.

The women and men in this study made assumptions based on their knowledge of my personal biography and had particular expectations that I felt I had to fulfil in order to preserve a meaningful relationship. To all intents and purposes, I firmly believe I was interrogated by most of those involved prior to any interviews taking place; quite rightly so, since my own expectation was for each of them to be as open, honest and candid as they possibly could be about living long-term with an HIV-positive diagnosis.

Just think about it! How on earth could I ask questions and delve into personal and intimate aspects of everyday life and expect frank, open and truthful responses if we did not have a meaningful relationship and genuine rapport at the onset? Displays of emotional exchanges during our conversations were frequent. I could no more have sat there and remained unmoved or detached whilst a person was sobbing and recounting painful memories, than I could watch someone on fire without attempting to put it out. Emotional neutrality during expressions of grief or indeed happiness was outside of my comfort zone; it would be inappropriate, cold, unnatural and disingenuous of me to perform and display such behaviours. I was at all times conscious of my own feelings and perceptions throughout every 'conversation with a purpose'; empathic understanding was something I had strived to achieve [not dispel] long before I embarked upon my PhD study. I am nevertheless aware that not all personal responses to any given situation are synonymous with empathic understanding in all contexts.

A forgotten generation: Long-term survivors' experiences of HIV and AIDS

Reflections on integrity and trust: keep your distance!

As with emotional detachment, the prevailing standpoint [there are exceptions] within research training suggests researchers maintain a professional distance between themselves and the story-tellers. How do you measure professional distance? Within the context of sensitive research, how is this to be put into practice? Surely this must depend on the type of research you are conducting. Researching sensitive topics such as HIV can render this approach impossible to attain. As I have mentioned on numerous occasions, it was important to build up a good working and personal relationship with the story-tellers who were willing to speak of their personal experiences. How will I know how to be?

We are talking here about matters and personal experiences centred on HIV and AIDS. I am asking questions about sexual practices, intimacy and sexual relationships, as well as matters regarding health and illness and relationships with the medical profession. Imagine how you might feel asking an almost total stranger about ways in which they practice sex within the context of HIV. How might the stranger react to this question? I became almost tormented by these deliberations.

Prior to the interview process, I became somewhat overwhelmed with questions emerging in my head about the actual doing of the research and was extremely apprehensive. Is professional distance a realistic expectation? How must I behave when I come face-to-face with people who are taking part in the study? What happens now since I am close to many of the story-tellers involved? How will I recognise an 'appropriate relationship'? How am I to know what is inappropriate? How do I maintain something I cannot conceptualise in this context? Meaningful relationships are built on mutual trust and confidence so I cannot maintain a professional distance and remain removed from the people and the issues and stay true to myself and others. By the very nature of the research, I become involved in their personal lives by asking very private and personal questions. Should the same distance be given to all involved? How much of myself should I give? Am I to change who I am for the purpose of this research?

The questions were complex and the answers did not flow freely. So I decided to make myself some promises and set my own ground rules based upon my own perceptions as well as my academic reading. I must do whatever I feel comfortable with in any given context and stay as true to myself and others as practicably possible. If I am to ask long-term survivors about personal and intimate experiences of living with HIV, they must surely be able to ask me questions about myself so that they themselves are relaxed, confident and willing to talk with me. So as long as I maintain my own integrity, remain true and be honest at all times, there should be few potential problems during any encounter. It is impossible to know where some boundaries begin or end within certain given social contexts.

On doing the interviews: long-term survivors as 'the makers of meaning'

As an individual unwilling to consider herself an 'expert' in this field, despite accumulating a vast wealth of HIV-related knowledge and understanding over time, I perceived women and men living with HIV, in particular those who were diagnosed prior to the advancement of effective HIV medicine as the 'expert': the 'makers of meaning'. Towards late 1980s, medical practitioners were still learning about HIV-related matters and were often reluctant to work within the HIV health community. Furthermore, I could not consider the medical profession as 'experts' due to the very nature of my enquiry. After all, where were medical and clinical practitioners obtaining much of their knowledge based on HIV and medicine? Where did prevailing sources of HIV-related matters initially emanate? Primarily from people living with HIV and AIDS-related illness including those actually swallowing the new medicines, naturally!

These were my thoughts and my contribution was to design a valid and comprehensive HIV research plan and then gather together significant HIV-related information by asking, listening, talking and hearing the personal accounts of lived experiences of people who have lived long-term with an HIV-positive diagnosis. Gathering information in order to intensify our understandings on essential HIV-related matters, however, did not include only the skills of talking and listening. By being a participant in each guided conversation that took place, I was simultaneously able to make crucial observations and personally experience feelings and emotions during each encounter. This is vitally important, I argue, for acquiring more in-depth insights into matters you are attempting to research. My own involvement, my feelings, observations and personal experiences whilst doing each interview enabled me to truly comprehend and grasp dominant HIV-related issues under scrutiny and these remain as lucid today as they did back in 2002.

Such valuable insights undoubtedly demonstrated huge gaps in our current knowledge of social aspects of HIV and illustrated how incomplete our awareness of dominant HIV-related issues had become since the advent of HAART from 1996-onwards. HIV research had been diverted and overshadowed by concentrating our gaze on medical and clinical matters pertaining to HIV. Where was funding for research proposals that focussed its gaze on social aspects of HIV and AIDS? In order to develop a more meaningful understanding of essential HIV-related matters, it is necessary to extend our gaze beyond HIV-medicine to discover what social factors might have changed since1996. How are we to understand the psychological and social aspects of HIV and AIDS 30 years down the road? Who better to ask than those women and men who have endured, experienced and managed HIV and AIDS-related illness from earlier times: enter the long-term survivors' perspective.

Scheduling, planning and preparing for interviews

Between ourselves, during 2002 we organised and successfully completed 28 in-depth interviews comprising 5 women and 23 men living across the UK who had been diagnosed HIV-positive. Twenty two long-term survivors had been diagnosed between 1981 and 1990 and the remaining six between 1991 and 1994. I asked everyone to choose their preferred method of interview: face-to-face or telephone interview. Surprisingly, twenty six people opted for the face-to-face interview however two of these scheduled meetings had to be altered due to repeated bouts of HIV-related illness and busy personal schedules. In total four telephone interviews and twenty four face-to-face interviews were accomplished during this period. We usually spent between one-and-a-half to two hours for each interview.

As the interview stage of the research progressed, it became easier to comfortably participate in each conversation with story-tellers. Prior to arranging and successfully completing 28 interviews, I had conducted two pilot interviews: one face-to-face and the other by telephone, as an exploratory test. Both of these were tremendously instructive and essential for the improvement of future interviews. Neither of these conversations was included in the original research or this story-of-stories as per our mutual agreement. Both interviews left me feeling nervous, anxious and slightly intimidated by the forthcoming interviewing process. I am delighted to report that such anxieties and negative feelings did not last too long into the journey.

Arranging interviews was, at times, complicated by problems associated with geographical location, individual time schedules and periods of ill health. On occasion pre-arranged interviews had to be postponed and re-scheduled on the account of my ill health. For example, if I had a sore throat, cold or symptoms suggesting the onset of influenza, it was inconceivable to conduct an interview with any person who lived with a compromised immune system. It was unethical and unfair. So I had to regularly check my health status prior to pre-arranged interviews. And by the very nature of our gaze, women and men involved in the research, at times, experienced periods of HIV-related and other ill health and therefore scheduled meetings could not occur. This was unavoidable and did not create any significant problems during the interview stage of the research plan.

Geographical location and planning: new learning experiences

The women and men involved in the study were to be found right across the UK and I was situated in West Yorkshire. Accordingly, there was a lot of travelling involved and I had to effectively plan and schedule face-to-face interviews in relation to geographical locality. For the most part I was pretty pleased with myself as I had always had a poor sense of direction: Geography has never been one of my stronger attributes. As many of our pre-arranged meetings took place at the person's home, this meant travelling across the North and South of the UK from my own location. It was an amazing learning experience: organising and planning our meetings involved either using public transport or driving my own car to get to my destination(s). I had to identify and situate towns, cities and counties in relation to each other; it sounds rather infantile but as my knowledge was limited, I had to learn about these matters. I travelled across Manchester and the Midlands driving my car, and went to London, Southampton, Portsmouth and Bournemouth to name a few places using public transport. Many of the most Southerly places I had never visited previously.

One rather embarrassing experience I had was when I was conducting interviews across the Midlands. I was in Birmingham and had arranged to interview two people who lived quite close to each other. Having taken my own car and interviewed the first person, I was to take a twenty minute journey to the next person's house and had clear and detailed instructions. This journey took me more than four hours and incorporated many frantic phone calls and eventual road side assistance before I managed to get to where I was supposed to be. Thankfully I was staying overnight and so I was offered a hot bath, a glass [or two] of wine and lovely home-cooked food and we decided to postpone our interview until morning. There was no satellite navigation technology at my disposal during this period and we still laugh about my poor sense of direction and my frantic state to this day.

My most southerly locations looked likely to be the most difficult to strategically plan and arrange at the beginning. I was not familiar with London at all. I had limited financial resources, and did not know anyone who lived in the London area during this period. By sheer chance, I asked a friend of mine who lived close to me if she knew anyone who lived in London. As luck would have it she told me her aunt resided in North London and would be only too pleased to help. She subsequently asked her Aunt if I could stay with her to conduct my HIV research and the rest is history. I set up base in North London where I stayed with Jane on a number of occasions whilst undertaking pre-arranged meetings with those story-tellers who lived within travelling distance of my base in London. I will be forever indebted to Jane for all her kindness, the use of her beautiful home and her endless love and understanding. I miss her every single day knowing that I can never pick up the phone and hear her voice. Bless you, you amazing human being!

London was an entirely new cultural experience for me, as I had only ever visited here once with my parents when I was young. It was a little daunting at first but I soon became well-rehearsed on the tube and took pleasure from many new and unusual experiences. When I was travelling outside the London area and if the story-teller personally suggested that I might stay overnight, this is what took place. Home-cooked food and amazing hospitality became the norm, which further nourished our already established personal relationships. It was an amazing experience for me.

Whilst in London during my frequent stays, Jane taught me so much and we spent a lot of time visiting the main tourist attractions and neighbouring locations. I certainly had no idea about travel permits, London zones and where places were situated in relation to each other. In reality I had difficulty identifying north from south and seriously struggled to read the A to Z. Jane gave me valuable cost-saving advice and I was able to obtain travel permits across the 4 zones I would be visiting during my work schedule. Having a London base meant I could arrange to comfortably travel to places like Reading, Southampton, Surrey and Bournemouth to interview story-tellers located in these regions. It was not only advantageous in terms of savings on time and costs but it was also a place of refuge; a safe haven where I could relax and unwind during my free time. I learned so much from Jane during my visits; she is one of the most remarkable women I have ever had the pleasure to meet.

Arranging, travelling and taking part in interviews every day was a surprisingly exhausting experience; what with my boundless nervous energy and the excitement too. I do remember it was incredibly hot during one of my scheduled visits to London. I had packed clothes for typical Yorkshire weather and was overcome with the heat for a few days. The unfamiliar surroundings and the meeting of people in their own environment was an overwhelming experience. Everyone was extremely hospitable, honest and open and some expressed such gratitude for my spending time exploring HIV-related matters with them. It was an incredibly humbling experience.

Before I went on my first trip to London, I took part in a one day workshop on 'Listening Skills' which was immeasurably valuable as it enhanced and polished some skills I had forgotten about and taught me new ones besides. Prior to leaving for London I meticulously planned my interview schedule for fear of making big blunders on the basis of my poor sense of direction. I learned a great deal about myself during this stage of the research. I wrote everything down: pre-arranged dates and times for meetings, names, addresses and clear directions for each visit. I entered all of these in my research diary and also took another small pocket-sized notepad with me with the same information written inside just in case I misplaced my diary. From home using the internet I found out train times and costs for travelling to, for example, Reading or Southampton in advance so I knew exactly what I was doing when in London. Jane had no internet access but there was an Internet Café close by. I asked each person to advise which tube stations to go from and gave Kings Cross as my point of reference. It was the only station I was familiar with in terms of getting to and from my North London base. Planning in advance saved me an enormous amount of time whilst I was in London and gave me free time to spend with Jane. It was a fabulous experience overall.

I am pleased to say my time keeping was surprisingly accurate too. I was on time for every interview with one exception. After an overnight stay with one story-teller and talking very late into the night, the following day I had an early afternoon interview with someone I was not familiar with. Following directions using the tube, I lost my sense of direction on foot and frustratingly was half an hour late. In my defence, once I left the tube station I did feel the 'on foot' directions were not as clear cut as they could have been. Furthermore, a half hour delay was a vast improvement on the Birmingham experience. In summary, detailed planning and preparation for travelling does take time but it is an absolute necessity and extremely worthwhile.

When staying away from home for prolonged periods, I had to ensure that I had all my necessary research documentation: personal information sheets, consent forms, interview schedule etc, in addition to recording equipment, telephone and other chargers, reusable batteries, sufficient tapes and so on. These were in addition to ensuring that I had clothes, toiletries and other creature comforts. Amazingly, I did not forget anything on any trip. It is a great pity that I did not have a laptop during this time; this would have been enormously useful.

Being unfamiliar with London did not pose any major problems for me and everybody involved made sure they gave me very clear and specific instructions to their homes. If a person lived in an area considered unsafe at certain times of the day or evening I was subsequently informed of this. I supposed that London and inner city areas were no different to many other cities and were perhaps no more or less safe than more familiar parts of West Yorkshire. I believe I took the necessary precautionary measures to be as 'safe' as practicably possible and I did have a personal safety system in place.

On the subject of safe practices, I did experience an incident quite early on whilst arranging an interview much closer to home. As a consequence, this led to my developing a security code alert system between me and my partner when conducting interviews with story-tellers I had not previously met who were new to the study. Having arranged by telephone a face-to-face interview in Manchester with a man I had not met previously, I mentioned to a friend that I was going to be in a certain area of Manchester to conduct an interview; I asked my friend if he would like to meet up beforehand. My friend became really anxious as he was familiar with the area and stated it was an extremely dangerous, murderous, rough no-go area even for the police. Alarm bells began to ring and I became somewhat nervous and agitated as the person I was to meet had failed to mention anything about the area.

Consequently, I asked my partner to accompany me in the car and sit in a nearby street in case of emergency. Our meeting was scheduled for early evening. When I examined the story-teller's personal information sheet, there was limited detail about the man I was going to visit. On it was written only his name, address and telephone number as he had only recently contacted me via an advertisement in the HIV press. It was noted, however, that he had recently moved from the South to the Manchester area. This might explain why nothing had been mentioned about the location of our meeting; he might be totally unaware of the reputation of his new home. All the same, I quickly designed a security code alert system so that my partner could check on my personal safety during our interview.

After being in the house for 10 minutes my partner was to call me. He would be sitting in the car located on the next street and I was to relay one of the following codes:

Code zero which means: 'I am not safe. Come to the house or call the police and give details of where I am.'
Code one which means: 'the situation is unclear so call me back in 5 minutes. If there is no response call the police.'
Code two which means: 'I am OK at present. Please call me back in 15 minutes to make sure.'
Code three which means: 'I feel fine and safe but to make sure call me back in half an hour.'
Code four which means: 'Everything is fine and safe. No need to call back as phone will be switched off after this security check.'

As it transpired, when my partner made the call I used *code four* and felt moderately guilty and embarrassed at my nervous panic and obvious distress. The man was a tremendously warm, accommodating human being who kindly offered me a welcome glass of wine to put me at ease prior to starting our conversation. I do believe that my personal distress was so clearly apparent to him that after the phone call I had to be totally honest and told him of the situation. He thought I was just nervous and clearly had no idea whatsoever of the area's reputation and was grateful for the information. He told me he might be thinking about moving pretty soon. We laughed about this and the atmosphere was brilliantly transformed into a calm and relaxed mood.

Whilst this was a false alarm it did bring to the forefront the notion that personal safety and security was a real issue which was addressed immediately. I must report that I did not feel the need to ever use this security alert code again but I was satisfied the system had been put in place. I did, however, telephone my partner after each interview once I was leaving the premises if I was not staying overnight. Indeed, I felt it necessary that my partner be aware of all the locations I was visiting whether I was staying away in London, the Midlands or driving to nearby areas where I lived for my own personal safety.

Reflections on being there: doing conversations with a purpose

Taking part in each of our conversations involved a certain kind of interpersonal interaction which differed from anything I had previously experienced. As a social form, experiencing the interview differed from other types of interactions I had become familiar with, for example: public lectures, student seminars, job interviews, board meetings, supervisory meetings and student and staff counselling sessions to name a few. Certainly we had already established a personal relationship between ourselves before our conversation but it was still a qualitatively different experience than any other that had gone before.

Between us we were engaging in a type of conversation that you might expect among very close friends; our conversations related to personal and lived experiences of HIV-related matters. Nonetheless these conversations were not the same as those of close friends because it was mutually assumed that each interaction was for a pragmatic purpose and not solely as a conversation in itself. In other words our personal interaction was understood to be a 'conversation with a purpose' that transcended beyond a friendship relationship. Understanding this was one thing, but actually experiencing these interactions was another.

The first few interviews were stressful and intimidating experiences for me which unleashed unexpected feelings of trepidation and led to my questioning my own competence. The telephone interview was more awkward than face-to-face conversations, and there were instances when I firmly believed I was unnecessarily intruding in the personal lives of the people concerned; I began to question my right to be doing this and felt out of my depth. Taking part in the first couple of interviews was a peculiar and surreal experience. No matter how much training, reading and preparation one might do around any area of study it is never the same as actually experiencing something first-hand. There appeared to be so many significant matters to take into account during every personal interaction.

As we now know, the research process in its entirety requires that you are multi-faceted. A researcher apparently has to be a 'Jack-or-Jill of all trades' and, without sounding like an incessant whinge bag, it is overwhelmingly demanding to begin with; especially if you seriously reflect on and critically take into account all aspects of the process. Our first few meetings demanded many considerations in addition to effectively listening and responding appropriately to the personal experiences of the story-tellers. At all times I was conscious of whether the tape recorder was working properly. It was imperative to conduct a sound check near the beginning of each conversation; this could be distracting for us both but then I had to ensure it was still working. Imagine if the tape recorder had not been working for the largest part of the interview… Was the recording of our conversations likely to distract story-tellers? Throughout the course of each lengthy interview I had to check that the tape had switched over to side B and nothing was lost. I was anxious to ensure the recording of the interview was not a distraction in itself; it appeared to be unproblematic for the story-tellers just problematic for myself.

Next I was worrying about if I was listening effectively and understanding what was being said. Equally, when responding was it in an appropriate manner? Was the story-teller still comfortable with the interview experience? Am I seeking clarification of certain issues at appropriate times? Am I distracting the story-teller's train of thought in any way? When asking questions or trying to seek clarification on an issue am I being too abrupt? Do I appear as if I have my own agenda and am not interested in what is currently being discussed? Are long silences an indication of discomfort? Is it my turn to speak? Am I maintaining a suitable conversational flow from one theme to another in a smooth and logical way or is it disjointed? Goodness me! The complexities involved with thinking critically and observing our situation in conjunction with talking, responding and listening was, at times, so intense. I was particularly keen to ensure the story-teller was comfortable and relaxed with our conversation. One of us had to be!

Over time, my anxious state diminished and I became mentally more confident, competent and prepared, thus feeling more relaxed and comfortable in doing what I was doing. Soon I started to genuinely enjoy our conversations, yet it is worthy to draw attention to the intensities of my feelings of incompetence and the negativities I experienced at the beginning. My knowledge of innumerable textbooks focussing on 'how to do' qualitative interviews was, to some extent, inadequate when it actually came to the doing of an interview.

Within the 'how-to-do' textbooks there is little space that seeks to explore differing perceptions of moral commitments, personal goals and primary objectives in the quest for knowledge from the perspective of the researcher. Equally, comprehensive ethical themes for consideration and how potentially powerful emotions of the researcher might emerge from conducting interviews are simply not dealt with. Consequently the intensity of emotions and perceptions of the researcher can be a shocking experience when you initially start interviewing story-tellers. Nevertheless, we all have to start somewhere and the whole adventure was an illuminating learning experience and one I would most definitely do again if necessary.

Telephone interviews: some reflections

As one might expect, telephone conversations are significantly different from face-to-face encounters and I am pleased that there were only four telephone interviews. For me, these interactions were the most demanding and I would not consider these the most effective method of interview for the purpose of a sensitive explorative study such as this. The sound quality when recording telephone conversations was, at times, problematic. Fortunately I conducted only one telephone interview with a story-teller I had not met beforehand. Unfortunately this was to be my first telephone interview and it was not a particularly rewarding experience from my point of view; I felt it went badly. As there is no visual contact between participants you cannot always determine how well proceedings are going and if you do not know the person you are speaking to, this creates further problems. Additionally, there is always a fear that the person you are calling might not answer. Thankfully this did not happen.

Whilst conducting my first telephone interview I was overcome with anxieties and fear. I recall being hesitant and unclear with my questions and wondered if I was making the right noises when the story-teller was describing some pretty horrific experiences related to his HIV-positive status. I was filled with self-doubt and left wondering if the responses and comments I made were patronising or demeaning in any way. Looking back at the transcript, whilst it felt like it was a terrifying experience at the time, it was not all that bad. The story-teller's experiences were quite different from many others; he lived with a debilitating mental health condition as well as HIV and took medication that left him confused and disorientated. He was helpful, kind and accommodating and upon reflection I could have explored issues in more detail had I been more competent at the time. I believe a face-to-face interview would have been more rewarding and less fearsome had this been possible.

The rest of the telephone interviews were more positive as we had already established strong personal relationships, exchanged numerous e-mails and had all met each other on previous occasions. My second telephone interview was with a man who had an extremely busy time schedule and this was his chosen method of interview. Unfortunately his telephone was cordless and this led to some sound quality problems which I later discovered whilst transcribing. Parts of our conversation centred on sensitive and distressing reflections of the past and his voice often became very quiet. This transcript took me three days and countless telephone calls before it was completed. Between us we filled in the gaps. Two days after the interview the man e-mailed me to say that the interview went well. He stated that I was 'sensitive in the right places without being over-the-top [to use his expression] and I made all the right noises at the right time. It was pitched just right.' I was over the moon with this feedback.

A forgotten generation: Long-term survivors' experiences of HIV and AIDS

The two remaining telephone interviews were not the chosen method of interview but as we had to reschedule our meetings due to illness this was our only option. Neither of these interviews was problematic as I knew each story-teller very well and we conducted these interviews towards the end of the interviewing process so I was well rehearsed by this time. There were no problems with transcribing our conversations and both interviews were extremely productive. On reflection I would not have liked to have conducted too many telephone interviews for the purpose of this study as apart from being beneficial in terms of time, costs and geographical location, the face-to-face interview was better suited to the focus of this study.

Face-to-face interviews: some reflections

Telling someone face-to-face about intimate characteristics of one's self and/or personal life is a complicated affair. As a form of confessional disclosure, sensitive conversations such as ours demand a guaranteed atmosphere of privacy, confidentiality and anonymity to maintain and further develop openness and mutual trust. To establish an even safer and protective environment, I believe it is imperative to be non-judgemental and not display condemnatory attitudes towards those telling their story or matters under discussion. I am not implying here that you have to continually express your approval without forms of (dis)agreement and further debate during such conversations. Instead I suggest it is possible to show support and a broad understanding of most given situations without unconditional approval by truly listening and effectively communicating with respect and genuine appreciation.

I believe a researcher should be constantly aware of her/his own attitudes, non-verbal behaviours and how she/he might be perceived by the story-teller so as not to affect the legitimacy and validity of any conversation in a detrimental way. In other words, we as researchers should always be aware of how we might affect or influence disclosures within a guided conversation, to avoid generating potential falsehoods or bias during conversation. I was continually aware of my self during each meeting; I tried to avoid any unwelcome outcomes during the entire interview process that might emanate from harmful behaviour. I acknowledge that this is not always attainable and I am equally aware that the story-teller can also have a detrimental effect on the interview process which can influence dialogue and social interaction.

A forgotten generation: Long-term survivors' experiences of HIV and AIDS

I recall an interview with one of my closest friends, who worked in the field, and who had initially inspired me to adopt a long-term survivors approach to my HIV study based on his personal experiences. During our conversation I became increasingly aware that his story was in fact indicative of his vast wealth of HIV-related knowledge as opposed to reflections of his own personal experiences of living with HIV over a long period of time. It soon became evident by his language and other certain irregularities, that he was making use of his HIV knowledge and experiences of others as the basis of his narrative. We had previously agreed we would be exploring his personal experiences of living with an AIDS-related illness and I knew these pretty well, as we had been close friends for many years.

As a consequence, I felt that the interview was being obscured and hijacked by his competitive desire to demonstrate his knowledge and awareness of HIV matters. His reluctance to concentrate on his own lived experiences when I raised my concerns during our conversation was becoming a source of frustration. That familiar glint in his eyes gave him away (I am smiling as I write this). We subsequently agreed to do the interview again at a later date; I could not include that particular conversation within the study. I learned a great deal from this experience and am so grateful that his competitive nature could not be quelled. It gave me a sense of awareness that I had not fully considered beforehand. If I had not been so familiar with this particular story-teller, would I have known what was going on? In truth, to a large extent, yes I think I would, but my awareness became more acute after this particular experience.

Whilst interviewer and interviewee effects and bias are widely acknowledged within academic textbooks, there are limited considerations on how uncomfortable the researcher might be about asking sensitive and personal questions during guided conversations. In my case, at the beginning I was extremely uncomfortable participating in our face-to-face conversations especially with people I did not know particularly well, despite discussing in detail the broad themes for exploration in terms of HIV-related matters. The more conversations I took part in, the more I achieved a sense of collaboration with the story-tellers; yet this only came to pass over time. I had purposely not prepared a rigid structure for our 'conversations with a purpose' so story-tellers would not be restricted. I did, nevertheless, have a semi-standardised system in place that sought to explore dominant themes in no particular order. It was suitably structured and organised sufficiently well enough to be a valid and robust HIV study, whilst simultaneously open and receptive to allow for the inclusion of other dominant themes that might emerge during our conversations.

A forgotten generation: Long-term survivors' experiences of HIV and AIDS

The power dynamics of face-to-face interviews was rather confusing and ambiguous at the start. As witnessed earlier, I had challenged notions of maintaining a 'professional distance' and emotional detachment in favour of developing a personal relationship based on mutual trust and openness by establishing a good rapport with as many story-tellers as practicably possible. I therefore held the belief that the power relationship between me and the story-tellers were of equal status. Whereas I did distinguish the story-teller as the 'expert' and myself as the 'student' I did not consider our conversations as an 'elite interview'. In other words, I did not consider my own status as lower than that of the story-teller – we were equals.

There were a few occasions when story-tellers perceived me as an 'expert' in HIV matters and sought guidance and advice which was a little tricky and awkward at first. But over time I was soon able to share information based on my own and other people's HIV knowledge and experiences. In some cases, after seeking appropriate consent from individuals, I was able to put people in touch with each other. That was gratifying! If someone was interested in finding out about current combination therapies and potential side effects, I could pass on useful websites or addresses for HIV, self-help or other-related voluntary organisations whereby they could access vital information. In other cases, if I knew a person who was currently taking a particular drug regimen, I was able to put them in touch with that person after seeking appropriate consent between the two parties. This was beneficial to us all.

My own willingness to self-disclose to story-tellers who wanted to know more about me as a person was essential to promote collaboration between us, allowing us to share power and develop a mutual understanding during our conversations. At the same time I was able to direct our conversational flow wherever necessary to explore those dominant themes previously agreed between ourselves. I was keen to show my genuine desire for understanding HIV-related matters by demonstrating my willingness to listen empathically and by expressing my own concerns and emotions. I was also willing, whenever necessary, to share similar personal experiences if it demonstrated mutual understanding. On the other hand, wherever demonstrations of understanding were not possible or in circumstances where I could not relate similar experiences, I did not pretend to understand how certain situations might have been perceived or experienced. It was vital to maintain a genuine and honest approach to maintain integrity without being hypocritical and disingenuous.

A forgotten generation: Long-term survivors' experiences of HIV and AIDS

In many cases the story-tellers had accumulated a vast wealth of knowledge pertaining to HIV-related matters over a prolonged period of time. There were a few people who worked in the field and some had been AIDS activists in earlier times. If I was unfamiliar with any issue under discussion I said so and I learned a great deal. At no time did I ever pretend to be familiar with any matter if this was not the case. I believe it is vital to be as honest and truthful as possible in such circumstances. Pretending to be aware of something can be potentially humiliating and hazardous to relationships you are attempting to develop. It was important not to pretend you knew things when you didn't, as it might be embarrassing if this eventually came to light. To be sure, if certain information or knowledge was unfamiliar, it was important to say so and was a clear indication of mutual honesty and integrity.

During a few of our conversations, it was evident that story-tellers wanted to share more than just HIV-related aspects of their personal lives. In some situations, people wanted to show me things in their homes, presents from their loved ones, even photographs of their family and close friends and we even shared certain activities outside of the interview process. On one occasion I went to play bingo (something I had never done before) with one story-teller. Whilst I found it fun and at times difficult to follow all the numbers at such speed, this was a serious hobby for those participating. On other occasions I went charity shopping and once people knew that I liked this type of shopping it became almost part of a ritual, especially amongst those who knew each other well. I shared many lunches and evening meals with people and, in some instances we went out again months later following our interviews. On more than a few occasions, story-tellers had invited their close friends around for meals in order to meet me after our scheduled meetings. These were very social occasions and I was privileged to be included in their friendship circles. Some people even gave me small presents and gifts so that I might always remember them. Priceless!

At times our conversations were interrupted by telephone calls, people knocking at the door, cats knocking my drink over, dogs licking my face and partners interrupting us by asking questions. These were all included in the typed transcript. On one occasion I had to reschedule another meeting to finish our conversation as the story-teller had other appointments and places to go. During our conversation he often lost his train of thought and was distracted by other things because he was quite ill. Fortunately he lived close by and so this was not problematic. We developed a good relationship after our interview until he sadly passed away months later. I was fortunate enough to be able to spend time with him and offer support until the end. I learned so much from this experience and he will never be forgotten.

During one interview in London, I arrived at the door of an address I had been given and it was answered by someone other than the story-teller I had met previously. I told the person my name and why I was there and he closed the door in my face. After a few minutes, the door opened and the story-teller appeared. He was very dishevelled and apologetic and had forgotten about our scheduled meeting. This experience brought to my attention the need to telephone in advance prior to our interviews, so that this did not happen again. This was my first first-to-face interview in London and I was quite taken aback for a few minutes.

During a conversation with one story-teller who worked in the field and was used to being interviewed, I felt that in places his story was well rehearsed and had been told before. I have no desire to demean or devalue those personal experiences, feelings and emotions that were conveyed during our conversation. I wish merely to acknowledge that these moments appeared less spontaneous and were more rehearsed than other stories I had previously heard. At times he broke down and cried when reflecting on past and current experiences and the loss of loved ones; this was by no means any less emotive or real than other narratives. Here my personal experiences raised my level of awareness that, in some instances, story-tellers had told their private stories in public on previous occasions. The story-teller confirmed that in the past, like a few others, he had accessed self-help groups and attended training courses which focussed on positive mental attitude and personal growth.

On numerous occasions I was told that our conversations had been extremely positive experiences for those who shared their stories. It was not uncommon for story-tellers to mention that having the opportunity to speak about their personal experiences and reflect on living with HIV had led to a sense of relief, individual personal satisfaction and in some situations was a form of closure. I received a letter from one man who told me that our interview had been an extremely positive and beneficial experience for him as it had helped him articulate things that he had not even thought through himself. He thanked me for my time and genuine interest. This was so reassuring.

Undoubtedly, the more interviews we accomplished between us the more competent I became in picking up and paying closer attention to detail. I was continually gaining confidence. Amazingly, many of the story-tellers themselves put me at ease although some were as nervous as I at the beginning. During one interview with a man, he was quite clearly more agitated and nervous than I had ever been during an interview. I became very aware of his nervousness and did not want to prolong his agony. He was twitching his leg and playing with a pen and was obviously apprehensive despite his friendly and accommodating approach and a desire to participate in the HIV study. We spoke about his nervousness during our conversation and I believe it did affect the content of our conversation. However, once I had left his home I kept in touch with him and we held further discussions by telephone to fill in the gaps.

I cannot ignore that during the interview process parts of our conversations were deeply emotional and moving and therefore did have an effect on me. From a psychological perspective, whilst I was gathering these personal experiences I sometimes felt quite sad and isolated. I had listened to the experiences and narratives of over 30 women and men during this period. My physical and emotional energies were beginning to deplete and it was mentioned by more than one person that I should seek appropriate counselling services for my own personal well-being. This was good advice. I certainly did feel the need to talk to someone so that I could off load my thoughts in a safe and professional environment for my own sanity and preservation. Unfortunately I did not actually pursue this in the end. I now realise that I should have made time for this, but time was something quite scarce. Sometimes we ought to practice what we preach.

The women and men who took part in this story-of-stories were so supportive of me and the HIV study. Their own courage and enthusiasm for the research made all the worry, stress and trauma, not to mention the long hours and the hard work of planning and preparation, very meaningful and worthwhile. This is why the completion of this story-of-stories in this particular format is paramount. It is not my intention here to sound artificial and insincere; it is the truth. For me, the entire experience with all the ups and downs has been and continues to be a worthwhile journey.

Transcribing our conversations: personal issues and reflections

The recording of audio taped conversations for the purpose of transcription is common practice in qualitative research. It is a method for collating information in textual form principally for coding and analysis by the researcher. Yet oddly the quality of the transcription process is not always afforded too much attention, methodologically speaking. Transcribing interviews is often a task relegated to others who might not have participated in the interview in the first instance. As the transcribing of interviews is an extremely time-consuming task, it is often considered acceptable to only write-up important features of the interview. It is common practice to ignore the ums and ahs if you are doing this task yourself. To be sure, I was advised to document the most interesting parts of each conversation that related to my themes, as the transcribing process was taking a long time to complete. I ignored this advice. I had made a promise to story-tellers that the interview was being recorded for a particular purpose; I had also made promises to myself to maintain accurate details of all recordings.

The quality of my transcripts was a verbatim facsimile of what was discussed during each conversation with a purpose. The accuracy of each transcript was paramount to depict and capture the social reality of each interview as it was experienced and expressed to me by the story-teller. Each transcript captured not only what was said, but often how it was said. For example, italics were often used in conjunction with brackets affirming the participant was laughing, sobbing, twitching, or when voices became quiet; even prolonged silences were recorded within each transcript. I believe the exactness of each conversation was paramount in order to facilitate a more reflective and critical analysis of each story afterwards. To be sure, I am more than grateful that I pursued such preciseness as when I read and re-read each transcript I am subsequently transported back to the time of our conversation yet again.

A one and a half hour interview took approximately 10 hours to transcribe [and the rest] and that was only if our voices were clear on the recording. As a qualified secretary in a previous life who could type at between 65 and 70 words per minute, this was an arduous and time-consuming task from an administrative point of view. I transcribed all the interviews myself because of the confidentiality issues involved in the sensitive research. Also, by transcribing the stories, it gave me an opportunity of encapsulating the experiences a second time. It should be mentioned here that I also took notes during each conversation in order to assist my memory, recall valuable information or elaborate on specific points and provide back up in case of any technical problems. Taking notes enhanced my listening skills and made room for identifying possible questions to ask later when appropriate. My pitman shorthand was a useful skill for this practice and having notes available to read shortly after each interview was extremely useful to identify and reconstruct significant points.

After completion of each transcript, I gave each story-teller the same opportunity to change or edit and add or remove any conversations that took place during our interview. In a few cases, people added and expanded upon issues and for the rest, the transcripts remained unchanged. One person I interviewed decided to opt out of the research after receiving the typed transcript. He believed that he was not always lucid and during our interview spoke of his forgetfulness in everyday life; he held the belief that he was living with the onset of AIDS-related dementia. The fact that he did not complete sentences during our conversation, confirmed this. I tried to reassure him by explaining that very few of us when speaking complete sentences and most people who told me their story had similar transcripts such as his own. He would not accept this and felt uncomfortable to proceed further with the research and so opted out. We still remained in close contact and I visited him again afterwards to make sure all was well and no harm had been done by his initial involvement in the research. I felt terrible but he was adamant that no harm had been done and was happy to have met me.

On a lighter note, one rather embarrassing mistake I made was not paying sufficient postage on some of the transcripts I sent out. Several people reported back that it had been necessary to collect their transcripts from the post office as insufficient postage had been paid and additional payment was required. Thankfully those few who experienced this oversight were laughing about this and were more than happy for me to buy them a beer when I next saw them. I am grateful for their understanding and good sense of humour.

The writing up process: reflections and challenges

I have no desire to reflect on too many matters here as the data analysis and writing up process of the PhD is so qualitatively different to the written layout of this story-of-stories. By the writing stage of the PhD journey I was disillusioned and found that I was beginning to lose the emotive, descriptive and valid content of the stories I had successfully accumulated during our guided conversations. The HIV study had amassed a huge amount of information which was far more than I was allowed to incorporate in the PhD thesis. To sort and manage the dominant themes into practical categories for theoretical exploration and critical analysis seemed unworkable without sufficient room for detailed descriptions of personal experiences.

There was insufficient space for me to include in-depth descriptions in the data analysis section after I had incorporated the literature review, numerous substantive chapters, the section on methodology, the bibliography and so on. I did not set out to test theories or preconceived ideas based on my research findings. This HIV study was, in some ways, rather unique and unlike any other HIV research post-1996. For me, the political objective of this HIV study was to be socially productive and useful and it was rapidly losing its edge.

As I had recently been in hospital, and had experienced prolonged episodes of chest infections and ill health I had to take sick leave. Due to continued ill health, necessary work commitments in order to live, and my changing personal circumstances, with regret I decided to leave the PhD programme of study before I had completed the writing up stage of my research. A couple of years later, I thought about writing a non-academic story-of-stories based on the findings of my HIV study from a long-term survivors' perspective. I felt by approaching it this way I could pay particular attention to and totally focus on the detailed personal experiences of living long-term with HIV and AIDS-related illness using the voices of the story-tellers. My political aim began to take shape once more and whilst it has taken me many years to successfully complete this book, I am now facing the end of my journey.

Writing the book in this particular layout has, in places, been challenging and difficult to complete. I have been academically trained and therefore spent many years reading and writing academic essays, dissertations and other texts, using: references and bibliographies, incorporating theories of other writers and adopting perspectives and disciplinary approaches within the social science, and adopting technical language which conveys specific meanings within particular academic disciplines that subsequently target academic, graduate and post-graduate audiences. By writing the book in this particular format, it has been a challenge for me. The importance of raising our awareness about fundamental concerns relating to HIV and long-term survival is paramount. It has therefore been necessary to write in such a way that will hopefully reach and inform a much wider audience.

To this end, I have had to entirely revisit my work, reconsider and write new chapters using language that seeks to explain and enhance our understanding using a more generalised approach. I have attempted to ensure that I pay particular attention to technical and medical language and terminology in order to explain wherever necessary what I am attempting to communicate in terms of meaning. At times, writing for a wider audience has made me think in more depth and it soon became crucial to involve the reader in this story-of-stories as much as possible. One of the reasons why I chose to include a glossary at the end of the book is because I cannot always avoid using technical or medical language.

I have had to go back and re-code some of the dominant themes and place these into different categories relating to similar and dissimilar personal experience. If there had been sufficient time to immerse myself in the data I had gathered during my research, and I had been given sufficient space to write more detailed descriptions within the PhD thesis it might have been a different story. Nevertheless, writing this book has enabled me to become more familiar with the stories and experiences that were shared. Having the space to revisit all the transcripts in my own time has subsequently shaped this story-of-stories into what we now see before us. This is now the end of my incredible journey and I would like to thank you, the readers, for sharing it with me.

GLOSSARY

∞

ACUTE INFECTION
A severe infection lasting for a short period of time (less than six months).

ADHERENCE
The act of taking medical treatment exactly as prescribed; this includes sticking closely to recommended ways of using HIV medication i.e. taking pills in accordance with dosage times and diet restrictions.

ADVERSE EVENT
An unwanted side-effect caused by a treatment and usually detected in a clinical trial with participants.

AIDS
Acquired Immune Deficiency Syndrome: A collection of specific illnesses and conditions that occur because the body's immune system has been damaged by HIV-infection.

AIDS-DEFINING ILLNESS
A serious opportunistic infection which would lead to a medical diagnosis of AIDS in an HIV-positive person.

AIDS DEMENTIA COMPLEX (ADC)
A degenerative neurological condition attributed to HIV infection and characterised by certain clinical presentations, such as: mood swings, loss of co-ordination, cognitive dysfunctions, and loss of inhibitions and is the most common central nervous system (CNS) complication of HIV infection.

AIDS-RELATED COMPLEX (ARC)
A term used by clinicians to describe a variety of symptoms and signs found in people living with HIV and AIDS including: recurrent fevers, weight loss, swollen lymph nodes, herpes, diarrhoea and fungal mouth infections.

ANAEMIA
A shortage or change in the size or function of red blood cells. These cells carry oxygen to cells in the body and leads to fatigue and skin turning pale.

ANERGY
A lack of reaction by the body's defence mechanisms when foreign substances come into contact with the body. This often indicates the inability of the immune system to mount a normal allergic response and can be thought of as the opposite of allergy, which is an overreaction to a substance.

ANOSCOPY
Examination of the anal canal and lower rectum using a short speculum.

ANTIBIOTIC
A substance that affects kills or inhibits the growth of micro organisms such as bacteria and fungi.

ANTIBODY
Protein substances produced by the immune system that tag, destroy or neutralise foreign organisms such as bacteria, viruses and other harmful toxins (antigens).

ANTIGEN
Any 'foreign' substance that stimulates or antagonises the immune system to produce antibodies.

ANTIOXIDANT
A vitamin, mineral or drug that reduces the activity of free radicals – the unpaired electrons that are produced as a result of burning energy in a cell.

ANTIRETROVIAL THERAPY (ART)
Any number of treatments designed to destroy retroviruses, such as HIV or interfere with their ability to replicate (reproduce).

ARV
A short term for antiretroviral therapy

ASSAY
A test used for measuring something.

ASYMPTOMATIC
Without having any symptoms; usually describes a person who has tested HIV-positive yet shows no clinical symptoms of the illness condition.

ATAXIA
A lack of muscular co-ordination.

ATROPHY
Wasting caused by nutritional imbalance e.g.: due to absorption problems caused by diarrhoea.

AZT
Zidovudine (ZDV): a nucleoside reverse transcriptase inhibitor (licensed in 1987) and initially used on its own and later in combination with other drug regimens. It is a failed chemotherapy drug.

BACTERAEMIA
The presence of bacteria in the blood.

BACTERIA
Tiny microscopic single-celled organisms often called germs. Many bacteria cause disease in humans.

BASELINE
The starting point or value with which an unknown is compared when measured or assessed.

BASOPHIL
A type of white blood cell, also called granular leukocyte, filled with granules of toxic chemicals that can digest micro organisms. Basophils, as well as other white blood cells, are responsible for some of the symptoms of an allergy.

B-CELLS
One of the two major classes of lymphocytes (immune cells) responsible for making antibodies. B cells are blood cells of immune system derived from the bone marrow and the spleen. During infections these cells are transformed into plasma cells which produce large quantities of antibody directed at specific pathogens.

BILE
A fluid produced by the liver. Partly a secretion of waste products and partly aids digestion by breaking down fats and assisting the absorption of nutrients.

BILIRUBIN
A red pigment occurring in liver bile, blood and urine. Its measurement can be used as an indication of the health of the liver. Bilirubin is the product of the breakdown of haemoglobin in red blood cells. It is removed from the blood and processed in the liver. If excretion is impaired by liver damage, bilirubin accumulates in the blood and can cause jaundice.

BIOAVAILABILITY
The extent to which an oral medication is absorbed in the digestive tract and reaches the bloodstream.

BIOPSY
A small sample of tissue removed from a living thing that may be examined microscopically to make diagnosis or determine the presence of abnormal cells.

BLOOD PRODUCTS
Blood itself and any other product derived from it, such as factor VIII and plasma.

BODY FLUIDS
Any fluid in the human body, such as blood, urine, saliva (spit), sputum, tears, semen, vaginal secretions or mother's milk. Only blood, semen, vaginal secretions and mother's milk have been directly linked to HIV transmission.

BONE MARROW
Soft tissue located in the cavities of the bones where blood cells such as erythrocytes, leukocytes and platelets are formed.

BOOSTER
A second or later dose of a vaccine given to increase the immune response to the original dose.

BRONCHOSCOPY
A visual examination of the bronchial passages of the lungs using the tube of an endoscope (a curved flexible tube containing fibres that carry light down the tube and project an enlarged image up the tube to the viewer). This tube is inserted in the upper lungs and can be used to take material from the lungs.

'BUFFALO HUMP'
Fat accumulation on the back of the neck and shoulders associated with hormonal changes and lipodystophy.

CAESAREAN SECTION
Method of birth where the child is delivered through a cut made in the womb.

CANDIDIASIS
A disease caused by a yeast-like fungus of the Candida family commonly found in the normal flora of the mouth, skin, intestinal tract and vagina which can be clinically infectious in immune-compromised persons. Candidiasis of the oesophagus, trachea, bronchi or lungs is an indicator disease of AIDS. Oral and recurrent vaginal Candida infection is an early sign of immune deterioration.

CARCINOMA
A malignant tumour that may spread throughout the body.

CATHETER
A tubular device that is implanted into canals, vessels, passageways or body cavities to permit injections (though an intravenous catheter into the vein) or to allow withdrawals of fluids out of the body or to keep a passage open.

CAT SCAN
Computerised Axial Tomography (CAT) scan. A type of specialised x-ray that allows a view of a 'slice' through the body and is used to detect tumours, infections and other changes in the anatomy.

CCR5 INHIBITORS
A new class of antiretrovirals which acts at a similar point in the HIV life cycle to Fusion Inhibitors by blocking HIV from entering a target cell and stopping it from making more copies of itself.

CD4 (CD4+) cells
A type of white blood T-cell involved in protecting against viral, fungal and protozoal infections. These cells normally start the immune response, signalling other cells in the immune system to perform their special functions. Also referred to as T-helper cells. The preferred target of HIV are cells that have a docking molecule called 'cluster designation 4' (CD4) on

their surfaces. Cells with this molecule are known as CD4-positive cells. Destruction of these lymphocytes is the major cause of the immunodeficiency observed in AIDS and decreasing CD4+ lymphocyte levels appear to be the best indicator for developing opportunistic infections.

CD8 (T8) cells
A protein encased in the cell surface of suppressor T-lymphocytes; also known cytotoxic T-cells. Some CD8 cells recognise and destroy cancerous cells and those infected by intracellular pathogens (some bacteria, viruses and mycoplasma).

CENTRAL NERVOUS SYSTEM (CNS)
The Central Nervous System (CNS) is composed of the brain, spinal cord and the meninges (protective membranes surrounding them). Although monocytes and macrophages can be infected by HIV they appear to be relatively resistant to destruction. However these cells do travel through the body and carry HIV to various organs (especially the lungs and the brain). People living with HIV and AIDS quite often experience abnormalities in the CNS.

CEREBRAL
Pertaining to the cerebrum: the main portion of the brain.

CERVIX
The neck of the womb at the top of the vagina.

CHLAMYDIA
A sexually transmitted disease that consists of bacterium (Chlamydia trachomatis) that infects the reproductive system. The infection is frequently asymptomatic and if left untreated can cause sterility in women.

CHOLESTEROL
A waxy substance mostly made by the body and used to produce steroid hormones. Popularly associated with atherosclerosis.

CHROMOSOME
A rod-like portion of the chromatin of a cell nucleus that performs an important part of the mimetic cell-division, and is also important in the transmission of hereditary factors.

CHRONIC INFECTION
An infection that tends to last for a long period of time (usually more than six months).

CIRRHOSIS
Fibrosis of the whole liver when it starts to look yellow and nodular and shrivels.

CLADES
The term for the different sub-types of HIV. A clade is a group of related HIV isolates classified in accordance to the degree of genetic similarity (such as the percentage of identity within their envelope genes).

CLAP CLINIC
See G U M clinic

CLINICAL
Founded on observation and treatment of patients as distinguished from theoretical and/or basic science. In other words the nursing or medical care of patients.

CLINICAL EVENT
The occurrence of a physical sign or symptom rather than an abnormality that can only be detected in a laboratory test.

CLINICAL TRIAL
A scientifically designed and executed investigation (or research study) examining the effects of a drug or medical regimen administered to people. The goal is to determine the safety, clinical efficacy and pharmacological effects (including toxicity, side effects, incompatibilities and interactions) of the drug or regimen.

CLOTTING FACTORS
Chemicals made in the liver to help stop bleeding.

COHORT
A group of people who share at least one common factor (eg: being HIV-positive) who are studied over a long period of time.

CO-INFECTION
The term given when a person is infected with two (or more) viruses. In this instance it refers to a hepatitis (B, C or both) infection in conjunction with HIV infection.

COMBINATION THERAPY
The use of two or more drugs or treatments used together to achieve optimum results against HIV infection or AIDS-related illness conditions.

COMPASSIONATE USE
A method of providing experimental drugs prior to FDA approval for use on sick people who have no other treatment options. Often case-by-case approval must be obtained for this type of therapy.

COMPLEMENTARY THERAPY
A whole range of therapies and services designed to complement traditional medical practices as part of a primary care plan for an individual.

COMPLIANCE
An alternative term for adherence.

CONCORDE STUDY
A controversial joint French/British clinical trial set out to examine the effectiveness of the drug AZT in asymptomatic HIV-infected individuals which started in 1988 for a three year period.

CONDOM
A sheath (often latex) to cover the penis during sexual practices: providing some protection against infection and pregnancy.

CONTAGIOUS
An infection that can spread easily by casual contact from one person to another. Casual contact can be defined as normal day-to-day contact among people at home, at school or at work. A contagious pathogen (eg: chicken pox) can be transmitted by casual contact. An infectious pathogen, on the other hand, is transmitted by direct or intimate contact (eg: sex). HIV is infectious not contagious.

CONTRAINDICATION
A specific circumstance when the use of certain treatments could be harmful.

CONTROLLED TRIALS
Control is a standard against which experimental observation can be evaluated. In clinical trials one group is given experimental drugs whilst another group (the control group) is given either standard treatment for a disease or a placebo.

CROSS-RESISTANCE
The mechanism by which HIV has acquired resistance to one drug by direct exposure and is also found to have resistance to other, similar drugs that it has not been exposed to. Cross-resistance arises because the biological mechanism of resistance to several drugs is the same and occurs through the identical genetic mutations.

CRYOTHERAPY
This is the use of liquid nitrogen to freeze and destroy growths and lesions, often used to induce scar formation and healing to prevent further spread of a particular condition, eg: warts.

CRYPTOCOCCAL MENINGITIS
A life-threatening infection of the membranes (meninges) that line the brain and the spinal cord caused by a fungus (Cryptococcus neoformans). This affects people that have immune systems that are damaged or suppressed by drugs.

CRYPTOSPORIDIUM
A relatively uncommon but worrisome opportunistic infection leading to chronic diarrhoea for people living with HIV and is an AIDS-defining infection.

CYTOMEGALOVIRUS (CMV)
A herpes virus which is a common cause of opportunistic diseases in persons with AIDS and others with immune suppression. Whilst CMV can infect most organs of the body, people living with HIV and AIDS are most susceptible to CMV retinitis and colitis (disease of the colon).

CYTOMEGALOVIRUS (CMV) RETINITIS
This is an eye disease common among people living with HIV and AIDS and remains in the body for life. Without treatment, persons with CMV retinitis can lose their vision and can affect both eyes. It is the most common cause of blindness among persons with AIDS.

CYTOTOXIC LYMPHOCYTE (CTL)
A lymphocyte (white blood cell) that is able to destroy foreign cells marked for destruction by the cellular immune system. CTLs, also known as killer T-cells carry the CD8 marker and can destroy cancer cells and cells infected with viruses, fungi and certain bacteria.

DATRI
Division of AIDS Treatment Research Initiative

DEMENTIA
Chronic intellectual impairment (ie: loss of mental capacity) with organic origins affecting people's ability to function in a social or occupational setting. These include changes in mental function, co-ordination and personality resulting from direct effects of HIV infection in the brain.

DERMATITIS
Inflammation of the skin.

DE-SENSITISATION
Gradually increasing the dose of a medicine in order to overcome severe reactions. An example has been when administering Bactrim to people with a history of adverse reactions to the drug. Bactrim is an important drug against PCP.

DIABETES
A condition characterised by raised concentration of sugar in the blood, due to problems with the production or action of insulin. Diabetes mellitus is a metabolic disease in which carbohydrate utilisation is reduced and that of lipid and protein utilisation is enhanced. It occurs when the body produces little or no insulin or cannot use the insulin that is produced. As a result, unused glucose collects in the blood; this leads to high blood-sugar levels. Insulin is the hormone that allows glucose to leave the bloodstream and enter body cells, where it is used for energy generation or stored for future use. In relation to HIV, long term complications include: the development of neuropathy (swelling and wasting of the nerves); retinopathy (non-swelling eye disorder); nephropathy (swelling or breakdown disorder of kidneys) generalised degenerative changes in large and small blood vessels, and increased susceptibility to infections.

DIAGNOSIS
A description of the causes of a patient's medical problems determined by the presence of a specific disease or infection, usually accomplished by evaluating clinical symptoms and laboratory tests.

DIARRHOEA
Abnormal or uncontrolled bowel movements characterised by watery or frequent stools. Severe or prolonged diarrhoea can lead to weight loss and malnutrition.

DISEASE PROGRESSION
The worsening of a disease.

DISLYPIDAEMIA
Abnormal blood lipid levels eg: decreased HDL and increased LDL cholesterol.

DNA
Deoxyribo**n**ucleic **a**cid: the material in the nucleus of a cell where genetic information is stored. DNA is the principal constituent of chromosomes, the structures that transmit hereditary characteristics.

DOSE-RANGING TRIAL
A clinical trial where two or more doses of a drug are compared to see which works best and is least harmful.

DOUBLE-BLIND STUDY
A clinical trial where neither the participating individuals nor the research staff know which patients are receiving the experimental drugs/treatments and which are receiving the placebo or other therapies. Double-blind trials are thought to produce the objective results since expectations do not affect the outcome.

DYSPLASIA
Any abnormal development of tissues or organs. In pathology, alteration in size, shape and organisation of adult cells.

EARLY INTERVENTION
Starting HIV treatment early in the course of the disease.

EFFICACY
The maximum ability of a drug or treatment to produce a result regardless of dosage. A drug treatment passes efficacy trials if it is effective at the dose tested and against the illness for which it is prescribed.

ELISA
Enzyme-Linked Immunosorbent Assay: a type of enzyme immunoassay (EIA) to determine the presence of antibodies to HIV in the blood or oral fluids. Repeatedly reactive (that is two or more) ELISA test results should be validated with an independent supplement test of high specificity.

EMPIRICAL
This is based on experimental data not on a theory.

ENCEPHALOPATHY
A disease or infection affecting the brain. Encephalitis is brain inflammation of viral or other microbial origin. Symptoms include: headaches, neck pain, fever, nausea, vomiting and nervous system problems. Several types of opportunistic infections can cause encephalitis.

ENDEMIC
This is pertaining to diseases associated with particular population groups or particular locales.

ENDOGENOUS
This relates to or is produced by the body, in other words, coming from within the body.

ENDOSCOPY
This involves viewing the inside of the body cavity (for example: the colon) with an endoscope: a flexible device using fibre optics.

ENDPOINT
An event used by a clinical trial to compare or evaluate whether a trial therapy is working, for example, developing AIDS or a rise in viral load above a certain level. Common endpoints are severe toxicity, disease progression or, in relation to HIV, surrogate markers such as CD4 count; sometimes death is used as an endpoint. It should be noted that this term is confusing because it often incorrectly implies that patients in a study are no longer followed after they experience an endpoint. Obviously when death occurs, this cannot be followed up; however non-fatal events may require continued treatments regardless of endpoints observed.

END-STAGE DISEASE
This is the final period of phase in the course of a disease leading to a person's death.

ENTERIC
Pertaining to the gut/intestines.

ENZYME
Proteins used by human cells, bacteria and viruses to speed up chemical reactions. Basically an enzyme acts as a catalyst.

EPIDEMIC
A disease that spreads rapidly through a demographic segment of the human population, such as everyone in a given geographical area; a military base or similar population unit. Epidemic diseases can be spread from person to person or from a contaminated source such as food or water.

EPIDEMIOLOGY
The study of incidence and distribution and control of diseases within a population.

EPIDERMIS
The outer layers of the skin.

EPITOPE
The unique shape or marker carried on an antigen's surface which the immune system recognises and triggers a response.

EPSTEIN-BARR VIRUS
The herpes-like virus that causes one of the two kinds of mononucleosis (the other caused by CMV). It infects the nose and throat and is contagious. EBV lies dormant in the lymph glands and has been associated with Burkitt's lymphoma.

ERYTHEMA
Redness, rash or inflammation of the skin or mucous membranes.

ERTHROPOIETIN
A natural hormone made in the kidneys to stimulate the production of red blood cells by the bone marrow.

ETHICS COMMITTEE
A panel of individuals who review any proposed clinical trial to ensure that the participants (those involved) are protected from any foreseeable exploitation or harm.

ETIOLOGY
The study or theory of the factors that cause disease.

EXCLUSION or INCLUSION CRITERIA
Medical or social conditions that would exclude or include a person from joining a clinical trial. For example, some trials may not include people with

chronic liver disease or those with certain drug allergies. Other trials may include people with a lowered CD4 cell count.

EXOGENOUS
Developed or originating from outside of the body.

EXPANDED ACCESS SCHEME
Refers to any of the FDA (Food and Drugs Administration) procedures, such as compassionate use, that distribute experimental drugs to people who are failing on currently available treatments for their condition and are unable to participate in ongoing clinical trials.

EXPERIMENTAL DRUG
A drug that is not FDA licensed for use in humans or as a treatment for a particular condition.

FDA
Food and Drug Administration. The US Department of Health and Human Services agency responsible for ensuring the safety and effectiveness of all drugs, biologics, vaccines and medical devices including those used in the diagnosis, treatment and prevention of HIV infection, AIDS and AIDS-related opportunistic infections.

FEMIDOM
Female version of the male condom inserted in the vagina.

FIBROSIS
Damaged liver cells are replaced by scar tissue: this is known as fibrosis.

FIRST-LINE THERAPY
The regimen used when starting treatment for the first time.

FOETUS
An unborn baby.

FORESKIN
The fold of the skin covering and protecting the head of the penis.

FUNCTIONAL ANTIBODY
An antibody that binds to an antigen and has an effect; for example: neutralising antibodies that inactivate HIV or prevent it from infecting other cells.

FUNGI
A group of organisms including the yeasts which cause candidiasis and cryptococcosis.

FUSION INHIBITOR
A class of antiretroviral agents that binds to the GP41 envelope protein and blocks structural changes necessary for the virus to fuse with the host CD4 cell. When the virus cannot penetrate the host cell membrane and infect the cell, HIV replication within that host cell is prevented.

GENE
A unit of DNA carrying information for the biosynthesis of a specific product in the cell. It is an ultimate unit by which inheritable characteristics are transmitted to succeeding generations in all living organisms.

GENERIC DRUG
A drug that is identical to a brand name drug in quality, performance, dose, strength, safety. Method of administration and the intended use. They are made by organisations that did not invent the drug or have a patent on the compound. For countries in the 'developing world', patented generic compounds are often manufactured and sold before a patent has expired. In countries in the 'developed world' there are often restrictions for manufacture even after the expiration date of the patent.

GENOME
The complete set of genes in the chromosomes of each cell of a particular organism.

GENOTYPE
The genetic make-up of an organism. Hepatitis B and C have many genotypes, each slightly different.

GENOTYPIC ASSAY
A test that determines whether HIV has become resistant to the antiviral drug(s) the patient is currently taking. The test analyses a sample of the

virus from the patient's blood to identify any mutations in the virus that are associated with resistance to specific drugs.

GLOBULINS
Simple proteins found in the blood serum and cerebrospinal fluid which contain various molecules central to the immune system function.

GONORRHEA
An infection caused by Neisseria gonorrhoeae (bacteria from the family Neisseriaceae containing gram-negative cocci). Although it is considered primarily a sexually transmitted disease, it can be transmitted during the birth process to new-borns.

GP41
Glycoprotein 41, a protein embedded in the outer envelope of HIV. It plays a key role in HIV's infection of CD4 cells by facilitating the fusion of the viral and the cell membranes.

G U M CLINIC
This stands for Genito Urinary Medicine clinic and is a NHS run clinic for all aspects of sexual health including sexually transmitted diseases (STD) or sexually transmitted infections (STI).

GYNAECOLOGICAL
This term relates to medical conditions which are specific only to women.

HAART
Highly **A**ctive **A**nti-**R**etroviral **T**herapy: the term given to the course of treatment to aggressively suppress viral replication and progression of HIV disease that includes the use of three or more drugs.

HAEMATOCRIT
Measurement of the proportion of red blood cells in the blood.

HAEMATOLOGY
Study of blood conditions and also used to describe a range of biochemical tests carried out on the blood.

HAEMOGLOBIN
Red coloured, iron-based, oxygen-carrying chemical in red blood cells.

HAEMOPHILIA
An inherited disorder that affects mostly males; it is a disorder of blood clotting. It is treated by lifelong injections of a synthetic version of clotting agents called *factors*. There are 12 factors and one of them is called factor VIII and the other is factor IX. It is the failure of the body to produce either normal factor VIII or factor IX that results in haemophilia. When factor VIII is not normal the disorder is called haemophilia A. When factor IX is abnormal, this disorder is called haemophilia B (Christmas disease). Haemophilia A is the most common type of haemophilia.

HBV
Hepatitis B Virus

HCV
Hepatitis C Virus.

HELPER T-CELLS
Lymphocytes bearing the CD4 marker that are responsible for many immune system functions including turning antibody production on and off.

HEPATIC
Pertaining to the liver.

HEPATITIS
An inflammation of the liver often caused by bacterial or viral infection; parasitic infestation; alcohol; drugs; toxins or transfusion of incompatible blood. Although most cases are not a serious threat to health, the disease can become chronic and can sometimes lead to liver failure and death. There are four major types of viral hepatitis: Hepatitis A virus spread by faecal-oral contact; Hepatitis B virus commonly passed on by sexual intercourse, anal sex, sharing needles and other drug paraphernalia and is highly infectious; non-A, non-B hepatitis caused by hepatitis C virus also spread via sexual contact, sharing needles, and so on. Hepatitis E virus is principally spread via contaminated water supply. Delta hepatitis (HDV) occurs only in persons already infected with HBV and occurs in persons frequently exposed to blood and blood products.

HEPATOTOXICITY
Side effects affecting the liver.

HERPES VIRUSES
A group of viruses that include: herpes simplex type1 (HSV-1); herpes simplex type 2 (HSV-2); cytomegalovirus (CMV); Epstein-Barr virus (EBV);

varicella zoster virus (VZV); human herpes virus type 6 (HHV-6) and HHV-8, a herpes virus associated with Kaposi's sarcoma.

HICKMAN LINE
A type of catheter that is surgically implanted with one end leading into the large vein in the chest and the other end remaining outside the chest.

HIGHLY TREATMENT EXPERIENCED
A person who has had more than three combination therapies for their HIV infection and have changed for many reasons and are more likely to have resistance to one or more components.

HISTOLOGY
Examining a sample of cells under a microscope to determine if they are normal or if there is evidence of infections or tumours.

HIV
Human Immunodeficiency Virus – the retrovirus that leads to AIDS. There are two variants: HIV-1 and HIV-2 and these are further divided into complex sub-types. HIV-1 Group M is the most common type of HIV with over 90 per cent of HIV infection deriving from this variant. The M group is further subdivided into Clades called subtypes which are also given a letter from A to K. Also in the same variant HIV-1 are three other groups: N, O and P and a further HIV-1 RCV group. Not widely seen outside of Africa is the variant HIV-2. Many test kits for HIV-1 will also detect HIV-2

HODGKIN'S DISEASE
A progressive malignant cancer of the lymphatic system. Symptoms include lymphadenopathy, wasting, weakness, fever, itching, night sweats and anaemia. Treatment includes radiation and chemotherapy.

HOLISTIC MEDICINE
Healing traditions promoting the protection and restoration of health through theories reputedly based on the body's natural ability to heal itself and through manipulation of various ways body components affect each other and are influenced by the external environment.

HOMEOPATHY
A therapy which aims to treat illness using tiny quantities of a substance that caused the illness or a substance that causes similar symptoms.

HORMONE
An active chemical formed in one part of the body and carried in the blood to other parts of the body where it stimulates or suppresses cell and tissue activity.

HTLV III
Human T-Cell Lymphotropic Virus Type III

HUMAN PAPILLOMA VIRUS (HPV)
A group of wart-causing viruses which are also responsible for cancer of the cervix and some anal cancers.

HYPER
Prefix meaning higher than usual.

HYPERGLYCAEMIA
An abnormally high concentration of sugar (glucose) in the circulating blood. This is common in persons with diabetes mellitus.

HYPERSENSITIVITY
An allergic reaction.

HYPO
Prefix meaning lower than usual.

HYPOTHESIS
A specific statement or proposition stated in a testable or researchable format which predicts a particular relationship or outcome amongst multiple variables.

HYPOXAEMIA
Reduced amount of oxygen in the blood usually caused by pneumonia.

IDIOPATHIC
Without a known cause.

IMMUNE COMPLEX
Clusters formed when antigens and antibodies bind together.

IMMUNE SYSTEM
The body's system for fighting off infection and eradicating dysfunctional cells.

IMMUNO-COMPROMISED
When the immune system is so weak it cannot offer resistance to infection.

IMMUNODEFICIENCY
A breakdown in immuno-competence when certain parts of the immune system no longer function. This makes a person more susceptible to certain disease that they would not ordinarily develop.

INCUBATION PERIOD
The time interval between the initial infection with a pathogen (eg: HIV) and the appearance of the first symptom or sign of disease.

INFECTION
The state or condition in which the body or part of the body is invaded by an infectious agent such as: bacterium, fungus or virus that then multiplies and produces active infection. In HIV, infection typically begins when HIV encounters a CD4+ cell.

INFORMED CONSENT
An agreement to take part in a clinical trial or to take a test after a full written or verbal explanation of the trial, including the risks and benefits of taking part, has been provided by researcher. This is a statement of trust between two parties and includes protection for those entering any drug trial.

INFUSION
A process of administering therapeutic fluid, other than blood, to an individual by slowly injecting a dilute solution of the compound into the vein. Infusions are often used when the digestive system does not absorb sufficient quantities of a drug or when a drug is too toxic or the volume is too large to be given by quick injection.

INSOMNIA
A state of sleeplessness.

INSULIN
A hormone produced by the pancreas that tends to lower blood sugar levels.

INTEFERON
One of a number of antiretroviral proteins which stimulates the immune system.

INTEGRASE
An enzyme that HIV uses to insert genetic material into an infected cell.

INTEGRASE INHIBITORS
Integrase inhibitors are a new class of ARV that block integrase and stop the HIV genetic material integrating into the host cell. They act after NRTIs/NNRTIs and before PIs in terms of HIV's lifecycle.

IN VITRO
Latin for experiments conducted in artificial environments outside a living organism used in experimental research to study a disease or process eg: in test tubes.

IN VIVO
Latin for experiments conducted on living organisms: animals and humans.

JAUNDICE
A yellowing of the skin and the whites of the eyes which is caused by raised levels of bilirubin in the blood associated with the liver and gall bladder.

KAPOSI'S SARCOMA (KS)
An AIDS-defining illness consisting of individual cancerous lesions caused by an overgrowth of blood vessels. KS typically appears as pink or purple painless spots or nodules on the surface of the skin or oral cavity. KS can also occur internally in the intestines, lymph nodes and lungs and in this case is life-threatening. The cancer may spread and also attack the eyes. There is speculation that KS is not a spontaneous cancer but is sparked by a virus.

KARNOFSKY'S SCORE
A number between 0 and 100 which is assigned by a clinician or doctor to describe a person's ability to function, as measured by the performance of common tasks.

KILLER T-CELLS
Because viruses exist inside human or host cells where antibodies cannot reach them, the only way of elimination is by killing the infected host cell. The immune system uses a white blood cell, called killer T-cells which act only when they encounter another cell that carries a 'marker' (a protein) that links it to a foreign protein (the invading virus). Killer T-cells can themselves become infected by HIV and other viruses or transformed by cancer.

LATENCY
This is the period when an infecting organism is in the body but is not producing any clinically noticeable ill effects or symptoms. In HIV disease clinical latency is an asymptomatic period in the early years of HIV infection. The period of latency is characterised in the blood by near normal CD4 counts. Cellular latency is the period after HIV has integrated its genome into a cell's DNA but has not yet begun to replicate.

LAV
Lymphadenopathy-associated virus associated with the Pasteur Institute believed to be the retroviral cause of the syndrome known as AIDS.

LESION
A general term to describe a damaged or altered area or abnormal body tissue such as an infected patch or sore on the skin or an internal organ caused by disease or injury.

LEUKOCYTES
A term used for white blood cells.

LIPID
A general term for fats.

LIPOATROPHY
A specific term concerned with the loss of body fat or fat wasting eg: hollow cheeks and thin limbs.

LIPODYSTROPHY
A medical condition characterised by abnormal and degenerative conditions of the body's adipose tissue. In other words it is a disruption to the way the body produces, uses, and distributes fat eg: thickening around the waist or 'buffalo hump'.

LIVER FUNCTION TEST
Tests, usually a blood test, to measure and evaluate the functioning of the liver by assessing proteins and enzymes that might be raised or lowered.

LOGARITHIM (LOG)
A (logarithmic) scale of measurement often used when describing 'viral load'. A one log change denotes a change in the value of what is being measured by a factor of 10 (such as from 100 to 10). A two log change is a one hundred-fold change such as from 1,000 to 10.

LONG-TERM NON-PROGRESSORS
Individuals who have been living with HIV for at least 7 to 12 years (different authors use different time scales) and have stable CD4+ T-cell counts of 600 or more cells per cubic millimetre of blood; no HIV-related diseases, and no previous antiretroviral therapy.

LUMBAR PUNCTURE
A small hole is made in the spinal column to take out cerebrospinal fluid for tests or to inject drugs. Also called a spinal tap. It involves the insertion of a needle through the tissue between the vertebrae to access the spinal canal.

LYMPH
A transparent, slightly yellow fluid that carries lymphocytes. Lymph is derived from tissue fluids collected from all parts of the body and is returned to the blood via lymphatic vessels.

LYMPHOCYTE
A type of white blood cell which is present in the blood, lymph and lymphoid tissue.

LYMPHOMA
A type of tumour affecting the lymph nodes. These are often described as being 'large cell' or 'small cell' types, cleaved or non-cleaved or diffuse or nodular. The different types often have a different prognosis that is the prospect of survival or recovery. The types of lymphomas associated with HIV infection are called non-Hodgkin's lymphomas or B cell lymphomas. In these types of cancers, certain cells of the lymphatic system grow abnormally, divide rapidly and grow into tumours.

LYMPH NODES
Special areas in the body where white blood cells and other important immune cells are located. Also referred to as glands.

LYMPHOPENIA
A relative or absolute reduction in the number of lymphocytes in the circulating blood.

MACROPHAGE
A large immune cell that roams the body tissues and devours foreign and invading organisms. These can harbour large quantities of HIV without being killed, acting as reservoirs of the virus.

MAI/MAC
Mycobacterium Avium-Intracellulare/Mycobacterium Avium Complex. A common opportunistic infection caused by two very similar organisms. It is a life threatening disease although new therapies offer promise for both prevention and treatment. MAC disease is extremely rare in persons who are not infected with HIV.

MAINTENANCE THERAPY
This involves taking drugs for a period of time after an infection has been treated in order to stabilise the condition or prevent a re-occurrence and deterioration.

MALIGNANT
Cells or tumours which may grow rapidly and infiltrate surrounding tissues and spread around the body in an uncontrolled way. This term 'malignancy' implies cancer.

MENINGITIS
An inflammation of the meninges (membranes surrounding the brain or spinal cord) which may be caused by bacterium, fungus or virus.

METABOLISM
The mechanisms which sustain life turning sugar and fat into energy.

MICROBES
Microscopic living organisms including bacteria, protozoa, viruses and fungi.

MICROBICIDE
An agent (chemical or antibiotic) that destroys microbes. Research into the use of rectal and vaginal microbicides to inhibit the transmission of sexually transmitted diseases including HIV is currently on-going.

MOLECULE
The smallest particle of a compound that has all the chemical properties of that particular compound. Molecules are made up of two or more atoms, either of the same element or of two or more different elements. Molecules differ in size and molecular weight as well as in structure.

MONOCYTE
A large white blood cell that ingests microbes or other cells and foreign particles. When a monocyte enters tissues it develops into a macrophage.

MONOTHERAPY
Taking a drug on its own as opposed to taking it with other drug combinations.

MORBIDITY
The condition of being diseased or sick; also the incidence of disease or rate of sickness.

MULTI-DRUG RESISTANCE
A term used when HIV has mutated so that two or more drugs no longer have an effect on its ability to replicate.

MUTATION
In biology a sudden change in a gene or unit of hereditary material that result in a new inheritable characteristic. In higher animals and plants, a mutation might be transmitted to future generations only if it occurs in germ (sex cell) tissue; body cell mutations cannot be inherited. Put simply, it is a single change in gene sequence. During the course of HIV disease, HIV strains may emerge in an infected person, which differs widely in their ability to infect and kill different cell types, as well as their rate of replication. HIV does not mutate into another type of virus.

MYOPATHY
Progressive muscle weakness or muscle wastage. Myopathy might arise as a toxic reaction to AZT or as a consequence of the HIV infection itself.

NADIR
The lowest point out of a series of measurements, such as the blood count after it has been depressed by chemotherapy. When applied to drugs, the lowest concentration of a drug in the body.

NATURAL KILLER CELLS
NK cells in the immune system which attack and destroy infected cells or tumour cells and protect against a wide variety of infectious microbes. They are 'natural' killers because they do not need additional stimulation or need to recognise a specific antigen in order to attack and kill. People with immunodeficiencies such as those caused by HIV infection have a decrease in 'natural' killer cell activities.

NAUSEA
Feeling sick.

NEOPLASM
An abnormal and uncontrolled growth of tissue; a tumour.

NEPHROTOXIC
Damage or poisoning to the kidneys.

NEURALGIA
A sharp or shooting pain along the path of a nerve.

NEUROLOGICAL
Relating to the brain or nervous system.

NEUTROPHILS
White blood cells that play a central role in defence of a host against bacteria and fungal infections. Neutrophils engulf and kill foreign microorganisms and are also called polymorphonuclear neutrophil (PMN).

NEUROPATHY
The name given to a group of disorders involving nerves. Symptoms range from a tingling sensation or numbness in the toes and fingers to paralysis.

NEW VARIANT CJD
New variant Creutzfeldt-Jakob disease (CJD) is a relatively new disease which was first reported in 1996. It is a rare, degenerative, fatal brain disorder in humans and is linked to bovine spongiform encephalopathy (BSE) in cattle.

NIGHT SWEATS
Extreme sweating during sleep and although they can occur with other conditions, night sweats are also a symptom of HIV disease.

NNRTI
Non-nucleoside reverse transcriptase inhibitors: known as 'non-nukes' or NNRTIs. These interfere with the HIV virus's ability to make more copies of itself by blocking the Reverse Transcriptase protein, but in another slightly different way to NRTIs. These are the family of antiretrovirals which include efavirenz, nevirapine and delavirdine.

NRTI
Nucleoside reverse transcriptase inhibitors: known as 'nukes' or 'NRTIs'. They interfere with the HIV virus ability to make more copies of itself by blocking the Reverse Transcriptase protein. These are the family of antiretrovirals which include AZT, ddI, 3TC, d4T, ddC and abacavir.

NON-HODGKIN'S LYMPHOMA (NHL)
A lymphoma made up of B cells and characterised by nodular or diffuse tumours that may appear in the stomach, liver, brain and bone marrow of persons with HIV. After Kaposi's Sarcoma, NHL is the most common opportunistic cancer in persons living with HIV.

NUCLEOSIDE
One of the basic substances or building blocks of nucleic acid that form RNA and DNA, the genetic material found in living organisms. Nucleosides are nucleotides without the phosphate groups.

NUCLEOSIDE ANALOGUE
An artificial copy of a nucleoside. When incorporated into a virus's DNA or RNA during viral replication, the nucleoside analogue acts to prevent production of new virus. Nucleoside analogues may take the place of natural nucleosides, blocking the completion of a viral DNA chain during infection of a new cell by HIV.

NUCLEOTIDE
Nucleotides are the building blocks of nucleic acids, DNA and RNA. Nucleotides are composed of phosphate groups, a five-sided sugar molecule (ribose sugars in RNA and deoxyribose sugars in DNA) and nitrogen containing bases. These fall into two classes: pyrimidines and purines.

NUCLEOTIDE ANALOGUE
Nucleotide analogues are drugs that are structurally related to nucleotides and are chemically altered to inhibit production or activity of disease-causing proteins. The chemical structures of these drugs may cause them to replace natural nucleotides in the viral DNA nucleic acid sequence.

Nucleotide analogues do not require as much phosphorylation in the host's cells as the nucleoside reverse transcriptase inhibitors to become active drugs. A chemical which resembles a nucleoside. The family of antiretrovirals include: cidofovir, adefovir and tenofovir.

NUCLEUS
The central controlling body within a living cell, usually spherical enclosed in a membrane and containing genetic codes for maintaining the life systems of the organism and for issuing commands for growth and reproduction. The nucleus of a cell is essential to such cell functions as reproduction and protein synthesis. It is composed of nuclear sap and a nucleoprotein-rich network from which chromosomes and nucleoli arise and is enclosed in a definite membrane.

OBSERVATIONAL STUDY
A clinical trial which reports on an unfolding situation.

OCULAR
Pertaining to the eye.

OEDEMA
An accumulation of fluid below the skin or in the cavities of the body.

OESOPHAGUS
The tube leading from the throat to the stomach.

ONCOLOGY
Study of cancers or other tumours.

OPPORTUNISTIC INFECTION
Specific infections or illnesses which cause disease in someone with a damaged immune system. Persons living with advanced HIV infection suffer opportunistic infections of the lungs, brain, eyes and other organs. Opportunistic infections in persons diagnosed with AIDS include: pneumocystis carinii pneumonia (PCP); Kaposi's Sarcoma (KS); cryptosporidiosis; histoplasmosis; other parasitic, viral and fungal infections and some types of cancers.

ORAL HAIRY LEUKOPLAKIA (OHL)
A whitish lesion which appears on the side of the tongue and inside the cheeks. The lesion appears raised with a ribbed or 'hairy' surface. OHL occurs mainly in persons with declining immunity and may be caused by

Epstein-Barr virus infection. OHL was not observed before HIV became widespread.

PALLIATIVE
A treatment that provides symptomatic relief but not a cure.

PANCREAS
A glandular organ situated near the stomach that secretes pancreatic digestive enzymes into the intestine through one or more ducts and also secretes the hormone insulin.

PANCYTOPENIA
Low numbers of all blood cells.

PARASITE
A plant or animal that lives and feeds on or within another living organism or host causing some degree of harm to the host organism.

PATHOGEN
Any micro-organism which can cause disease. There are four main types: bacteria; fungi; protozoa; viruses.

PCP
Pneumocystis Carinii Pneumonia

PCR
Polymerase chain reaction: a diagnostic technique or method of amplifying fragments of genetic material so that they can be detected. Some viral load tests use this method.

PERIANAL
Around the anus.

PERINATAL TRANSMISSION
Transmission of a pathogen, such as HIV, from mother to baby before, during and after the birth process.

PERIPHERAL NEUROPATHY
Damage to nerves usually resulting in numbness to the feet and hands which can also lead to excruciating pain.

PESSARY
A solid medication or device which can be inserted into the vagina either as a support for the uterus or to deliver a drug.

PHAGOCYTE
A cell that is able to ingest and destroy foreign matter including bacteria.

PHENOTYPE
Trait or behaviour which results from a particular genotype.

PLACEBO
A pill or liquid which looks and tastes exactly like a real drug but contains no active substance.

PLACEBO EFFECT
A physical or emotional change which occurs after a substance is taken or administered that is not the result of any special property of the substance. The change may be beneficial, reflecting the expectations of the person concerned and often the expectations of the person giving the substance.

PLASMA
A clear substance in which cells float.

PLATELETS
Active agent of inflammation when damage occurs to a blood vessel. They are not actually cells but fragments released by megakaryocyte cells. Megakaryocyte is a large cell in the bone marrow whose function is to produce platelets. When vascular damage (ie: damage to blood vessels) occurs, the platelets stick to the vascular walls, forming clots to prevent the loss of blood. Thus, it is important to have adequate numbers of normally functioning platelets to maintain effective coagulation (clotting) of the blood. There are drugs that can potentially alter the platelet count, making it necessary to monitor the count. Also, some persons living with HIV develop thrombocytopenia – a condition characterised by a platelet count of less than 100,000 platelets per cubic millimetre of blood.

PML
Progressive Multifocal Leukoencephalopathy: a rapidly debilitating opportunistic infection caused by the JC virus that infects the brain tissue and causes damage to the brain and spinal cord. Symptoms vary from person to person but include loss of muscle control, paralysis, blindness, problems with speech and altered mind states. PML can lead to coma and

death. In some cases, HAART regimens using medications known to cross the blood-brain barrier are used to treat PML.

PRECLINICAL
This refers to the testing of experimental drugs in the test tube or in animals – the testing that occurs before trials in humans may be carried out.

PREVALENCE
A measure of the proportion of people in a population affected with a particular disease at a given time.

PROGNOSIS
This is a likely outcome such as the risk of disease progression.

PROPHYLAXIS
Treatment to prevent the onset of a particular disease ('primary' prophylaxis) or the recurrence of symptoms in an existing infection that has been brought under control ('secondary' prophylaxis or maintenance therapy).

PROTEASE
An enzyme that breaks down proteins into their component peptides. HIV's protease enzyme breaks apart long strands of viral protein into the separate proteins making up the viral core. The enzyme acts as new virus particles are budding off a cell membrane. Protease was the first HIV protein whose three-dimensional structure had been characterised.

PROTEASE INHIBITORS
Also known as 'PIs', these antiretroviral drugs interfere with the HIV virus's ability to make more copies of itself by blocking the function of protease, a protein which is needed for the task. Specifically, these drugs block the protease enzyme from breaking apart long strands of viral proteins to make the smaller, active HIV proteins that comprise the virion. If the larger HIV proteins are not broken apart, they cannot assemble themselves into new functional HIV particles.

PROTEINS
Highly complex organic compounds found in all living cells. Protein is the most abundant class of all biological molecules comprising fifty percent of cellular dry weight. Structurally, proteins are large molecules composed of one or more chains of varying amounts of the same 22 amino acids that are linked by peptide bonds. Each protein is characterised by a unique and invariant amino acid sequence. The information for the synthesis of the

specific amino acid sequence in a protein from free amino acids is carried by the cell's nucleic acid.

PROTHROMBIN TIME
A test to ensure your liver is successfully making chemicals that help you stop bleeding if you have a cut.

PROTOCOL
The detailed plan for conducting a clinical trial. It states the trial's rationale, purpose, drug or vaccine dosages, length of study, routes of administration, who may participate (inclusion and exclusion criteria) and other aspects of trial design.

QUASISPECIES
Small genetic variations in a population of viral particles but too minor to qualify as a different strain or genotype.

RADIOTHERAPY
A treatment using radiant energy or other radioactive matter: it includes X-rays, CT scans and the destruction of tumours by radiation.

RECEPTOR
A molecule on the surface of a cell that serves as a recognition or binding site for antigens, antibodies or other cellular or immunological component.

REFLEXOLOGY
A type of complementary therapy which involves the massaging of the feet.

REGIMEN
This applies to a treatment combination and the way it is taken.

REGRESSION
An improvement in a tumour.

REMISSION
It is the lessening of the severity or duration of outbreaks of a disease or the reduction in degree or intensity of symptoms altogether over a period of time

RENAL
Relating to the kidneys.

REPLICATION
The process of cell or viral reproduction.

RESISTANCE
This is the term given when HIV has mutated so that the drug has reduced or no activity in stopping the replication process.

RETINITIS
Inflammation of the retina (light sensitive tissue at the back of the eye that transmits visual impulses via the optic nerve to the brain) linked in AIDS to CMV. Untreated it can lead to blindness.

RETROVIRUS
A type of virus that, when not infecting a cell, stores its genetic information on a single-stranded RNA molecule instead of a more usual double-stranded DNA. HIV is an example of a retrovirus. After a retrovirus penetrates a cell, it constructs a DNA version of its genes using a special enzyme called reverse transcriptase. This DNA then becomes part of the cell's genetic material.

REVERSE TRANSCRIPTASE
This enzyme of HIV converts the single-stranded viral RNA into DNA, the form in which the cell carries its genes. Some antiviral drugs work by interfering with this stage of the viral life cycle (referred to as reverse transcriptase inhibitors RTIs). These include: AZT, ddC, ddI, 3TC, D4T and abacavir).

RIBAVIRIN
One of the treatments used for people with hepatitis C. It must be used in combination with interferon alfa.

RNA (RiboNucleic Acid)
A nucleic acid found in the cytoplasm rather than the nucleus of cells, which is important in the synthesis of proteins. The amount of RNA varies from cell to cell. RNA like the structurally similar DNA is a chain made up of sub units called nucleotides. In protein synthesis, messenger RNA replicates the DNA code for a protein and moves to sites in the cell called ribosomes. Most forms of RNA consist of a single nucleotide strand but a few forms of viral RNA that function as carriers of genetic information are double-stranded. The HIV virus carries RNA instead of the more usual genetic material DNA.

SALVAGE THERAPY
This is any treatment regimen used for someone who is resistant to, or does not respond to most of the currently licensed antiretroviral medications from all classes. People are usually dependent on drugs in clinical trials (alongside drugs from the existing classes that they have limited or no resistance to) to manage their HIV infection.

SARCOMA
A malignant (cancerous) tumour of the skin and soft tissue.

SEROCONVERSION
The time at which a person's antibody status changes from negative to positive.

SERONEGATIVE
A negative result from a blood test.

SEROPOSITIVE
A positive result from a blood test.

SERUM
Clear, sticky, thick, non-cellular portion of the blood containing antibodies and other proteins and chemicals and remains after coagulation (clotting). Serum contains no blood cells, platelets or fibrinogen.

SEXUALLY TRANSMITTED INFECTIONS (STI)
Also referred to as sexually transmitted diseases (STDs): these are infections spread by the transfer of organism from person to person during sexual contact. In addition to the traditional infections such as syphilis and gonorrhoea, the spectrum of STIs now includes HIV infection.

SHIATSU
A complementary therapy using massage.

SIDE EFFECTS
The actions or effects of a drug or vaccine other than those desired. The term usually refers to undesired or negative effects, such as headaches, skin irritation or liver damage. Experimental drugs must be evaluated for both immediate and long-term side effects.

SPECULUM
An instrument for enlarging the opening of any canal or cavity in order to inspect its interior eg: vagina, rectum, ear or nose.

SPERMICIDE
A cream or jelly that kills sperm and is sometimes used as a contraceptive.

STEM CELLS
Cells from which all blood cells derive. Bone marrow is rich in stem cells. Clones of stem cells may become any one of the repertoires of immune cells depending upon which cytokines and hormones they are exposed to.

SVR – SUSTAINED VIROLOGICAL RESPONSE
This relates to a person remaining clear of a virus (usually hepatitis C) after treatment has finished. This time period is often six months after treatment.

SYMPTOMS
Any perceptible, subjective change in the body or its functions that indicates disease or phases of an illness or disease as reported by the patient.

SYMPTOMATIC
Experiencing symptoms associated with a disease.

SYNDROME
A group of symptoms and diseases that when put together are characteristic of a specific condition.

SYNERGY
An interaction between two or more drugs or treatments that produce an effect greater than adding their separate effects by the individual treatments.

SYPHILIS
A disease, primarily sexually transmitted, resulting from infection with the spirochete (a bacterium), Treponema pallidum. Syphilis can also be acquired in the uterus during pregnancy.

SYSTEMIC
Acting throughout the body rather than locally.

TB – TUBERCULOSIS
A disease caused by the bacterium Mycobacterium tuberculosis. TB bacteria are spread by airborne droplets expelled from the lungs when a person with active TB coughs, sneezes or speaks. Exposure to these droplets can lead to infection in the air sacs of the lungs. The immune defences of healthy people usually prevent TB infection from spreading beyond a very small area of the lungs. If the body's immune system is impaired because of infection with HIV, ageing, malnutrition or other factors, the TB bacterium may begin to spread more widely in the lungs or to other tissues. TB is seen with increasing frequency among persons infected with HIV. Most cases of TB occur in the lungs (pulmonary TB); however, the disease may also occur in the larynx, lymph nodes, brain, kidneys or bones (extrapulmonary TB). Extrapulmonary TB infections are more common among persons living with HIV.

T-CELLS
A type of immune cell which is targeted and damaged in the course of HIV infection. CD4 and CD8 cells are both sub-types of T-cell.

T4 CELLS
Antibody-triggered immune cells that seek and attack invading organisms. Macrophages summon T4 cells to the infection site and these cells then reproduce and secrete its potent lymphokines that stimulate B cell production of antibodies; signal natural killer or cytotoxic (cell killing) T-cells and summon other macrophages to the infection site. In healthy immune systems, T4 cells are twice as common as T8 cells.

T8 CELLS
These cells are also known as 'killer cells' that shut down the immune response after it has effectively wiped out invading organisms. Sensitive to high concentrations of circulating lymphokines, T8 cells release their own lymphokines when an immune response has achieved its goal signalling all other participants to cease their co-ordinated attack. With HIV however, the immune system response does not work. T4 cells are dysfunctional, lymphokines proliferate in the bloodstream and T8 cells compound the problem by misreading the over production of lymphokines as meaning that the immune system has effectively eliminated the invader. Thus, whilst HIV is multiplying, T8 cells are simultaneously attempting to further shut down the immune system.

TERATOGENIC
Causing physical birth defects in a foetus. Teratogenicity is a potential side effect of some drugs, such as thalidomide.

TESTICLES
Male reproductive glands found in the scrotum.

THROMBOCYTOPENI
A decreased number of specific cells in the blood responsible for blood clotting.

THRUSH
A fungal infection of the mouth, throat or genitals marked by white patches. Also called candidiasis. Thrush is one of the most frequent early symptoms or signs of an immune disorder. The fungus commonly lives in the mouth but only causes problems when the body's resistance is reduced by either antibiotics that have reduced the number of competitive organisms in the mouth or by an immune deficiency such as HIV infection.

THYMUS
A mass of glandular tissue found in the upper chest where T-cells produced in the bone marrow mature into effective immune system components. The thymus is essential to the development of the body's system of immunity beginning in foetal life

TISSUE
A collection of similar cells acting together to perform a particular function. There are four basic tissues in the body: epithelial; connective; muscle and nerve.

TOPICAL
Applied directly to the affected area, as opposed to systemic.

TOXICITY
The extent or ways in which a drug is harmful or poisonous to the body.

TOXIN
A poisonous substance.

TRANSAMINASE
A liver enzyme that can be measured in a blood sample to indicate the health of the liver.

TRANSFUSION
The process of transfusing fluid, such as blood, into a vein or the transfer of hole blood or blood products from one individual to another.

TRANSMISSION
In the context of HIV infection, HIV is spread most commonly by sexual contact with an infected person. The virus can enter the body through the mucosal lining of the vagina, vulva, penis, rectum or rarely the mouth during sex. The likelihood of transmission is increased by factors that may damage these linings, especially other sexually transmitted infections that cause ulcers or inflammation. HIV is also spread through contact with infected blood, most often by the sharing of drug needles or syringes contaminated with quantities of blood containing the virus. Children can contact HIV from their infected mothers during either pregnancy or birth or post-natally through breast feeding. In addition, HIV can be transmitted via blood transfusions or blood products, such as clotting agents.

TREATMENT EXPERIENCED
The term given for a person who has undergone a treatment combination for HIV infection.

TREATMENT NAÏVE
The term given for a person who has not had any treatment for HIV infection.

TRIGLYCERIDES
The basic 'building blocks' from which fats are formed.

TUMOUR
Uncontrolled new tissue growth in which cells multiply rapidly.

ULCER
A break in the skin or mucous membrane which involves the loss of the surface tissue.

UNDETECTABLE VIRAL LOAD
A level of viral load that is too low to be picked up by the particular viral load test being used.

URETHRA
The tube that carries urine from the bladder to the outside of the body.

VACCINE or VACCINATION
A substance that contains antigenic components from an infectious organism. By stimulating an immune response (but not disease) it protects against subsequent infection by that organism.

VAGINA
The passage that extends from the neck of the uterus to the external genitals.

VERTICAL TRANSMISSION
Transmission, for example of HIV, from mother-to-baby.

VIRAEMIA
The presence of virus in the blood.

VIRAL LOAD
A measurement of the amount of virus in a sample. HIV viral load indicates the extent to which HIV is reproducing in the body. Results are expressed as the number of copies per millilitre of blood plasma. Research indicates that the viral load is a better predictor of the risk of HIV disease progression than the CD4 count. The lower the viral load the longer the time to a possible AIDS diagnosis and the longer the survival time.

VIRION
A virus particle existing freely outside of a host cell.

VIROLOGICAL RESPONSE
The effect of treatment on viral load.

VIROLOGY
The study of viruses and viral disease.

VIRULENCE
The power of bacteria or viruses to cause a disease. Different strains of the same micro-organism can vary in virulence.

VIRUS
A microscopic germ which reproduces within the living cells of the organism it infects. When viruses enter a living plant, animal or bacterial cell, they make use of the host cell's chemical energy and protein (and nucleic acid) synthesising ability to replicate themselves. Some viruses do not kill cells

but transform them into a cancerous state. Others cause illness and then seem to disappear whilst remaining latent and later causing another disease.

VISCERAL
Of or pertaining to the internal organs.

VULVA
The external female genitals.

WESTERN BLOT
A laboratory test for specific antibodies to confirm repeatedly reactive results on the HIV ELISA tests.

WHITE BLOOD CELLS
The cells of the immune system including basophils, lymphocytes, neutrophils, macrophages and monocytes.

WILD-TYPE VIRUS
The original type of HIV virus that has not been exposed or changed by having developed resistance to anti-HIV drugs before.

WINDOW PERIOD
Time from infection with HIV until detectable.

WORKS
This is a general term for the injecting equipment (usually syringes) used by injecting drug users.

Made in the USA
Columbia, SC
22 April 2020